Neuromodulation

Editors

WENDELL LAKE
ASHWINI SHARAN
CHENGYUAN WU

NEUROSURGERY
CLINICS OF NORTH AMERICA

www.neurosurgery.theclinics.com

Consulting Editors
RUSSELL R. LONSER
DANIEL K. RESNICK

April 2019 • Volume 30 • Number 2

ELSEVIER

1600 John F. Kennedy Boulevard • Suite 1800 • Philadelphia, Pennsylvania, 19103-2899

http://www.theclinics.com

NEUROSURGERY CLINICS OF NORTH AMERICA Volume 30, Number 2
April 2019 ISSN 1042-3680, ISBN-13: 978-0-323-67852-0

Editor: Stacy Eastman
Developmental Editor: Laura Fisher

Neurosurgery Clinics of North America (ISSN 1042-3680) is published quarterly by Elsevier Inc., 360 Park Avenue South, New York, NY 10010-1710. Months of issue are January, April, July, and October. Business and Editorial Offices: 1600 John F. Kennedy Blvd., Suite 1800, Philadelphia, PA 19103-2899. Customer Service Office: 11830 Westline Industrial Drive, St. Louis, MO 63146. Periodicals postage paid at New York, NY, and additional mailing offices. Subscription prices are $430.00 per year (US individuals), $748.00 per year (US institutions), $470.00 per year (Canadian individuals), $928.00 per year (Canadian institutions), $513.00 per year (international individuals), $928.00 per year (international institutions), $100.00 per year (US students), and $255.00 per year (international and Canadian students). International air speed delivery is included in all *Clinics* subscription prices. All prices are subject to change without notice. **POSTMASTER:** Send address changes to *Neurosurgery Clinics of North America*, Elsevier Periodicals Customer Service, 11830 Westline Industrial Drive, St. Louis, MO 63146. **Customer Service: 1-800-654-2452 (US and Canada). From outside the US and Canada, call: 1-314-453-7041. Fax: 1-314-453-5170. E-mail: JournalsCustomerService-usa@elsevier.com (for print support) and journalsonlinesupport-usa@elsevier.com (for online support).**

Reprints. For copies of 100 or more, of articles in this publication, please contact the Commercial Reprints Department, Elsevier Inc., 360 Park Avenue South, New York, NY 10010-1710. Tel. 212-633-3874; Fax: 212-633-3820; E-mail: reprints@elsevier.com.

Neurosurgery Clinics of North America is covered in *MEDLINE/PubMed (Index Medicus), EMBASE/Excerpta Medica, and Current Contents/Clinical Medicine (CC/CM).*

Contributors

CONSULTING EDITORS

RUSSELL R. LONSER, MD
Professor and Chair, Department of Neurological Surgery, The Ohio State University Wexner Medical Center, Columbus, Ohio, USA

DANIEL K. RESNICK, MD, MS
Professor and Vice Chairman, Program Director, Department of Neurosurgery, University of Wisconsin-Madison School of Medicine and Public Health, Madison, Wisconsin, USA

EDITORS

WENDELL LAKE, MD, FAANS
Assistant Professor, Department of Neurosurgery, University of Wisconsin-Madison, University of Wisconsin Hospitals and Clinics, Madison, Wisconsin, USA

ASHWINI SHARAN, MD
Professor, Department of Neurological Surgery, Thomas Jefferson University Hospitals, Philadelphia, Pennsylvania, USA

CHENGYUAN WU, MD, MSBME
Assistant Professor, Department of Neurological Surgery, Thomas Jefferson University Hospitals, Philadelphia, Pennsylvania, USA

AUTHORS

GARRETT P. BANKS, MD
Resident, Department of Neurosurgery, Columbia University, New York, New York, USA

MICHAEL F. BARBARO, BA
Department of Neurological Surgery, Keck School of Medicine of USC, University of Southern California, USC Neurorestoration Center, Los Angeles, California, USA; T&C Chen Brain Machine Interface Center, California Institute of Technology, Pasadena, California, USA

MARK CORRIVEAU, MD
Department of Neurosurgery, University of Wisconsin Hospitals and Clinics, Madison, Wisconsin, USA

NICHOLAS DIETZ, BS
Research Fellow, Department of Neurosurgery, University of Louisville School of Medicine, Louisville, Kentucky, USA

DARIO J. ENGLOT, MD, PhD
Surgical Director of Epilepsy, Assistant Professor, Department of Biomedical Engineering, Vanderbilt University Institute of Imaging Science, Assistant Professor, Departments of Neurological Surgery and Radiology and Radiological Sciences, Vanderbilt University Medical Center, Nashville, Tennessee, USA

MEGAN M. FILKOWSKI, PhD
Postdoctoral Fellow, Department of Neurosurgery, Baylor College of Medicine, Houston, Texas, USA

CHRISTY GOMEZ, APN
Nurse Practitioner, Department of Neurosurgery, The University of Illinois at Chicago, Chicago, Illinois, USA

HERNÁN F.J. GONZÁLEZ, MS
Graduate Student, Department of Biomedical Engineering, Vanderbilt University Institute of Imaging Science, Vanderbilt University Medical Center, Nashville, Tennessee, USA

AMGAD HANNA, MD
Associate Professor, Department of Neurosurgery, University of Wisconsin Hospitals and Clinics, Madison, Wisconsin, USA

PETER HEDERA, MD, PhD
Associate Professor, Department of Neurology, Vanderbilt University Medical Center, Nashville, Tennessee, USA

EMIL D. ISAGULYAN, MD, PhD
Section Head, Burdenko Neurosurgical Institute, Moscow, Russian Federation, Russia

SPENCER KELLIS, PhD
USC Neurorestoration Center, Keck School of Medicine of USC, Los Angeles, California, USA; Department of Biology and Biological Engineering, T&C Chen Brain Machine Interface Center, California Institute of Technology, Pasadena, California, USA

MICHAEL KOGAN, MD, PhD
Resident Physician, Department of Neurosurgery, University at Buffalo, Buffalo, New York, USA

PETER KONRAD, MD, PhD
Professor, Department of Neurosurgery and Biomedical Engineering, Vanderbilt University Medical Center, Nashville, Tennessee, USA

DANIEL R. KRAMER, MD
Department of Neurological Surgery, Keck School of Medicine of USC, University of Southern California, USC Neurorestoration Center, Los Angeles, California, USA; T&C Chen Brain Machine Interface Center, California Institute of Technology, Pasadena, California, USA

WENDELL LAKE, MD, FAANS
Assistant Professor, Department of Neurosurgery, University of Wisconsin-Madison, University of Wisconsin Hospitals and Clinics, Madison, Wisconsin, USA

BRIAN LEE, MD, PhD
Department of Neurological Surgery, Keck School of Medicine of USC, University of Southern California, USC Neurorestoration Center, Los Angeles, California, USA; T&C Chen Brain Machine Interface Center, Department of Biology and Biological Engineering, California Institute of Technology, Pasadena, California, USA

MORGAN B. LEE, BS
Department of Neurological Surgery, Keck School of Medicine of USC, University of Southern California, USC Neurorestoration Center, Los Angeles, California, USA; T&C Chen Brain Machine Interface Center, California Institute of Technology, Pasadena, California, USA

CHARLES Y. LIU, MD, PhD
Department of Neurological Surgery, Keck School of Medicine of USC, University of Southern California, USC Neurorestoration Center, Los Angeles, California, USA; T&C Chen Brain Machine Interface Center, California Institute of Technology, Pasadena, California, USA

CAIO M. MATIAS, MD, PhD
Postdoctoral fellow, Department of Neurological Surgery, Thomas Jefferson University Hospitals, Philadelphia, Pennsylvania, USA; Neurosurgeon, Department of Surgery and Anatomy, Ribeirão Preto Medical School, University of São Paulo, Ribeirão Preto, São Paulo, Brazil

MATTHEW McGUIRE, BS
MD-PhD Candidate, Department of Neurosurgery, Jacobs School of Medicine and Biomedical Sciences, University at Buffalo, Buffalo, New York, USA

JOSEPH NEIMAT, MD, MS
Department Chair, Department of Neurosurgery, University of Louisville School of Medicine, Louisville, Kentucky, USA

YUNSEO LINDA PARK
Summer Research Fellow, Department of Neuroscience and Experimental Therapeutics, Albany Medical College, Albany, New York, USA

TERRANCE PENG, BS, MPH
Department of Neurological Surgery, Keck School of Medicine of USC, University of Southern California, USC Neurorestoration Center, Los Angeles, California, USA; T&C Chen Brain Machine Interface Center, California Institute of Technology, Pasadena, California, USA

JULIE G. PILITSIS, MD, PhD
Professor, Department of Neurosurgery, Chair, Department of Neuroscience and Experimental Therapeutics, Albany Medical College, Albany, New York, USA

JONATHAN RILEY, MD
Assistant Professor, Department of Neurosurgery, Jacobs School of Medicine and Biomedical Sciences, University at Buffalo, Buffalo, New York, USA; Medical Director, Functional Neurosurgery, Kaleida Health System, Orchard Park, New York, USA

ANDREW K. ROCK, MD, MHS
PGY-1 Resident, Department of Neurosurgery, Albany Medical College, Albany, New York, USA

HAMID SHAH, MD, FAANS
Assistant Professor, Department of Neurosurgery, Vanderbilt University, Nashville, Tennessee, USA

ASHWINI SHARAN, MD
Professor, Department of Neurological Surgery, Thomas Jefferson University Hospitals, Philadelphia, Pennsylvania, USA

SAMEER A. SHETH, MD, PhD
Associate Professor, Department of Neurosurgery, Baylor College of Medicine, Houston, Texas, USA

KONSTANTIN V. SLAVIN, MD
Professor, Department of Neurosurgery, The University of Illinois at Chicago, Chicago, Illinois, USA

VISHAD V. SUKUL, MD
Assistant Professor, Departments of Neurosurgery and Neuroscience and Experimental Therapeutics, Albany Medical College, Albany, New York, USA

HUY TRUONG, MD
Functional Neurosurgery Fellow, Department of Neurosurgery, Albany Medical College, Albany, New York, USA

CHRISTOPHER J. WINFREE, MD
Assistant Professor of Neurological Surgery, Department of Neurosurgery, Columbia University, New York, New York, USA

CHENGYUAN WU, MD, MSBME
Assistant Professor, Department of Neurological Surgery, Thomas Jefferson University Hospitals, Philadelphia, Pennsylvania, USA

AARON YENGO-KAHN, MD
Resident, Department of Neurological Surgery, Vanderbilt University Medical Center, Nashville, Tennessee, USA

DALI YIN, MD, PhD
Assistant Professor, Department of Neurosurgery, The University of Illinois at Chicago, Chicago, Illinois, USA

Contents

Preface: Neuromodulation: Successful Treatments, Future Opportunity, and Challenges xiii

Wendell Lake, Ashwini Sharan, and Chengyuan Wu

Deep Brain Stimulation for Parkinson Disease 137

Michael Kogan, Matthew McGuire, and Jonathan Riley

Parkinson disease (PD) is the second most common neurodegenerative disorder and affects more than 1 million individuals in the United States. Deep brain stimulation (DBS) is one form of treatment of PD. DBS treatment is still evolving due to technological innovations that shape how this therapy is used.

Deep Brain Stimulation for Treatment of Tremor 147

Wendell Lake, Peter Hedera, and Peter Konrad

Deep brain stimulation is now the most common surgical treatment of tremor. Tremor can be classified as action or resting tremor and is one of the most common movement disorders. Initial treatment of tremor should focus on medical treatment but, if patients fail medical therapy, deep brain stimulation should be considered with likely success. The usual target is the ventral intermediate nucleus of the thalamus. Common side effects of treatment include paresthesias, dysarthria, and less often ataxia. Future directions of research and development, including directional leads and closed-loop stimulation, may eventually lead to additional improvement in patient outcomes.

Neuromodulation: Deep Brain Stimulation for Treatment of Dystonia 161

Nicholas Dietz and Joseph Neimat

Dystonia is a heterogeneous, hyperkinetic movement disorder with sustained or intermittent abnormal postures, hyperkinetic muscle contractions, or repetitive movements. Classification of dystonia involves 2 axes: axis I and axis II, defining relevant clinical features and etiology, respectively. Medical therapy varies based on subtype and includes intramuscular botulinum toxin injections and oral anticholinergic pharmaceuticals. Deep brain stimulation became widely incorporated in 1999 after several landmark studies and has been effectively used in targets of the thalamus, pallidum, and subthalamic nucleus. New insights into pathophysiology of dystonia and genetic analysis continue to guide surgical technique toward ever-effective treatment.

Spinal Cord Stimulation 169

Andrew K. Rock, Huy Truong, Yunseo Linda Park, and Julie G. Pilitsis

Spinal cord stimulation (SCS) has been well established as a safe and effective treatment of pain derived from a wide variety of etiologies. Careful patient selection including a rigorous trial period and psychological evaluation are essential. When patients proceed to permanent implantation, various considerations should be made, such as the type of lead, type of anesthesia, and waveform patterns for SCS. This article discusses the common indications for SCS, patient selection criteria, and pertinent outcomes from randomized clinical trials related to common indications treated with SCS. Technical considerations, such as type of implant, anesthesia, and programming, are also discussed.

Intrathecal Pain Therapy for the Management of Chronic Noncancer Pain **195**

Vishad V. Sukul

Intrathecal drug delivery has been well established an effective and safe method for the treatment of pain, including palliative cancer-related and chronic nonmalignant pain. In this article, we discuss the role of intrathecal pain therapy in the management of chronic, refractory nonmalignant pain. Common indications, patient selection criteria, medication options, complications, and adverse events are discussed within the context of results from randomized controlled trials, clinical consensus guidelines, and best available literature to date.

Intrathecal Baclofen Infusion for the Treatment of Movement Disorders **203**

Wendell Lake and Hamid Shah

Intrathecal baclofen infusion is an accepted treatment for spasticity. Evidence also exists for the treatment of secondary generalized dystonia with intrathecal baclofen infusion. Benefits include decreased tone, improved positioning, and decreased decubitus ulcers. Despite these benefits, there are significant complications that can occur with this therapy, including drug withdrawal, catheter infection, drug overdose, failure, and pump failure. In some cases, practitioners encourage a trial dose of intrathecal baclofen by injection or catheter infusion before pump implantation. To improve patient selection and outcomes many centers offering intrathecal baclofen therapy use a multidisciplinary team composed of physicians, surgeons, and physical therapists.

Occipital Nerve Stimulation **211**

Konstantin V. Slavin, Emil D. Isagulyan, Christy Gomez, and Dali Yin

Although the first publications on clinical use of peripheral nerve stimulation for the treatment of chronic pain came out in the mid-1960s, it took 10 years before this approach was used to stimulate the occipital nerves. The future for occipital nerve stimulation is likely to bring new indications, devices, stimulation paradigms, and a decrease in invasiveness. As experience increases, one may expect that occipital nerve stimulation will eventually gain regulatory approval for more indications, most likely for occipital neuralgia, migraines and cluster headaches. This process may require additional studies, at least for approval from the US Food and Drug Administration.

Vagus Nerve Stimulation for the Treatment of Epilepsy **219**

Hernán F.J. González, Aaron Yengo-Kahn, and Dario J. Englot

Vagus nerve stimulation (VNS) was the first neuromodulation device approved for treatment of epilepsy. In more than 20 years of study, VNS has consistently demonstrated efficacy in treating epilepsy. After 2 years, approximately 50% of patients experience at least 50% reduced seizure frequency. Adverse events with VNS treatment are rare and include surgical adverse events (including infection, vocal cord paresis, and so forth) and stimulation side effects (hoarseness, voice change, and cough). Future developments in VNS, including closed-loop and noninvasive stimulation, may reduce side effects or increase efficacy of VNS.

Responsive Neurostimulation for the Treatment of Epilepsy **231**

Caio M. Matias, Ashwini Sharan, and Chengyuan Wu

There are a significant number of patients with epilepsy who are drug-resistant and for whom resective procedures are not an option. For these patients, neuromodulation may be an option, including closed-loop stimulation, such as responsive neurostimulation (RNS). The RNS System is a programmable and responsive device that consists of leads, a pulse generator, and an external programmer. An algorithm detects specific patterns of epileptogenic activity and triggers focal stimulation to interrupt a seizure. RNS is an effective and safe adjunctive therapy that in addition to seizure frequency reduction may have other applications, such as drug-response evaluation and long-term electrocorticography recording.

Deep Brain Stimulation for Depression: An Emerging Indication **243**

Megan M. Filkowski and Sameer A. Sheth

Depression is a heterogenous disorder, with roughly 30% of patients deemed resistant to conventional treatments. In these cases, neurosurgical interventions such as lesion procedures or deep brain stimulation offer possible therapeutic options. Here, we review neurosurgical interventions for treatment-resistant depression, focusing on the recent advancements and future directions of deep brain stimulation.

Nerve Stimulation for Pain **257**

Mark Corriveau, Wendell Lake, and Amgad Hanna

Nerve stimulation is a reversible technique that is used successfully for the treatment of traumatic neuropathic pain, complex regional pain syndrome, and craniofacial neuropathic pain. Nerve field stimulation targets painful regions rather than a single nerve and has expanded indications, including axial low back pain. Appropriate patient education and motivation are crucial prior to surgery. Ongoing research is necessary to provide high-level evidence for the use of nerve stimulation. Most electrodes are primarily designed for spinal cord stimulation, hence the need to develop nerve electrodes dedicated for nerve stimulation.

Evolving Techniques and Indications in Peripheral Nerve Stimulation for Pain **265**

Garrett P. Banks and Christopher J. Winfree

Peripheral nerve stimulation is the direct electrical stimulation of named nerves outside the central neuraxis to alleviate pain in the distribution of the targeted peripheral nerve. These treatments have shown efficacy in treating a variety of neuropathic, musculoskeletal, and visceral refractory pain pathologies; although not first line, these therapies are an important part of the treatment repertoire for chronic pain. With careful patient selection and judicious choice of stimulation technique, excellent results can be achieved for a variety of pain etiologies and distributions. This article reviews current and past practices of peripheral nerve stimulation and upcoming advancements in the field.

Brain-Computer Interfaces in Quadriplegic Patients **275**

Morgan B. Lee, Daniel R. Kramer, Terrance Peng, Michael F. Barbaro, Charles Y. Liu, Spencer Kellis, and Brian Lee

Brain-computer interfaces (BCI) are implantable devices that interface directly with the nervous system. BCI for quadriplegic patients restore function by reading motor

intent from the brain and use the signal to control physical, virtual, and native prosthetic effectors. Future closed-loop motor BCI will incorporate sensory feedback to provide patients with an effective and intuitive experience. Development of widely available BCI for patients with neurologic injury will depend on the successes of today's clinical BCI. BCI are an exciting next step in the frontier of neuromodulation.

NEUROSURGERY CLINICS OF NORTH AMERICA

FORTHCOMING ISSUES

July 2019
Lumbar Spondylolisthesis
Zoher Ghogawala, *Editor*

October 2019
Pituitary Adenoma
Manish K. Aghi and Lewis S. Blevins, *Editors*

January 2020
NewTechnologies in Spine Surgery
Nathaniel P. Brooks and Michael Y. Wang, *Editors*

RECENT ISSUES

January 2019
Low-Grade Glioma
Guy M. McKhann and Hugues Duffau, *Editors*

October 2018
Coagulation and Hematology in Neurological Surgery
Shahid M. Nimjee and Russell R. Lonser, *Editors*

July 2018
Degenerative Spinal Deformity: Creating Lordosis in the Lumbar Spine
Sigurd Berven and Praveen V. Mummaneni, *Editors*

Preface

Neuromodulation: Successful Treatments, Future Opportunity, and Challenges

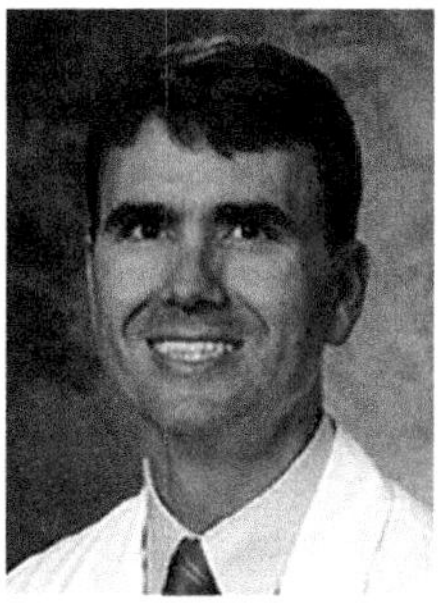
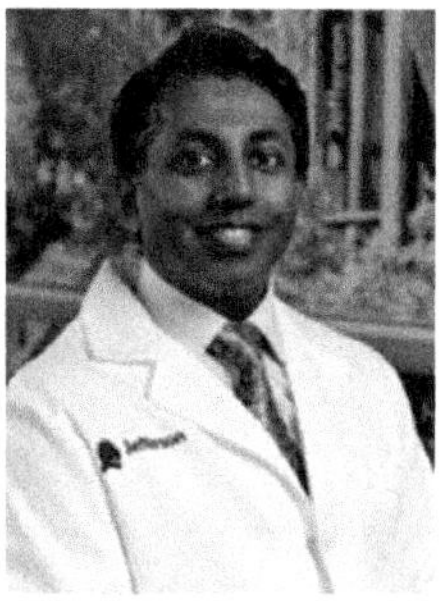
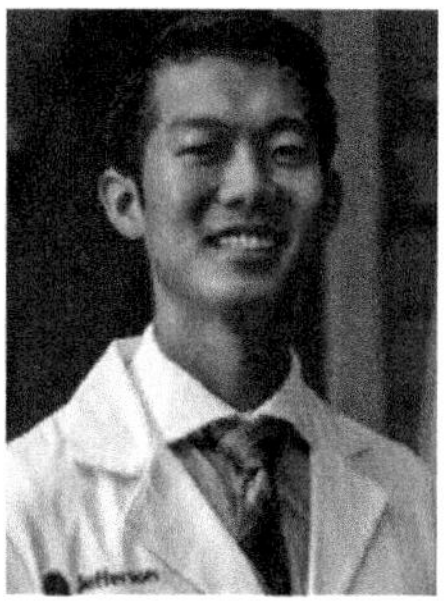

Wendell Lake, MD   Ashwini Sharan, MD   Chengyuan Wu, MD, MSBME

Editors

This issue of *Neurosurgery Clinics of North America* focuses on neuromodulation, one of the most exciting and rapidly growing areas of neurosurgery. Both physicians and patients have increasingly looked toward implantable electronic technologies to treat a multitude of conditions, including neurodegenerative diseases, movement disorders, psychiatric disorders, pain, and epilepsy.

In the current issue of *Neurosurgery Clinics of North America*, we seek to address the practical issues faced by clinicians implanting neuromodulatory devices for common indications, such as medically refractory tremor, Parkinson disease, and pain. With an eye toward the future, we also discuss emerging technologies, such as the use of neuromodulation for psychiatric indications, brain-computer interfaces, and the use of closed loop stimulation. Exciting advancement in our field will occur in two arenas: an expansion of neuromodulation technologies for new indications; and substantial improvement in existing neuromodulation technology for illnesses currently being treated.

While there is good reason to be excited about our field, there are also concerns that physicians must continue to address. We must continue to pursue high-quality clinical studies demonstrating the efficacy of these treatments and use basic science to elucidate mechanisms of action for these treatments. Understanding these mechanisms of action will allow us to further improve and advance the technology. As devices become increasingly interconnected, contain more data, and continue to provide ongoing therapy, issues of privacy and data management will arise. Finally, as physicians and patient advocates, we must assure that as these devices become accessible to patients from a variety of socioeconomic backgrounds. We hope this issue enhances your current clinical practice while encouraging you to think about the exciting future of neuromodulation.

Wendell Lake, MD
Department of Neurosurgery
University of Wisconsin-Madison
600 Highland Avenue, Box 8660
Madison, WI 53792, USA

Ashwini Sharan, MD
Department of Neurological Surgery
Thomas Jefferson University Hospitals
909 Walnut Street, Third Floor
Philadelphia, PA 19107, USA

Chengyuan Wu, MD, MSBME
Department of Neurological Surgery
Thomas Jefferson University Hospitals
909 Walnut Street, Third Floor
Philadelphia, PA 19107, USA

E-mail addresses:
lake@neurosurgery.wisc.edu (W. Lake)
ashwini.sharan@jefferson.edu (A. Sharan)
chengyuan.wu@jefferson.edu (C. Wu)

Neurosurg Clin N Am 30 (2019) xiii
https://doi.org/10.1016/j.nec.2019.01.003

Deep Brain Stimulation for Parkinson Disease

Michael Kogan, MD, PhD[a], Matthew McGuire, BS[b], Jonathan Riley, MD[c,*]

KEYWORDS

- Parkinson disease • Deep brain stimulation • Levodopa

KEY POINTS

- Parkinson disease (PD) is the second most common neurodegenerative disorder and affects more than 1 million individuals in the United States.
- Deep brain stimulation (DBS) is one form of treatment of PD.
- DBS treatment is still evolving due to technological innovations that shape how this therapy is used.

INTRODUCTION

Parkinson disease (PD) is the second most common neurodegenerative disorder and affects more than 1 million individuals in the United States; 75% of patients are afflicted with the cardinal disease feature of a resting tremor.[1] Several treatment options have been developed over the preceding decades to treat the motor complications of PD, which significantly affect quality of life and psychosocial well-being.[2] There is a rich experience in the early stereotactic neurosurgical literature with use of lesion-based interventions to ameliorate the motor manifestations of PD. The introduction of levodopa (L-dopa) and subsequently dopaminergic agonists quickly became the cornerstone of treatment. Seminal work by pioneers, such as Dr Mahlon DeLong[3,4] and Dr Alim Benabid,[5–7] expanded on the early stereotactic experience. Their work, respectively, further delineated the role of the basal ganglia in physiology (and pathology) and explored high-frequency deep brain stimulation (DBS) as an emerging therapeutic modality. This article explores the context for utilization of DBS as a treatment of PD viewed through the lens of historically available treatments. This foundation is used to explore the currently evolving role for implementation of DBS and technological innovations that continue to shape how this therapy is used.

MEDICAL MANAGEMENT AND DEEP BRAIN STIMULATION: A SHIFTING DYNAMIC

Early Interventions and Stereotactic Lesioning

During the 1950s and 1960s, stereotactic surgery lesioning the globus pallidus internus (GPi) (pallidotomy) or the ventralis intermedius (Vim) nucleus of the thalamus (thalamotomy) was the primary surgical treatment of PD.[8] These procedures were applied as treatment of symptoms in refractory cases and little was available in the way of medical management for motor complications in patients with advanced PD. Stereotactic ablations focused on the pallidothalamic pathway, including the globous pallidus, its outflow pathways, and the thalamus. Lesions in the GPi improved dyskinesias and parkinsonian motor symptoms.[9] Overall, these procedures often resulted in an improvement of motor symptoms but at the risk of irreversible and severe side effects like dysarthria or hemiparesis.[10] Performance of bilateral surgical

Disclosure: The authors have nothing to disclose.

[a] Department of Neurosurgery, University at Buffalo, 100 High Street Section B, 4th Floor, Buffalo, NY 14203, USA; [b] Department of Neurosurgery, Jacobs School of Medicine and Biomedical Sciences, University at Buffalo, 875 Ellicott Street, 6071 CTRC, Buffalo, NY 14203, USA; [c] Department of Neurosurgery, Jacobs School of Medicine and Biomedical Sciences, University at Buffalo, Functional Neurosurgery Kaleida Health System, 5959 Big Tree Road, Orchard Park, NY 14207, USA
* Corresponding author.
E-mail address: jriley@ubns.com

Neurosurg Clin N Am 30 (2019) 137–146
https://doi.org/10.1016/j.nec.2019.01.001
1042-3680/19/

lesions dramatically increased complications and, therefore, was rarely performed.[11]

Levodopa and a Shift Toward Medical Management

When L-dopa, an effective medical treatment of PD, was introduced in 1967, the following decade saw a reduction in the number of surgical interventions for PD.[8,12–14] L-dopa, the metabolic precursor to dopamine, is an oral medication that uses the aromatic amino acid transport system in the gut to enter the bloodstream. From here, the drug can enter into the central nervous system by crossing the blood-brain barrier via active transport from aromatic amino acid transporters. Once in the central nervous system, L-dopa can be taken up by presynaptic dopaminergic neurons and metabolized into dopamine via decarboxylation. Dopaminergic conversion is responsible for the therapeutic actions of L-dopa therapy as well as its side effects. After release from the dopaminergic neurons, dopamine can then be either reabsorbed by the presynaptic terminal or metabolized by monoamine oxidase A and B and catechol O-methyltransferase into inactive metabolites.

Clinically, L-dopa is often administered with a concurrent L-amino acid decarboxylase inhibitor, carbidopa. The combination of carbidopa–L-dopa is known by the trade name, Sinemet. The L-amino acid decarboxylase inhibitor prevents the metabolism of L-dopa into dopamine within the systemic circulation and liver.[15] Without this coadministration, less than 1% of the given L-dopa arrives at the target dopaminergic neurons in the substantia nigra. Additionally, the peripheral conversion to dopamine can produce the side effects of nausea, vomiting, and orthostatic hypotension. More severe adverse reactions to L-dopa therapy may occur in patients and can include confusion, hallucinations, delusions, agitation, psychosis, and orthostatic hypotension.

Prolonged administration of increasing doses of L-dopa formulations promote the development of motor fluctuations, known as the wearing off phenomenon. This commonly manifests as return of tremor, akinesia, rigidity, and dystonia. The risk of motor complications increases with a younger age at PD onset and with an increasing L-dopa dosing regimen.[16] The increasing motor fluctuations over time most likely are due to progressive degeneration of nigrostriatal dopamine terminals, which increasingly limits the normal physiologic uptake and release of dopamine, thereby leading to reduced buffering of the natural fluctuations in plasma L-dopa.

A longstanding clinical concern is that L-dopa has the potential to promote oxidative stress from dopaminergic metabolism and cause accelerated neurodegeneration. Clinically, a common strategy is to delay the initiation of L-dopa until symptoms significantly interfere with patient function. A concern is that prolonged use of L-dopa may directly hasten the degeneration of dopamine neurons in the substantia nigra by promoting the generation of free radicals and oxidative stress. Conversely, the Earlier vs Later L-DOPA (ELLDOPA) study data suggested that L-dopa may either slow the progression of PD or even be neuroprotective, leading other investigators to argue that a delay in treatment unnecessarily deprives patients of therapeutic benefit early in the disease course.[17]

Re-emergence of Surgical Intervention, the Contemporary Role for Deep Brain Stimulation

Subcortical neurostimulation historically was used to localize the area to be lesioned during an ablative procedure, such as a thalamotomy,[18] and later became an adjustable and reversible alternative procedure to stereotactic lesioning procedures.[5] In randomized controlled trials, DBS showed a better functional outcome with fewer side effects[19] and, therefore, has largely replaced lesional surgery in the United States as a first-line surgical therapy.[11] A broad consensus now exists among neurologists and neurosurgeons that DBS results in improved quality-of-life measures for movement disorder patients. Nevertheless, relative to the number of PD diagnoses made each year, DBS for PD is likely underutilized as a therapeutic intervention.[20]

Goals of intervention

Improved motor control is the main goal of surgical treatment of PD. Factors guiding consideration of surgery include symptoms, age, degree of functional disability, comorbidities, patient preference, and likelihood of overall benefit.[20]

Symptoms that are resistant to dopaminergic medications are typically also resistant to DBS; therefore, candidates should achieve an improvement of at least 30% in the preoperative L-dopa test measurement measured by the United Parkinson's Disease Rating Scale (UPDRS) motor score.[11] Preoperative evaluation of cognitive function and neuropsychiatric symptoms is of importance. Manifestations of dementia and/or psychiatric disorders like psychosis or depression that are persistent during ON phases and uncompensated personality disorders are potential contraindications for DBS.[11] Consideration of patients' social support network is also of importance, given the need for postoperative care and DBS programming that allow optimal results for this therapy.

The efficacy of bilateral DBS for the treatment of motor symptoms and L-dopa–induced dyskinesias in PD patients is well established. Symptoms that are best controlled by DBS can be classified as L-dopa-sensitive OFF symptoms, L-dopa-induced dyskinesias (such as peak-dose hyperkinesia and biphasic dyskinesia), OFF-dystonia, and tremor.[11,21] As discussed later, recent investigations are challenging the early pattern of practice that DBS should be reserved for late-stage patients.

Considerations of target choice for different subpopulations

Management of individual patients with PD requires careful consideration of multiple factors. The clinical heterogeneity of individual cases of PD can complicate the selection of the appropriate target for DBS. Factors influencing target selection include preference and experience of the surgical center, predominance of dyskinesias and dystonia, risk of future cognitive or psychiatric comorbidity, and preoperative L-dopa requirements.[20,22–24] Currently there are no definitive objective data that guide specific target selection in DBS for PD, but many practitioners seek to tailor DBS target selection to the unique needs of the individual patient.

The 2 prevailing targets used for DBS treatment of PD include the subthalamic nucleus (STN) and the GPi.[11] A large randomized controlled trial (Veterans Affairs Cooperative Studies Program [CSP]) compared DBS outcomes using either the STN or the GPi target. The study found that patients undergoing STN stimulation needed lower L-dopa doses but had worsening of visuomotor processing, worsening of depressive symptoms, and poorer scores on dementia rating scales as well as verbal learning tests. Cognitive findings may have been affected by slightly poorer preoperative cognitive function in the STN group.[20,25] Assessments of cognitive function included the Mattis Dementia Rating Scale and the Hopkins Verbal Learning Test. These findings initially indicated that GPi targeting was better tolerated from cognitive and psychiatric standpoints and that the STN targeting is preferable if a significant reduction in medication requirement is sought. Longer follow-up studies bring into question whether clear differences exist between the STN and GPi regarding these findings.[26,27]

Targeting of locomotor-related brain stem nuclei, such as the pedunculopontine nucleus, has shown benefit for some patients with PD; however, in several randomized trials, the results have been variable across patients.[20,28–30]

Reimagining the Role for Deep Brain Stimulation

DBS has traditionally been considered for patients with intermediate to late motor complications of PD, and many patients were diagnosed with the illness 10 years or more prior to their consideration for DBS. Consequences of this include both an older chronologic age at time of implantation and having dealt with stimulation-responsive symptomatology for a longer period of time through medication adjustments alone. Implications for the former are the possibility for increased frailty and development of comorbidities, and implications of the latter include having endured more medication adjustments and medication-related side effects earlier in the disease course. These observations and small-scale prospective studies[31] prompted completion of the Controlled Trial With Deep Brain Stimulation in Patients With Early Parkinson's Disease (EARLYSTIM) study.[32] This was an investigator-initiated, parallel-group, multicenter, prospective study that considered implantation of patients with motor complications of PD for a duration of 4 or more years. The mean age was 52 years (range 18–60 years) and mean disease duration was 7.5 years. Patients were followed for 2 years and blinded analysis supported that both groups conformed to the standard of care for medical therapy. At trial conclusion, the neurostimulation group had improved motor complications and activities of daily living, reduced L-dopa-induced dyskinesias, increased time with good mobility. These data were further supported by follow-up analyses, indicating the cost-effectiveness of early intervention in with PD-related motor complications in patients who fit the criteria of the EARLYSTIM trial (eg, <61 years old).[33] A further note is that this study was conducted in Germany and France; validity of economic analyses, therefore, should be used only for qualitative inference.

Although EARLYSTIM has provided clinical data supporting earlier implementation of neurostimulation after development of PD-related motor complications, parallel lines of inquiry have explored a role for early neurostimulation as modifying the course of disease progression. Preclinical studies have demonstrated a neuroprotective effect for STN stimulation with regards to nigral protection.[34–36] These preclinical data provided the basis for a pilot investigation comparing optimal drug therapy (ODT) to ODT + DBS.[37] Enrolled patients (50–75 years old) were on medication (6 months to 4 years) but without dyskinesias or other motor fluctuations. All patients underwent weeklong inpatient stays at baseline and at 6-month intervals during the study to allow a monitored washout of all PD-related therapies; 28 of 30 enrolled patients were included in the final analysis. Medication requirements were reduced in the DBS + ODT group. Expectedly, given the early intervention, UPDRS total and UPDRS-III scores did not differ between groups at the study conclusion. Detailed subsequent analysis, however, yielded findings of UPDRS-III subscore worsening for resting tremor and findings of an increasing number of limbs affected by resting tremor in the ODT group compared with the DBS + ODT group.[38] These findings provide the basis for an upcoming Food and Drug Administration (FDA)-approved multicenter pivotal trial that will assess the role for STN stimulation as a possible PD-modifying therapy.

ONGOING PROCEDURAL ENHANCEMENTS

Iterative technological advances have resulted in ongoing improvements in both patient customized target identification as well as novel surgical approaches for electrode placement. These ongoing technological improvements have allowed new working paradigms to emerge. Recent advances in microelectrode recording (MER)-based targeting techniques and imaging-based targeting techniques are reviewed. Direct comparisons between various methodological approaches are sparse. Excellent results have been shown, however, for both enhanced MER-based techniques and evolving imaging-based targeting paradigms. Additionally, selected hardware-based and software-based advances are reviewed.

Microelectrode Targeting–based Enhancements

At the inception of stereotactic targeting, standardized coordinates were used to localize targets for PD based on consensus measurements obtained from early stereotactic atlas analysis. A coordinate system generated from the midpoint of the anterior commissure–posterior commissure line allowed standardization between patients. In combination with rigid external frame use, this method allowed for more precise targeting than previously possible. Interindividual patient variation was too great, however, to target based solely on standardized coordinates.[39] In this setting, electrophysiologic techniques, including MER and either stimulation through the microelectrode or the DBS lead, became important tools to customize standardized coordinates to individual patients.[40]

The application of novel analytics to the MER waveform is providing new insights into electrode placement. For example, although the dorsal aspect of the STN border may be easy to identify using MER, the ventral STN/substantia nigra pars reticulata (SNr) border may be difficult to distinguish given a close physical proximity and similar recording features.[41] Furthermore, a trajectory that misses the STN but reaches SNr may seem well localized using MER alone. Spectral analysis of MER has been used effectively and holds promise for potential intraoperative use.[42,43] In 1 study, investigators used a supervised machine learning protocol to differentiate between STN and SNr in prior electrode recordings.[44] In this setting, the ratio of high-frequency (100–150 Hz) to low-frequency (5–25 Hz) power was able to differentiate between the 2 nuclei and delineate the start and end of the STN along the trajectory. Quantitative confirmation of the length of the trajectory through subcortical nuclei provides a powerful adjunctive tool to the prior qualitative confirmation of an adequate run that sometimes can vary upwards of 1 mm with determination of the entrance and exit.

Direct Imaging–based Targeting Advances

The introduction of improved MRI techniques has seen the reliance on anatomic atlases give way to increasingly refined patient specific imaging-based targeting techniques. MRI has made it possible to directly visualize deep structures, such as the GPi and STN. T2, Fast Gray Matter Acquisition T1 Inversion Recovery, Quantitative Susceptibility Mapping, Susceptibility weighted imaging, Diffusion Tensor Imaging (DTI)-based techniques have been investigated for DBS planning.[45–50] Although no consensus currently exists for optimal targeting based on this newly available imaging, these capabilities have led to improved understanding of the anatomy targeted in DBS that extends beyond defined structural anatomy.

In light of variations in patient anatomy, recent efforts have yielded deformable atlases that may be used in conjunction with MRI to aid target selection. Such deformable atlases also hold significant promise for research application by bringing individual patient imaging into a normalized image space. Standard printed atlases, based on anatomic and histologic studies, have been used to guide stereotactic procedures for decades.[51,52] Many of these resources have now been digitized and can be superimposed onto patient-specific anatomy, which further augments DBS targeting.[53–55] These digitized anatomic representations may aid target selection in cases where deep nuclei are difficult to visualize.

In addition to traditional MRI sequences, DTI has emerged as an alternative for visualization of deep structures. DTI technology is based on the brownian motion of hydrogen, presumed to follow axonal pathways. This imaging can produce accurate connectivity maps between cortical and nuclear regions.[56,57] In DBS, DTI has found multiple uses: visualization of targets not seen on traditional T1-weighted and T2-weighted MRI, retrospective analysis of effective lead placement and connectivity, and revision of electrode position for patients not receiving clinical benefit.[58,59] Retrospectively, effects of stimulation may be estimated by tract stimulation modeling or tract proximity analysis, which respectively seek to either estimate the affected tracts from specific contact stimulation or evaluate the distance of a specific tract of interest to a lead. Direct tract targeting allows for planning a trajectory of interest based on a selected tract.

Retrospective analysis has shown compelling evidence that tract stimulation does relate to clinical outcome in DBS for PD. In 1 study, effective lead stimulation was found to also activate dentatorubrothalamic tract (DRT).[60] The distance of the DRT has also been shown to be close to effective electrode contacts across multiple PD patients.[61,62] Likewise, in a case study of a PD patient with initial suboptimal lead placement, subsequent successful lead revision surgery was shown to place the now effective lead in closer proximity to DRT.[63] Similar findings showed conserved fiber network activation in 12 VIM patients who underwent DBS for tremor-predominant PD.[64] In 1 patient with gait-predominant PD, long-term follow-up of successful DBS demonstrated restoration of normal connectivity. Although there is little prospective evidence that direct tract targeting improves clinical outcome in DBS for PD, several findings suggest that such approaches hold promise for future DBS target localization.[65] In 2 patients with tremor-predominant PD, DTI was used to allow for electrode spanning both DRT and STN with good clinical results.[66] Because direct targeting has also been successfully used to target tracts in numerous other pathologies, it is likely that further targeting studies will be undertaken for PD.[58] The success of DTI in these instances, along with findings that anatomic nuclear targets do not always correlate to maximal effect, have even led to theories that tract stimulation may account for the therapeutic effect seen in DBS.[58]

Direct Imaging–Based Targeting and Intraoperative Lead Confirmation

Compared with the use of intraoperative electrophysiology and patient assessment to assist with confirmation of lead positioning, direct imaging–based lead placement commonly is completed under general anesthesia. Common practice, therefore, is to obtain intraoperative 3-D confirmation of lead placement. Two common approaches are commonly used. In the first method, lead position is confirmed by using image processing software to merge an intraoperative CT (Ceretom [NeuroLogica, Danvers, Massachusetts], or O-arm [Medtronic, Minneapolis, Minnesota]) with a preoperative MRI to verify that the lead position is acceptably close to the planned target. The 2 commonly available systems for intraoperative CT scanning have various benefits and disadvantages. The O-arm offers a larger working area, allowing imaging with frame in place, whereas the Ceretom offers improved soft tissue visualization and is considered to provide images of diagnostic quality. Alternatively, in the second strategy commonly used for asleep DBS lead placement, the procedure may completed in an intraoperative or interventional MRI (iMRI) with a specialized MRI compatible frame that allows stereotactic lead placement (ClearPoint [MRI Interventions, Irvine, California]).[67] Because this approach requires the use of nonferromagnetic operating room instruments and often a dedicated MRI scanner, comparatively few hospitals have been able to implement this technology. Intraoperative MRI (iMRI), however avoids the added error of CT/MRI coregistration and also may compensate for brain shift–related error.

The availability of intraoperative imaging has raised debate about the necessity of intraoperative recording. Although not directly compared with (Electrophysiology) EP-based placement, asleep CT-based and MRI-based techniques have yielded results that are comparable to awake surgeries. A case series of 66 PD and ET patients using Ceretom and Nexframe (Medtronic) yielded reliable accuracy under 2 mm.[68] Furthermore, of 119 electrodes placed, only 1 required revision. After a review of factors affecting electrode deviation, proximity to ventricle (under 4 mm) was the most significant factor in trajectory error. Subsequent analysis of 160 leads in 94 patients has also demonstrated that medial shift is likely when targeting STN and VIM, and coronal approach angle may affect VIM placement.[69] Similarly, iMRI-based DBS for PD has shown trajectory error magnitude comparable to that of intraoperative CT and lower procedure times than traditional awake

MER, although it is not clear that there is any superiority of outcome for asleep DBS procedures.[70,71] In light of these results and the increased risk of intracranial hemorrhage with the multiple passes associated with MER,[72,73] some investigators have suggested making asleep DBS routine. Direct comparisons are likely needed between asleep image–guided and awake methodologies. Furthermore, the role of limited MER in awake or asleep setting with image navigation has yet to be rigorously evaluated.

SELECTED ADVANCES IN DEEP BRAIN STIMULATION HARDWARE AND PROGRAMMING

The advent of DBS for PD has led to improved quality of life for many patients. Nonetheless, significant opportunities remain for improvement in this therapy.[74] Patients who have elevated energy requirements to obtain effective therapy may require frequent battery changes. Furthermore, many patients have optimal settings that are task-specific, necessitating a manual change in programming in preparation for a specific activity. The concept of closed-loop DBS holds promise to improve therapy administration by providing a mechanism to automatically detect changes in physical activity or state and then delivering customized stimulation only at the appropriate time and at optimized settings. In general, there are 2 approaches to closed-loop stimulation: invasive and noninvasive. Invasive methods involve placement of a permanent detector to communicate with an implantable pulse generator (IPG) device, whereas noninvasive techniques involve fixation of external devices that can be worn and wirelessly communicate with an IPG. NeuroPace (Mountain View, California), the first commercial closed-loop system for neuromodulation, created currently available for epilepsy applications.[75] For PD, Medtronic produces an investigational device, the Activa PC + S, an IPG capable of both signal detection and stimulation therapy. This system may be used in conjunction with sophisticated methods, such as an external computer signal processing, by using a wireless interface (Nexus-D system, Medtronic).

Invasive signals have been acquired in PD populations from a variety of intracranial sources, such as cortical strip (electrocorticography [EcOG)][76–80]; subcortical electrode, such as the DBS electrode itself (local field protentional [LFP])[81–87]; and other experimental recordings. For example, direct dopamine sampling has been suggested as a marker for basal ganglia activity[88]; however, the efficacy of this approach remains to be shown in humans. EcOG is relatively noninvasive and has the advantage of allowing for simultaneous recording and stimulation, which is not possible when both are done though 1 DBS lead. Noninvasive methods may detect state changes. This has been accomplished with PD patients using external scalp electroencephalogram,[89] electromyogram,[90,91] or peripheral motion sensors.[90,92] Although requiring no additional hardware placement, the practical feasibility of these external devices for long-term treatment is a barrier to their use. Both LFP and EcOG-based approaches have been shown to detect state changes in PD patients.[76,78,84,85] Based on these detected states, a variety of program strategies have been developed. This remains an active area of investigation.[93,94] Closed-loop strategies have been shown to reduce the needed battery power in PD patients and have shown excellent clinical results compared with the standard open-loop approach.[95,96]

Both MER-guided and image-guided asleep techniques for DBS lead placement commonly produce clinically acceptable electrode placement,[71] but in some cases there is a need to optimize stimulation for electrodes that are not placed in an ideal location. Furthermore, some patients have multiple settings and may use different electrodes for various tasks.[97] The proximity to off-target sites may limit the possible therapeutic voltage that is possible for a given lead site. New research has demonstrated that directing current selectively to the site of therapeutic interest is feasible.[98,99] A pilot study of 14 STN patients using the Vercise PC (Boston Scientific, Valencia, California) system demonstrated significant improvements compared with nondirectional stimulation.[100] Larger improvements were seen in electrodes that were ineffective with traditional radial stimulation, suggesting that patients with suboptimal electrodes are most likely to benefit from directional stimulation as a form of salvage therapy.

SUMMARY

Since FDA approval in 1997, DBS has revolutionized the treatment of PD. Within the past decade, the technology has seen an explosion of ideas in both surgical targeting and more nuanced stimulation delivery with new devices. The ability to use intraoperative imaging, as well as DTI, has made it possible to target deep nuclei more accurately, perhaps without the need for MER. DTI targeting also may allow for electrode placement that incorporates or avoids specific fiber tracts. Furthermore, electrodes placed in proximity to otherwise typically avoided structures may be salvaged with directional stimulation. The ability to use multiple sites, in combination with automated state detection may, also may provide more nuanced closed-loop stimulation paradigms. Although more work is needed to show the clinical utility of many new treatment strategies, DBS for PD is an established treatment, and techniques and devices for implementing this treatment are certain to increase in coming decades.

REFERENCES

1. Heusinkveld LE, Hacker ML, Turchan M, et al. Impact of tremor on patients with early stage Parkinson's disease. Front Neurol 2018;9:628.
2. Hariz GM, Limousin P, Hamberg K. "DBS means everything - for some time". Patients' perspectives on daily life with deep brain stimulation for parkinson's disease. J Parkinsons Dis 2016;6(2): 335–47.
3. Wichmann T, DeLong MR. Pathophysiology of parkinsonian motor abnormalities. Adv Neurol 1993;60:53–61.
4. Mitchell SJ, Richardson RT, Baker FH, et al. The primate globus pallidus: neuronal activity related to direction of movement. Exp Brain Res 1987;68(3): 491–505.
5. Benabid AL, Pollak P, Gervason C, et al. Long-term suppression of tremor by chronic stimulation of the ventral intermediate thalamic nucleus. Lancet 1991;337(8738):403–6.
6. Benabid AL, Pollak P, Louveau A, et al. Combined (thalamotomy and stimulation) stereotactic surgery of the VIM thalamic nucleus for bilateral Parkinson disease. Appl Neurophysiol 1987;50(1–6):344–6.
7. Krack P, Pollak P, Limousin P, et al. Stimulation of subthalamic nucleus alleviates tremor in Parkinson's disease. Lancet 1997;350(9092):1675.
8. Rodriguez-Oroz MC, Moro E, Krack P. Long-term outcomes of surgical therapies for Parkinson's disease. Mov Disord 2012;27(14):1718–28.
9. Lang AE, Lozano AM. Parkinson's disease. First of two parts. N Engl J Med 1998;339(15):1044–53.
10. Fasano A, Daniele A, Albanese A. Treatment of motor and non-motor features of Parkinson's disease with deep brain stimulation. Lancet Neurol 2012; 11(5):429–42.
11. Groiss SJ, Wojtecki L, Sudmeyer M, et al. Deep brain stimulation in Parkinson's disease. Ther Adv Neurol Disord 2009;2(6):20–8.
12. Speelman JD, Schuurman PR, de Bie RM, et al. Thalamic surgery and tremor. Mov Disord 1998; 13(Suppl 3):103–6.
13. Hariz MI. From functional neurosurgery to "interventional" neurology: survey of publications on thalamotomy, pallidotomy, and deep brain stimulation for Parkinson's disease from 1966 to 2001. Mov Disord 2003;18(8):845–53.
14. Yahr MD, Duvoisin RC, Schear MJ, et al. Treatment of parkinsonism with levodopa. Arch Neurol 1969; 21(4):343–54.
15. Di Stefano A, Sozio P, Cerasa LS, et al. L-Dopa prodrugs: an overview of trends for improving Parkinson's disease treatment. Curr Pharm Des 2011; 17(32):3482–93.
16. Kadastik-Eerme L, Taba N, Asser T, et al. Factors associated with motor complications in Parkinson's disease. Brain Behav 2017;7(10):e00837.
17. Fahn S, Oakes D, Shoulson I, et al. Levodopa and the progression of Parkinson's disease. N Engl J Med 2004;351(24):2498–508.
18. Albe-Fessard D. Electrophysiological methods for the identification of thalamic nuclei. Z Neurol 1973;205(1):15–28.
19. Schuurman PR, Bosch DA, Bossuyt PM, et al. A comparison of continuous thalamic stimulation and thalamotomy for suppression of severe tremor. N Engl J Med 2000;342(7):461–8.
20. Rowland NC, Sammartino F, Lozano AM. Advances in surgery for movement disorders. Mov Disord 2017;32(1):5–10.
21. Limousin-Dowsey P, Pollak P, Van Blercom N, et al. Thalamic, subthalamic nucleus and internal pallidum stimulation in Parkinson's disease. J Neurol 1999;246(Suppl 2):II42–5.
22. Fasano A, Lozano AM. Deep brain stimulation for movement disorders: 2015 and beyond. Curr Opin Neurol 2015;28(4):423–36.
23. Siegfried J, Lippitz B. Bilateral chronic electrostimulation of ventroposterolateral pallidum: a new therapeutic approach for alleviating all parkinsonian symptoms. Neurosurgery 1994;35(6):1126–9 [discussion: 1129–30].
24. Bergman H, Wichmann T, DeLong MR. Reversal of experimental parkinsonism by lesions of the subthalamic nucleus. Science 1990;249(4975):1436–8.
25. Follett KA, Weaver FM, Stern M, et al. Pallidal versus subthalamic deep-brain stimulation for Parkinson's disease. N Engl J Med 2010;362(22): 2077–91.
26. Weaver FM, Follett KA, Stern M, et al. Randomized trial of deep brain stimulation for Parkinson disease: thirty-six-month outcomes. Neurology 2012; 79(1):55–65.
27. Odekerken VJ, Boel JA, Geurtsen GJ, et al. Neuropsychological outcome after deep brain stimulation for Parkinson disease. Neurology 2015;84(13): 1355–61.
28. Ferraye MU, Debu B, Fraix V, et al. Effects of pedunculopontine nucleus area stimulation on gait disorders in Parkinson's disease. Brain 2010; 133(Pt 1):205–14.
29. Moro E, Hamani C, Poon YY, et al. Unilateral pedunculopontine stimulation improves falls in Parkinson's disease. Brain 2010;133(Pt 1):215–24.

30. Collomb-Clerc A, Welter ML. Effects of deep brain stimulation on balance and gait in patients with Parkinson's disease: a systematic neurophysiological review. Neurophysiol Clin 2015;45(4–5):371–88.
31. Schupbach WM, Maltete D, Houeto JL, et al. Neurosurgery at an earlier stage of Parkinson disease: a randomized, controlled trial. Neurology 2007;68(4):267–71.
32. Schuepbach WM, Rau J, Knudsen K, et al. Neurostimulation for Parkinson's disease with early motor complications. N Engl J Med 2013;368(7):610–22.
33. Dams J, Balzer-Geldsetzer M, Siebert U, et al. Cost-effectiveness of neurostimulation in Parkinson's disease with early motor complications. Mov Disord 2016;31(8):1183–91.
34. Musacchio T, Rebenstorff M, Fluri F, et al. Subthalamic nucleus deep brain stimulation is neuroprotective in the A53T alpha-synuclein Parkinson's disease rat model. Ann Neurol 2017;81(6):825–36.
35. Wallace BA, Ashkan K, Heise CE, et al. Survival of midbrain dopaminergic cells after lesion or deep brain stimulation of the subthalamic nucleus in MPTP-treated monkeys. Brain 2007;130(Pt 8): 2129–45.
36. Spieles-Engemann AL, Steece-Collier K, Behbehani MM, et al. Subthalamic nucleus stimulation increases brain derived neurotrophic factor in the nigrostriatal system and primary motor cortex. J Parkinsons Dis 2011;1(1):123–36.
37. Charles D, Konrad PE, Neimat JS, et al. Subthalamic nucleus deep brain stimulation in early stage Parkinson's disease. Parkinsonism Relat Disord 2014;20(7):731–7.
38. Hacker ML, DeLong MR, Turchan M, et al. Effects of deep brain stimulation on rest tremor progression in early stage Parkinson disease. Neurology 2018;91(5):e463–71.
39. Nestor KA, Jones JD, Butson CR, et al. Coordinate-based lead location does not predict Parkinson's disease deep brain stimulation outcome. PLoS One 2014;9(4):e93524.
40. Amirnovin R, Williams ZM, Cosgrove GR, et al. Experience with microelectrode guided subthalamic nucleus deep brain stimulation. Neurosurgery 2006;58(1 Suppl):ONS96–102 [discussion: ONS96–102].
41. Hutchison WD, Allan RJ, Opitz H, et al. Neurophysiological identification of the subthalamic nucleus in surgery for Parkinson's disease. Ann Neurol 1998;44(4):622–8.
42. Moran A, Bar-Gad I, Bergman H, et al. Real-time refinement of subthalamic nucleus targeting using Bayesian decision-making on the root mean square measure. Mov Disord 2006;21(9):1425–31.
43. Wong S, Baltuch GH, Jaggi JL, et al. Functional localization and visualization of the subthalamic nucleus from microelectrode recordings acquired during DBS surgery with unsupervised machine learning. J Neural Eng 2009;6(2):026006.
44. Valsky D, Marmor-Levin O, Deffains M, et al. Stop! border ahead: Automatic detection of subthalamic exit during deep brain stimulation surgery. Mov Disord 2017;32(1):70–9.
45. Polanski WH, Martin KD, Engellandt K, et al. Accuracy of subthalamic nucleus targeting by T2, FLAIR and SWI-3-Tesla MRI confirmed by microelectrode recordings. Acta Neurochir (Wien) 2015;157(3): 479–86.
46. Chandran AS, Bynevelt M, Lind CR. Magnetic resonance imaging of the subthalamic nucleus for deep brain stimulation. J Neurosurg 2016; 124(1):96–105.
47. Rasouli J, Ramdhani R, Panov FE, et al. Utilization of quantitative susceptibility mapping for direct targeting of the subthalamic nucleus during deep brain stimulation surgery. Oper Neurosurg (Hagerstown) 2018;14(4):412–9.
48. Sudhyadhom A, Haq IU, Foote KD, et al. A high resolution and high contrast MRI for differentiation of subcortical structures for DBS targeting: the Fast Gray Matter Acquisition T1 Inversion Recovery (FGATIR). Neuroimage 2009;47(Suppl 2):T44–52.
49. Liu T, Eskreis-Winkler S, Schweitzer AD, et al. Improved subthalamic nucleus depiction with quantitative susceptibility mapping. Radiology 2013;269(1):216–23.
50. Coenen VA, Jenkner C, Honey CR, et al. Electrophysiologic validation of diffusion tensor imaging tractography during deep brain stimulation surgery. AJNR Am J Neuroradiol 2016;37(8):1470–8.
51. Talairach J, Tournoux P. Co-planar stereotaxic atlas of the human brain: 3-dimensional proportional system : an approach to cerebral imaging. New York: Georg Thieme; 1988.
52. Schaltenbrand G, Bailey P. Einführung in die stereotaktischen Operationen, mit einem Atlas des menschlichen Gehirns. Introduction to stereotaxis, with an atlas of the human brain. Stuttgart (Germany): G. Thieme; 1959.
53. Nowinski WL. Anatomical targeting in functional neurosurgery by the simultaneous use of multiple Schaltenbrand-Wahren brain atlas microseries. Stereotact Funct Neurosurg 1998;71(3):103–16.
54. Nowinski WL, Yang GL, Yeo TT. Computer-aided stereotactic functional neurosurgery enhanced by the use of the multiple brain atlas database. IEEE Trans Med Imaging 2000;19(1):62–9.
55. St-Jean P, Sadikot AF, Collins L, et al. Automated atlas integration and interactive three-dimensional visualization tools for planning and guidance in functional neurosurgery. IEEE Trans Med Imaging 1998;17(5):672–80.
56. Calabrese E, Badea A, Cofer G, et al. A diffusion MRI tractography connectome of the mouse brain

and comparison with neuronal tracer data. Cereb Cortex 2015;25(11):4628–37.
57. Thomas C, Ye FQ, Irfanoglu MO, et al. Anatomical accuracy of brain connections derived from diffusion MRI tractography is inherently limited. Proc Natl Acad Sci U S A 2014;111(46):16574–9.
58. Calabrese E. Diffusion tractography in deep brain stimulation surgery: a review. Front Neuroanat 2016;10:45.
59. See AAQ, King NKK. Improving surgical outcome using diffusion tensor imaging techniques in deep brain stimulation. Front Surg 2017;4:54.
60. Coenen VA, Madler B, Schiffbauer H, et al. Individual fiber anatomy of the subthalamic region revealed with diffusion tensor imaging: a concept to identify the deep brain stimulation target for tremor suppression. Neurosurgery 2011;68(4):1069–75 [discussion: 1075–6].
61. Pouratian N, Zheng Z, Bari AA, et al. Multi-institutional evaluation of deep brain stimulation targeting using probabilistic connectivity-based thalamic segmentation. J Neurosurg 2011; 115(5):995–1004.
62. Sweet JA, Walter BL, Gunalan K, et al. Fiber tractography of the axonal pathways linking the basal ganglia and cerebellum in Parkinson disease: implications for targeting in deep brain stimulation. J Neurosurg 2014;120(4):988–96.
63. O'Halloran RL, Chartrain AG, Rasouli JJ, et al. Case Study of image-guided deep brain stimulation: magnetic resonance imaging-based white matter tractography shows differences in responders and nonresponders. World Neurosurg 2016;96:613.e9-e16.
64. Klein JC, Barbe MT, Seifried C, et al. The tremor network targeted by successful VIM deep brain stimulation in humans. Neurology 2012;78(11): 787–95.
65. Schweder PM, Joint C, Hansen PC, et al. Chronic pedunculopontine nucleus stimulation restores functional connectivity. Neuroreport 2010;21(17): 1065–8.
66. Coenen VA, Rijntjes M, Prokop T, et al. One-pass deep brain stimulation of dentato-rubro-thalamic tract and subthalamic nucleus for tremor-dominant or equivalent type Parkinson's disease. Acta Neurochir (Wien) 2016;158(4):773–81.
67. Vega RA, Holloway KL, Larson PS. Image-guided deep brain stimulation. Neurosurg Clin N Am 2014;25(1):159–72.
68. Burchiel KJ, McCartney S, Lee A, et al. Accuracy of deep brain stimulation electrode placement using intraoperative computed tomography without microelectrode recording. J Neurosurg 2013; 119(2):301–6.
69. Ko AL, Ibrahim A, Magown P, et al. Factors affecting stereotactic accuracy in image-guided deep brain stimulator electrode placement. Stereotact Funct Neurosurg 2017;95(5):315–24.
70. Ostrem JL, Ziman N, Galifianakis NB, et al. Clinical outcomes using ClearPoint interventional MRI for deep brain stimulation lead placement in Parkinson's disease. J Neurosurg 2016;124(4):908–16.
71. Kochanski R, Sani S. Awake versus asleep deep brain stimulation surgery: technical considerations and critical review of the literature. Brain Sci 2018;8(1) [pii:E17].
72. Zrinzo L, Foltynie T, Limousin P, et al. Reducing hemorrhagic complications in functional neurosurgery: a large case series and systematic literature review. J Neurosurg 2012;116(1):84–94.
73. Hariz MI. Safety and risk of microelectrode recording in surgery for movement disorders. Stereotact Funct Neurosurg 2002;78(3–4):146–57.
74. Hamani C, Richter E, Schwalb JM, et al. Bilateral subthalamic nucleus stimulation for Parkinson's disease: a systematic review of the clinical literature. Neurosurgery 2005;56(6):1313–21 [discussion: 1321–4].
75. Morrell MJ, RNS System in Epilepsy Study Group. Responsive cortical stimulation for the treatment of medically intractable partial epilepsy. Neurology 2011;77(13):1295–304.
76. de Hemptinne C, Ryapolova-Webb ES, Air EL, et al. Exaggerated phase-amplitude coupling in the primary motor cortex in Parkinson disease. Proc Natl Acad Sci U S A 2013;110(12): 4780–5.
77. Rowland NC, De Hemptinne C, Swann NC, et al. Task-related activity in sensorimotor cortex in Parkinson's disease and essential tremor: changes in beta and gamma bands. Front Hum Neurosci 2015;9:512.
78. Kondylis ED, Randazzo MJ, Alhourani A, et al. Movement-related dynamics of cortical oscillations in Parkinson's disease and essential tremor. Brain 2016;139(Pt 8):2211–23.
79. Swann NC, de Hemptinne C, Miocinovic S, et al. Gamma oscillations in the hyperkinetic state detected with chronic human brain recordings in Parkinson's disease. J Neurosci 2016;36(24):6445–58.
80. Qasim SE, de Hemptinne C, Swann NC, et al. Electrocorticography reveals beta desynchronization in the basal ganglia-cortical loop during rest tremor in Parkinson's disease. Neurobiol Dis 2016;86: 177–86.
81. Priori A, Foffani G, Pesenti A, et al. Rhythm-specific pharmacological modulation of subthalamic activity in Parkinson's disease. Exp Neurol 2004; 189(2):369–79.
82. Brown P, Williams D. Basal ganglia local field potential activity: character and functional significance in the human. Clin Neurophysiol 2005; 116(11):2510–9.

83. Wingeier B, Tcheng T, Koop MM, et al. Intra-operative STN DBS attenuates the prominent beta rhythm in the STN in Parkinson's disease. Exp Neurol 2006;197(1):244–51.
84. Niketeghad S, Hebb AO, Nedrud J, et al. Single trial behavioral task classification using subthalamic nucleus local field potential signals. Conf Proc IEEE Eng Med Biol Soc 2014;2014:3793–6.
85. Mamun KA, Mace M, Lutman ME, et al. Movement decoding using neural synchronization and inter-hemispheric connectivity from deep brain local field potentials. J Neural Eng 2015;12(5):056011.
86. Quinn EJ, Blumenfeld Z, Velisar A, et al. Beta oscillations in freely moving Parkinson's subjects are attenuated during deep brain stimulation. Mov Disord 2015;30(13):1750–8.
87. Abosch A, Lanctin D, Onaran I, et al. Long-term recordings of local field potentials from implanted deep brain stimulation electrodes. Neurosurgery 2012;71(4):804–14.
88. Kishida KT, Sandberg SG, Lohrenz T, et al. Sub-second dopamine detection in human striatum. PLoS One 2011;6(8):e23291.
89. Swann N, Poizner H, Houser M, et al. Deep brain stimulation of the subthalamic nucleus alters the cortical profile of response inhibition in the beta frequency band: a scalp EEG study in Parkinson's disease. J Neurosci 2011;31(15):5721–9.
90. Shukla P, Basu I, Graupe D, et al. A neural network-based design of an on-off adaptive control for Deep Brain Stimulation in movement disorders. Conf Proc IEEE Eng Med Biol Soc 2012;2012:4140–3.
91. Basu I, Graupe D, Tuninetti D, et al. Pathological tremor prediction using surface electromyogram and acceleration: potential use in 'ON-OFF' demand driven deep brain stimulator design. J Neural Eng 2013;10(3):036019.
92. Malekmohammadi M, Herron J, Velisar A, et al. Kinematic adaptive deep brain stimulation for resting tremor in Parkinson's disease. Mov Disord 2016;31(3):426–8.
93. Kuo CH, White-Dzuro GA, Ko AL. Approaches to closed-loop deep brain stimulation for movement disorders. Neurosurg Focus 2018;45(2):E2.
94. Parastarfeizabadi M, Kouzani AZ. Advances in closed-loop deep brain stimulation devices. J Neuroeng Rehabil 2017;14(1):79.
95. Little S, Beudel M, Zrinzo L, et al. Bilateral adaptive deep brain stimulation is effective in Parkinson's disease. J Neurol Neurosurg Psychiatry 2016;87(7):717–21.
96. Little S, Tripoliti E, Beudel M, et al. Adaptive deep brain stimulation for Parkinson's disease demonstrates reduced speech side effects compared to conventional stimulation in the acute setting. J Neurol Neurosurg Psychiatry 2016;87(12):1388–9.
97. Maks CB, Butson CR, Walter BL, et al. Deep brain stimulation activation volumes and their association with neurophysiological mapping and therapeutic outcomes. J Neurol Neurosurg Psychiatry 2009;80(6):659–66.
98. Contarino MF, Bour LJ, Verhagen R, et al. Directional steering: A novel approach to deep brain stimulation. Neurology 2014;83(13):1163–9.
99. Pollo C, Kaelin-Lang A, Oertel MF, et al. Directional deep brain stimulation: an intraoperative double-blind pilot study. Brain 2014;137(Pt 7):2015–26.
100. Steigerwald F, Muller L, Johannes S, et al. Directional deep brain stimulation of the subthalamic nucleus: a pilot study using a novel neurostimulation device. Mov Disord 2016;31(8):1240–3.

Deep Brain Stimulation for Treatment of Tremor

Wendell Lake, MD[a], Peter Hedera, MD, PhD[b], Peter Konrad, MD, PhD[c,*]

KEYWORDS

• Essential tremor • Thalamic • Deep brain stimulation • Microelectrode • Image guided
• Closed loop

KEY POINTS

- Tremor is the most common movement disorder.
- A considerable proportion of patients with essential tremor develop medically refractory tremor; the clinically diagnosed movement disorder is often heritable and tends to increase in incidence with age.
- Thalamic deep brain stimulation provides a durable and marked improvement of tremor for patients with essential tremor.
- Other conditions resulting in tremor may not respond as reliably or substantially to thalamic deep brain stimulation.
- Closed-loop stimulation systems and directional deep brain stimulator leads may have the potential to improve deep brain stimulation treatment of essential tremor.

INTRODUCTION

Deep brain stimulation (DBS) for treatment of tremor was the first US Food and Drug Administration–approved use of intracranial neuromodulation. Since 1997, DBS for treatment of tremor has continued as a safe, widely used therapy that can significantly affect this disabling condition. This article provides clinicians with a brief review of the salient clinical and surgical features for this disease.

History of Deep Brain Stimulation for Tremor

Tremor is an involuntary, rhythmic, oscillatory movement of a body part.[1] The original article describing high-frequency stimulation as a therapeutic option for controlling tremor was published by Benabid and colleagues[2] in 1987. They raised the notion that long-term stimulation (>90 Hz) may be a reasonable alternative to lesioning. The idea is a natural extension of the previously used method of creating a temporary "test" lesion by preforming a short period of test stimulation at high frequency. This elegant method of confirming the exact location for optimal lesions in awake patients led to the idea that continuous high-frequency stimulation may be a safer alternative to lesioning. Lesions of small targets surrounded by critical pathways or structures that must be protected required a method to ensure the precision of the intended therapy. Furthermore, bilateral lesions were almost uniformly fraught with much worse morbidity than unilateral lesions, thereby making surgical treatment of bilateral homologous

Disclosure: W. Lake has no financial disclosures. P. Konrad has consulting agreements without honorarium with Medtronic and Neuropace and research support from Medtronic and Microtransponder Inc. P. Hedera has no financial disclosures.
[a] University of Wisconsin-Madison, 600 Highland Avenue, Box 8660, Madison, WI 53792, USA; [b] Vanderbilt University Medical Center, 645 21st Avenue South, Nashville, TN 37240, USA; [c] Vanderbilt University Medical Center, Room 4333, VAV, 1500 21st Avenue, Nashville, TN 37212, USA
* Corresponding author.
E-mail address: peter.konrad@vumc.org

Neurosurg Clin N Am 30 (2019) 147–159
https://doi.org/10.1016/j.nec.2019.01.002

structures less desirable. Use of DBS afforded a reversible method of treating the bilateral symptoms of essential tremor while minimizing the risks of morbidity associated with bilateral lesioning procedures.[3–5] The role of DBS versus thalamotomy for unilateral tremor was more debated initially,[6] but in general DBS is viewed as safer for most practitioners because of the reversibility of the treatment.[7–9]

Over the past 2 decades that DBS has been used for treatment of tremor, it has afforded a reversible, adjustable therapy that can be modified to a significant degree without additional surgery, by adjusting the implants' programmed settings. Parameters that can be adjusted include contacts stimulated, pulse width, frequency, and current amplitude.

Use of unilateral DBS for tremor-predominant Parkinson disease was the first clinical indication for DBS in the United States. Use of this therapy in essential tremor was also applied at that time, but approved only as a unilateral implant. It is still considered by many payors unapproved for bilateral implantation during the same setting, necessitating 2 separate procedures for treatment of bilateral disabling tremor. Other forms of disabling tremor, such as those types caused by multiple sclerosis, stroke, or trauma, are much more rare and only reported in small numbers in the literature. Efficacy for DBS for these indications may vary.

Disabling tremor, associated with Parkinson disease or essential tremor, remains the predominant use of DBS today. To understand the appropriate patient selection and targeting of this therapy, the anatomy and pathophysiology of tremor should be considered.[10]

Tremor: Pathology and Anatomy

Tremor is the most common manifestation of involuntary movement. Tremor is defined as a rhythmic oscillatory movement that occurs at rest or during activity; all tremors cease during sleep. Tremor is thought to arise in patients when there is a failure in the motor system's ability to close the loop between intended limb location and existing limb location. The normal physiology of limb movement involves a premotor command that contains a virtual target in space to which the limb should reach. Subconsciously, the motor system has an assessment of the existing position of the limb through proprioception of the limb. There is then an error or mismatch of the intended position versus existing position, and movement is created three-dimensionally to correct the error until it reaches zero (ie, the limb reaches the intended target). Correction of the limb in 3 dimensions continues until the error signal is reduced; the larger the error signal, the larger the correction signal to bring the limb back to target. When there is a failure to close the error signal, or failure to recognize when the target location is reached, oscillating limb movements occur and can be seen as tremor.

The anatomy involved in movement initiated tremor production (so-called action tremor) therefore involves limb proprioception pathways, intended motor planning pathways, and the circuitry involved in signal mismatch closure. **Fig. 1** shows the general anatomic concepts related to tremor production. The pathway that is central to this concept is the dentatorubrothalamic (DRT) pathway, and it is thought to be a central common pathway involved in virtually all forms of tremor.[9,11] For patients with essential tremor, this pathway is thought to be where the primary disorder lies in the form of hyperactive circuitry. Although the thalamus has traditionally been the focus of either lesioning or neuromodulation therapy, it is known that other points (zona incerta and posterior subthalamus where this pathway traverses) are also effective therapy points.[12]

Tremor that occurs with Parkinson disease is thought to involve the motor system's resting state. Classic tremor present with Parkinson is manifest as a so-called pill-rolling tremor that is asymmetric and often starts out unilaterally. Usually this form of tremor disappears with kinetic movement and resumes slowly when the limb reaches a new resting position (reemergent tremor). It is also significantly affected by attention and can be voluntarily controlled for short periods. Newer imaging and functional connectivity studies suggest that primary motor cortex (M1) and the general cortical-thalamic network of motor initiation is the source of this dysfunctional state. Although the DRT pathway may also be involved, it seems that treatment of the thalamus through lesioning or DBS is effective through a different mechanism. Nonetheless, disabling tremor from Parkinson disease can be effectively controlled by Vim thalamic lesions or DBS. However, zona incerta and superior subthalamic pathways are also significantly involved in the pathophysiology of this disease and may just represent another point along the DRT as it curves superiorly from the red nucleus. A unilateral lesion is more often performed in patients when treating tremor-predominant Parkinson disease when ablative surgical management is desired.[11,13]

This conceptual model allows clinicians to understand why tremor may manifest differently with distinct diseases and even in some normal

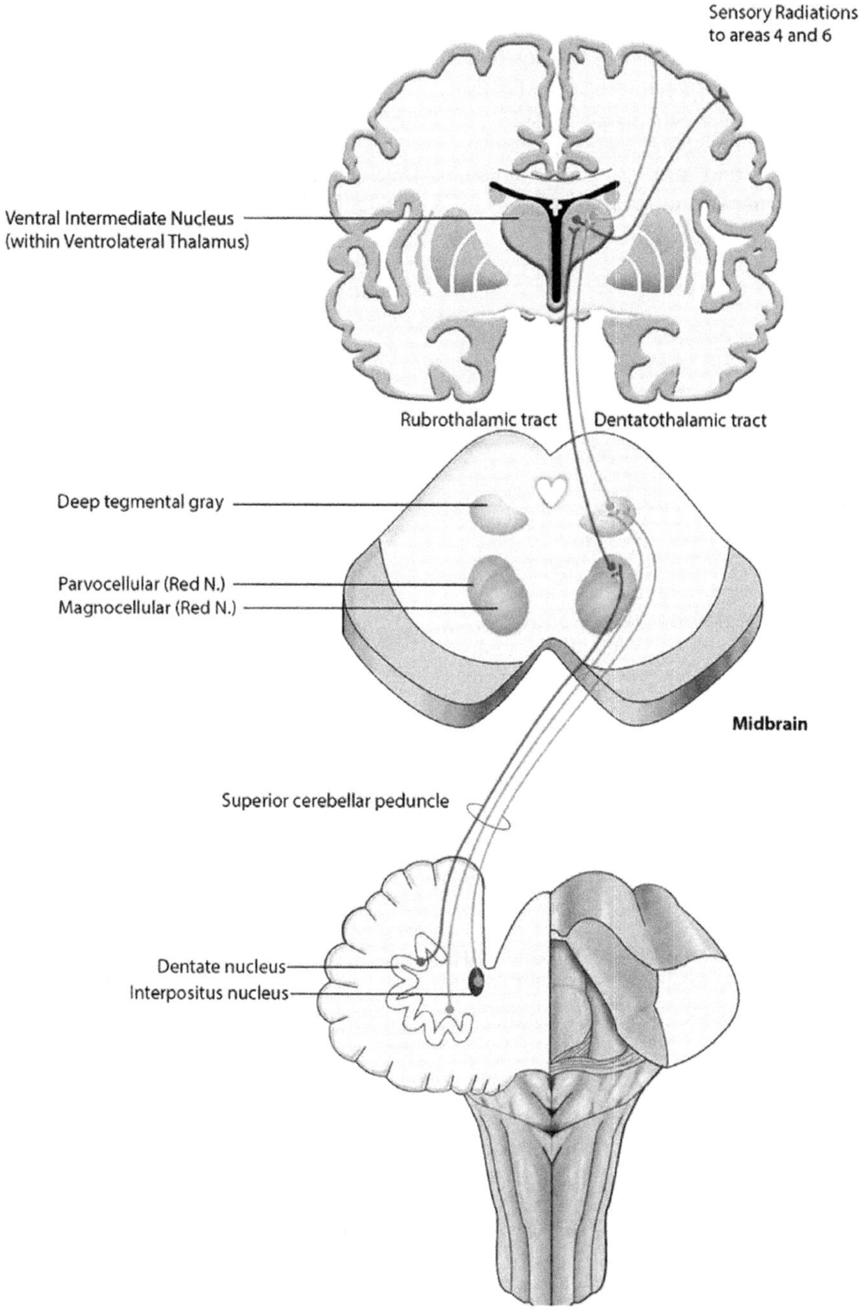

Fig. 1. Primary pathways involved in the regulation of tremor. The pathway critically involved in correction for intended versus existing limb position is thought to arise from the cerebellum (dentate nucleus) and travel to the contralateral thalamus via the red nucleus. Treatment of tremor is most effective presently by targeting the insertion point of this pathway into the inferior, lateral thalamus (Vim). N, nucleus. (*From* Dallapiazza RF, Lee DJ, De Vloo P, et al. Outcomes from stereotactic surgery for essential tremor. J Neurol Neurosurg Psychiatry 2018. [Epub ahead of print]; with permission.)

physiologic states.[10] A review by Bhatia and colleagues[1] in 2018 has surgical importance when understanding the pathologic anatomy of tremor and its surgical treatment options. Although tremor classification in the past involved both anatomic and clinical descriptions (eg, cerebellar tremor vs parkinsonian tremor), a newer classification scheme attempts to normalize the description of tremor based on clinical and causative factors. The International Parkinson and Movement Disorder Society recently proposed an update to the 1998 tremor classification to now include a 2-axis description: axis I is a clinical descriptor involving historical features (age at onset, family history, and temporal evolution), tremor characteristics (body distribution, activation condition), associated signs (systemic, neurologic), and laboratory tests (electrophysiology, imaging); and axis 2 is an cause descriptor (acquired, genetic, or idiopathic).[1]

Axis I: Clinical

Age of onset

Age of onset can be roughly divided into 6 major time periods: infancy (birth to 2 years), childhood (3–12 years), adolescence (13–20 years), early adulthood (21–45 years), middle adulthood (46–60 years), and late adulthood (>60 years).

Anatomic distribution

Anatomic distribution may be focal (eg, head, jaw, arm), segmental (2 or more connected regions; eg, head and arm, or both arms), hemibody (limited to 1 side of body), or generalized (upper and lower body).

Activation conditions

Activation conditions may be rest or action. Three additional descriptors are used for action tremor: kinetic (involves intentional movement-induced tremor as well as task-specific induced tremor), postural (position specific or more general when maintaining antigravity posture, such as arms extended).

Frequency

Most pathologic tremors of extremities range from 4 to 8 Hz. Physiologic tremor has a higher range of 8 to 12 Hz, which matches the central neurogenic component.

Isolated versus additional clinical signs

Tremors may be the sole isolated clinical concern, whereas others, like Parkinson disease, are also associated with other signs, such as rigidity, dystonic posture, or bradykinesia.

Axis 2: Cause

The cause may be genetic, acquired, or idiopathic.

How does this definition fit into the surgical treatment of tremor, especially use of DBS? Although this is a newly proposed classification, it embodies the core features of what defines tremor syndromes that are successfully treated with DBS and those that are not, or have less ideal results.

When tremor onset occurs in middle and late adulthood, has a focal or segmental nature, is not postural, and lies within 4 to 8 Hz, this responds well to DBS in our experience. It involves patients with genetic or idiopathic causes. This type of tremor is traditionally associated with essential tremor and Parkinson disease and historically responds well to DBS of the thalamus.

When the tremor has postural component; is associated with trauma, stroke, or multiple sclerosis; and/or has an associated dystonia, then DBS typically has less optimal outcomes or even minimal impact on the overall tremor.

This new classification scheme has not been used in classifying outcomes for DBS as yet. However, this simple feature-rich description should allow for easier validation with future DBS outcome studies. The authors expect the next 5 years to shift in the use of this internationally recommended tremor classification scheme as a benchmark to report patient selection and efficacy of DBS for tremor. As yet, selection and outcomes criteria still use a traditional mixture of anatomy and disease classification when reporting DBS as a therapy for tremor.

PATIENT SELECTION FOR DBS

Adequate patient selection depends on correlating the clinical findings with the correct anatomic-pathologic target. Also knowing whether the tremor will be significantly affected by neuromodulation allows patients and physicians to select whether the risk/benefit ratio is acceptable. **Table 1** lists the features and presentation of several common tremor conditions that surgeons may be asked to treat.

Some clinical features of tremor have excellent prognosis with neuromodulation of the thalamus. The best responders to DBS of the Vim are those with distal tremor (predominantly hand) and a history consistent with essential tremor. The classic presentation of someone with essential tremor is that of an action tremor that is notably absent at rest. Patients may appear completely normal when sitting, but, on performing a movement of the hand to a target-driven task, the tremor worsens the closer the hand or the finger is to the final target position. The tremor usually emerges over years and is symmetric. It can become severe and disabling to the point where the patients can no longer feed themselves or perform activities of daily living because of inability to control the tremor with any common task, such as holding a spoon or cup, or brushing teeth, or grooming, or dressing. This stage is usually what brings patients to surgical attention. There is also a strong autosomal dominant family history of tremor in about 70% of all patients. Medications that should be tried initially include β-blockers and primidone. Other possible therapies include topiramate or pregabalin (for review see **Table 1**). Patients often endorse that alcohol reduces the tremor significantly. However, as the tremor progresses in some patients, medication side effects (such as somnolence or fatigue

Table 1
Clinical features and pathophysiology of various forms of tremor

	Essential Tremor	Parkinson Disease	Cerebellar Tremor	Physiologic Tremor
Present at Rest	+	++++	+	+
Activated by Motion	+++	++	+++	++
Limb Location	Distal>proximal	Distal	Proximal>distal	Distal
Frequency (Hz)	6–11	3–7	3–5	6–12
Amplitude	Variable	Moderate	Large	Small
Symmetry	Yes	No, asymmetry persists in bilateral disease	No in structural causes, yes in neurodegenerative causes	Yes
Hereditary	Autosomal dominant	Rare	—	No
Disabling	Yes	Yes	Yes	No
Medication Response	β-Blockers, primidone, topiramate	Anti-PD meds (eg, L-DOPA agonists)	Acetazolamide, but overall poor response	β-Blockers, anxiolytics

Abbreviation: PD, Parkinson disease.

from β-blocker use) also limit their activities, especially during the working years of life.

In contrast, patients with Parkinson disease usually have a very different presentation of tremor. The tremor for patients with Parkinson disease emerges as a unilateral rest tremor also associated commonly with other cardinal features of Parkinson disease such as postural instability, bradykinesia, and rigidity. Other motor symptoms, such as slowness or clumsiness, may be subtle in the tremor-dominant subtype of Parkinson disease and these patients are mostly disabled from tremor. The rest tremor is slower in frequency (3–7 Hz) and typically starts out as a pill-rolling of the thumb and second and third fingers.[11] Eventually it becomes worse, involving supination-pronation tremor and more amplitude over time. The tremor initially may go away easily with movement or focused attention by the patient. Response to dopaminergic medications (levodopa or dopaminergic agonists) can confirm the diagnosis of Parkinson disease but many patients require high doses that are not well tolerated, and some patients with tremor-predominant idiopathic Parkinson disease have no improvement in their tremor symptoms with levodopa medications. Surgical treatment of tremor-predominant Parkinson disease for many centers always entails a discussion of whether treatment of the tremor alone is better than treating the eventual progression of other features of Parkinson disease, such as bradykinesia, rigidity, and/or dyskinesia. Understanding the complete risk/benefit profile of these patients can be challenging and often there is no single correct choice for target and treatment. Anatomic targets for treatment of Parkinson disease–related tremor include the subthalamic nucleus, the globus pallidus interna, and the Vim nucleus of the thalamus. In recent years there has been a greater tendency to target the subthalamic nucleus and globus pallidus interna because stimulation of these areas may result in improvement of the other cardinal symptoms of Parkinson disease in addition to tremor improvement.[14]

Cerebellar tremor needs to be identified and distinguished clinically from the other forms of tremor. Cerebellar tremor, also known as Holmes or outflow tremor, is characterized by a low-frequency high-amplitude tremor that is mostly generated in proximal limb segments during postural or kinetic tasks. Intention tremor with increased frequency before reaching the target is another feature of cerebellar tremor. Patients with advanced essential tremor may develop tremor with cerebellar features, but other signs of cerebellar dysfunction, such as limb dysmetria, dysdiadochokinesis, gaze-evoked nystagmus, and cerebellar dysarthria, are absent in essential tremor. This type of tremor may be a unique disabling complaint or a component of other forms of tremor.[15]

Dystonic tremor refers to the coexistence of tremor and dystonia in the same body segment. Dystonic tremor is further characterized by directionality, with the increasing amplitude in 1 particular direction, and by the null point phenomenon, resulting in diminished or absent tremor in certain limb positions. This distinction is clinically relevant because dystonic tremor usually does not respond to typical essential tremor medications, and its pharmacologic and surgical therapies are similar to the treatment of generalized or focal dystonia.[1,15,16]

It is also worth mentioning the diagnosis of physiologic tremor. It is a low-amplitude, higher-frequency tremor that is brought out mostly by fatigue and stress. It usually responds well to oral β-blockers. This tremor is not disabling and not considered a surgically treatable tremor.[10,11]

Regardless of the type of tremor present, it is common practice and informative to the surgical team to benchmark the severity of the tremor before and following any intervention. Several common tremor rating scales are used. The Fahn-Tolosa-Marin (FTM) tremor rating scale has been used for many years as a standard tremor severity score in routine clinical as well as research studies. A newer tremor severity rating scale, The Essential Tremor Rating Assessment Scale (TETRAS), has shown improved range of severity scoring and more inter-rater robustness, and may also supplant the FTM.[17] Typically surgical candidates should have moderate to severe tremor severity before consideration for DBS surgery. This severity usually amounts to an FTM total score greater than 50 (116 maximum) on average in several studies.[18–20]

Role of the Multidisciplinary Conference

Most DBS centers that perform more than 20 DBS implants per year have naturally evolved a clinical process of discussion of candidates for therapy among the specialists involved in the selection, surgery, and postimplant care of the patient. Probably one of the most important criteria for success of DBS surgery is the process of vetting appropriate candidates for DBS surgery through a multidisciplinary conference.[19–22] The purpose is to consolidate and describe a range of treatment options and outcomes that can be considered for patients with disabling tremor. The authors review what is disabling to the patient, medication failures, other medical concerns that may influence surgical candidacy, target selection, type of device to implant, and postoperative expectations. These discussions are all critical to the successful selection of patients undergoing surgical treatment of tremor.[21]

SURGICAL TECHNIQUE

Awake Surgery

After a patient has been appropriately selected for tremor surgery, the surgical process commences. Thalamic DBS is the most common surgical treatment of tremor at many medical centers. The specific technique used for implantation of the DBS system varies from center to center. In the past, awake surgery in which test stimulation with or without microelectrode recording has been used to appropriately place the leads in the Vim nucleus of the thalamus. However, recently some groups have begun to use asleep surgery with image guidance to place DBS leads for treatment of tremor.[22,23] Whether or not the center then proceeds with placement of lead extenders and the internal pulse generator at the time of the lead placement or proceeds with this portion of the procedure at a later date is also variable between different practitioners. Also, unilateral, bilateral single stage (both sides implanted at same surgery), or bilateral staged (each side implanted at different times) varies among different centers and with the clinical scenario. If the patient has the most significant symptoms in the dominant hand or if the tremor is symmetric but the patient would be happy with only symptom control in the dominant hand, then the more conservative approach of unilateral lead placement may be considered. If the patient has symmetric tremor and desires bimanual control of the tremor (particularly for hobbies or occupation), then bilateral lead placement during 1 surgery or staged into 2 surgeries can be considered. Nuances for both asleep and awake treatments are discussed later.

During awake surgery for tremor, it is important that the patient be prepared ahead of time by discussing expectations for participation in surgery and stimulation side effects that may be encountered and should be reported by the patient (ie, paresthesias, muscle contraction, or dysarthria). To maximize the effect of stimulation, it is helpful to have patients off of any antitremor medications beginning the evening before surgery. In the operating room, monitored anesthesia with a short-acting agent such as remifentanil or propofol allows the clinical team to easily visualize the impact of stimulation on the tremor. If microelectrode recording is to be performed, the anesthetic agent may affect firing rate if it is not allowed to dissipate.[24] Local anesthetic incorporating both a short-acting and long-acting agent administered to the scalp (lidocaine-Marcaine mixture) reduces need for systemic medications and typically lasts for the duration of the procedure.

Use of a stereotactic frame allows precise targeting of the Vim nucleus of the thalamus based on consensus coordinates developed from anatomic atlases. These atlases base their coordinates on a system classically referencing the midpoint of the anterior and posterior commissures, also known as the midcommisural point (MC). A common starting point for targeting Vim is 11 mm lateral to the wall of the third ventricle, 6 mm posterior to the MC (or 6–8 mm in front of the posterior commissure), and 0 mm below the MC. **Fig. 2** shows a typical entry and target.

The stereotactic frame or other targeting system can be set to the Vim target. The scalp is marked at the entry point and the skin opened in a bicoronal or linear fashion. A bur hole may then be created at the entry point or points and the dura is opened on the desired side or sides. At this point, the surgeon may consider placing microelectrodes singly or in an array. Alternatively, some surgeons place the lead to target. At this point the practitioner can make neurophysiologic recordings, often beginning either 10 of 15 mm above the target and/or perform test stimulation. If the lead alone is placed and no microelectrodes are placed, then the practitioner may proceed directly to test stimulation without microelectrode recording. If microelectrode recordings are made, they often show thalamic activity; possibly tremor cells; and, in a more posterior pass, somatosensory thalamus (known as Vc in Hassler terminology) may be shown by increased the firing rate with tactile stimulus, particularly in the hand or face contralateral to the recording electrodes. Microelectrodes within the Vim respond with increased firing to passive movement of the joints (kinesthetic response). The dorsal portion of Vc responds to muscle belly pressure, whereas the Vc centrally responds to light tactile stimulation in a small somatotopic region; again, the hand and face often have large representation and are most easily elicited.[25]

With microelectrode recording complete, the practitioner now has a good idea of where to begin test stimulation with a macroelectrode. Often a microelectrode concentric within a macroelectrode is used. Therefore, the microelectrode can be withdrawn into the macroelectrode and then the macroelectrode is positioned using a Microdrive. The region thought to encompass the Vim thalamus is stimulated at 2 or 3 points 3 mm apart. Stimulation parameters are usually square wave, biphasic frequency 150 Hz, and pulse width 100 microseconds. Test stimulation current ranges up to 4 mA. Clinical response is recorded. The ideal scenario is a patient that develops tremor arrest or significant reduction at 1 to 2 mA and no persistent side effects at currents less than 4 mA. Transient paresthesias can be tolerated and generally go away after 30 seconds or less. Persistent paresthesias require an anterior repositioning of the electrode. Capsular side effects are noted with an electrode positioned too laterally and loss of efficacy is noted with electrodes positioned too medially or too anteriorly.[25]

Once the correct lead location is determined with microelectrode recording and macrostimulation, the final DBS lead can be implanted. This lead is implanted with the contact span centered in the area where the Vim is localized. Each contact of the final DBS lead is then tested to verify normal impedance and to verify that the lead produces the intended clinical effect of tremor arrest with a therapeutic window that avoids persistent

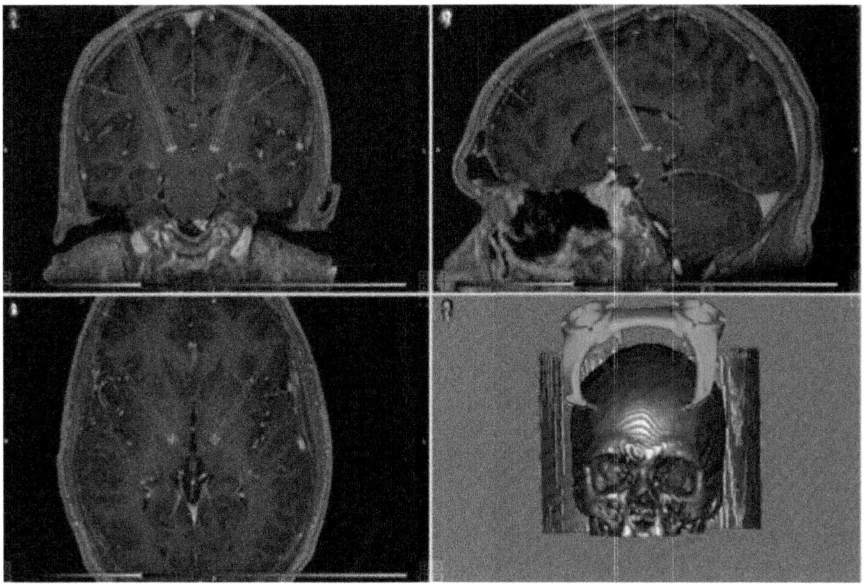

Fig. 2. Typical trajectories for bilateral thalamic DBS placement in the treatment of essential tremor. A virtual model of a rapid prototype stereotactic frame (Waypoint System, FHC, Inc, Bowdoin, ME) used by the authors is shown in the (*lower right*) frame.

side effects at efficacious currents. The lead is secured in place with a cap provided by the manufacture or with cement. The lead or leads are then tunneled under the scalp and incisions are closed.

Asleep Surgery

Although traditionally most tremor surgery has been done in awake patients with intraoperative testing, several groups have begun to routinely offer asleep surgery for placement of deep brain stimulator leads.[22,26,27] Many of the data published for these cases focuses on the treatment of Parkinson disease or dystonia, but asleep surgery for essential tremor is now being described in the literature as well.[22] Performing asleep surgery to treat tremor represents a special challenge because, unlike the globus pallidus interna or subthalamic nucleus (targets commonly used for Parkinson and dystonia), the target for tremor, Vim nucleus of the thalamus, cannot be visualized easily on 1.5-T or 3-T MRI. Therefore, the Vim must be targeted indirectly.

Image-guided targeting for Vim DBS lead placement commonly proceeds by 2 different methods, one using intraoperative computed tomography (CT) scan to confirm proper lead placement and the other using intraoperative MRI scanning to confirm lead placement. The most common method is using the intraoperative CT scan to confirm lead placement. In this technique, the patient undergoes preoperative CT scan and MRI. These 2 images are merged and the Vim nucleus is targeted. The patient comes to the operating room and is placed under general anesthesia. The stereotactic frame is applied and the Vim nucleus is targeted. Approximate coordinates for the Vim nucleus are 11 mm lateral to the wall of the third ventricle, 6 mm posterior to the MC, and 0 mm below MC. Some groups consider the use of tractography for delineating the dentatorubrothalamic tract (DRTT) and seek to place the electrode either within the DRTT or in a position posterior, inferior, or lateral to the DRTT. The scalp and skull are opened, the lead is placed through the stereotactic frame, and an intraoperative CT scan is performed to verify lead placement. If the lead has a vector error of less than 3 mm from the intended target, it is left in place. Errors in lead placement from intended target to lead are routinely less than 1.5 mm.[22,27] Once the lead is placed, it is secured with a plastic cap or cement. The distal end of the lead is tunneled under the scalp and the incisions are closed. The patient is allowed to awaken.

The alternative to asleep placement with intraoperative CT is the use of intraoperative MRI. Few centers have adopted this technique for tremor cases because the Vim nucleus is not directly visible on MRI and the logistics of performing surgery within an MRI scanner can be daunting. Briefly, for this technique the patient is placed under general anesthesia and positioned in the bore of the MRI magnet. The scalp entry point is marked appropriately using a gadolinium-containing grid adhered to the patient's head. The scalp is opened at the correct location or locations. Bur holes are created and the securing caps are placed. Special stereotactic frames with gadolinium-containing cannulas are mounted on the patient's head and iterative MRI takes place to align the stereotactic frames to the correct target. Then peel-away sheaths with ceramic stiffening stylets are placed to target.[26] MRI verifies appropriate placement and no hemorrhages. **Fig. 3** shows a view of the ceramic stylet placement in a Vim DBS procedure. The ceramic stylets are removed and the leads are placed. Leads are secured in place and further MRI verifies appropriate placement. Frames are removed and the surgery is closed in a routine fashion.

Postoperative Care

Regardless of the technique used to place the patient's DBS system, postoperative care involves an adequate period of observation for immediate postoperative complications. For patients undergoing DBS for essential tremor, medication adjustments are less critical in the immediate postoperative period than for patients with Parkinson disease. Nonetheless, the most serious complication, hemorrhage, is usually present within the first 24 to 48 hours of DBS lead insertion.[28,29] Consequently most patients are admitted and observed following DBS lead placement. Furthermore, postoperative imaging (usually CT) within the first few hours following DBS lead insertion is routinely done at most centers.[28,30] If the postoperative image shows no hemorrhage or if the patient has no new deficits, the patient can likely be observed on a regular ward. If there are any new deficits postoperatively, regardless of imaging findings, the authors advocate having the patient under closer neurologic observation. Other reasons for concern in the immediate postoperative period are seizures (<1%) and nonhemorrhagic new deficit (transient or permanent) with or without an associated new brain lesion. Management of a hemorrhage related to DBS insertion usually requires supportive care only and rarely reoperation for evacuation. The

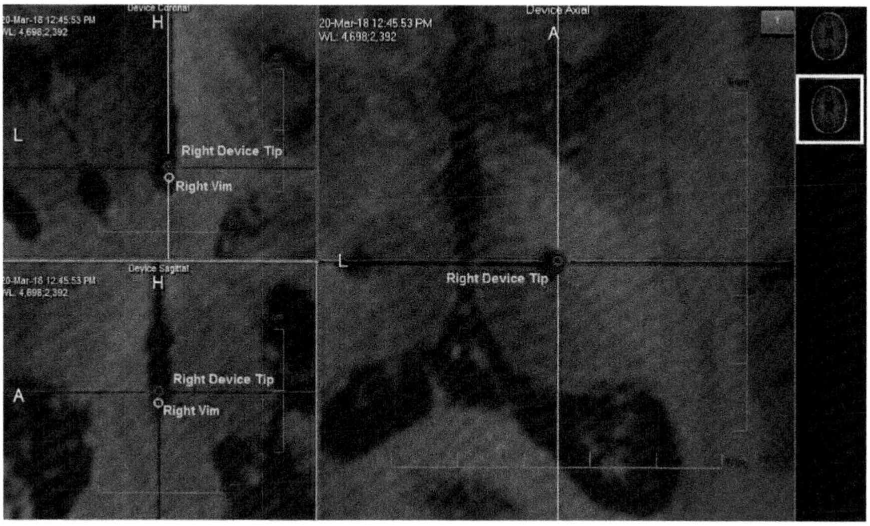

Fig. 3. Clearpoint Vim trajectory. Trajectory plan for DBS electrode placed using intraoperative MRI navigation (Clearpoint system, MRI Interventions, Inc, Irvine, CA). Coronal (*left upper*), sagittal (*left lower*) and axial (*right*) T1 MRI images shown with DBS lead and intended target.

same is true of focal edema surrounding a newly inserted DBS lead.[31,32] Seizures that present in the initial postoperative period should be managed with anticonvulsants and followed by a neurologist.

For historical reasons related to the concept of trialing leads before generator insertion, lead extender and internal pulse generator placement often occurs as a separate procedure at a future date (typically a week after lead implantation). Typically, patients can be mobilized early and placed back on the appropriate tremor medications immediately after surgery. When anticoagulants are held before DBS surgery, there are no clear data on resuming anticoagulation. At our centers, we typically restore anticoagulation within a week or two after DBS leads have been inserted and no documentation of postoperative hemorrhage is present. Prolonged inpatient stay is rare but reasons include postoperative nausea, difficulty mobilizing because of balance problems, and postoperative headache or pain.

After the patient has undergone placement of the DBS system, the device needs to be appropriately programmed. The system is often left in the off position for the first month postoperatively to allow any edema surrounding the lead to resolve. Programming begins at the 1-month postoperative appointment and usually starts with a monopolar survey and then proceeds to delineate an optimal program. Most patients have at least 4 postoperative programming visits scheduled, each 2 weeks apart initially. However, some data indicate that optimization of programming takes greater than 3 months in many cases.[33]

After the DBS program has been optimized, the patients need to be instructed on how to monitor their battery life. In general, primary cell internal pulse generators are placed for initial implantation and rechargeable internal pulse generators are placed for patients requiring frequent battery replacement. Patients may require battery replacement on average every 3 to 5 years, but this varies depending on programmed settings.[34]

OUTCOMES AND AVOIDING COMPLICATIONS

Complications Avoidance

Deep brain stimulator placement for the treatment of tremor is generally well tolerated and efficacious in appropriately selected patients. However, complications can and do occur. These complications may be acute in the hours to weeks following placement of the implants, or chronic, persisting in the months or years following implantation. Although avoidance of all complications is unrealistic, some basic principles are often followed to mitigate the risk of complications.

Discuss the patient's treatment plan with a multidisciplinary team, including neurologists, neuropsychologists, physical therapists and so forth. This discussion encourages appropriate patient selection and optimizes risk-benefit analysis.

Obtain appropriate preoperative clearance from medical specialists such as primary care physicians, pulmonologists, or cardiologists for patients with medical comorbidities.

Administer preincision antibiotics in a timely fashion.

Place incisions in such a fashion that the amount of implant underlying the incision is minimized and the profile of implants is kept smooth and low. This precaution may minimize acute infections and chronic instances of hardware erosion.

Consider intraoperative test stimulation and/or intraoperative imaging (MRI or CT) to ensure appropriate lead revision. These methods minimize the prevalence of stimulation-related side effects such as capsular side effects or sensory side effects that may result in acute or delayed need for lead revision.

Obtain postoperative or intraoperative imaging to rule out hemorrhage. Patients with intracranial hemorrhage need to be observed closely for any sign of neurologic decline.

Carefully evaluate the risk/benefit ratio for resuming any antiplatelet or anticoagulant medications in patients who have undergone recent placement of intracranial leads.[35]

Outcomes

In general, surgical treatment of disabling tremor has an excellent prognosis for patients. Both action and rest tremor respond well to DBS of the Vim region of the thalamus.

DBS targeting the Vim thalamic nucleus is an established therapy for patients with medically refractory and debilitating tremor (see **Table 2**). The first systemic analysis of surgical outcomes in patients with essential tremor showed that either complete tremor control or major improvement was observed in 88% of patients and these benefits were sustained up to 19 months.[4] A follow-up study by the same group confirmed that DBS remained effective in most of the patients more than 10 years after surgery.[36] The long-term benefits of Vim DBS surgery were also confirmed by several other groups and clinically meaningful tremor control was achieved in more than 80% of patients with essential tremor, and most patients enjoy a sustained benefit from DBS.[37–41]

Dysarthria is the most commonly observed adverse effect and it is problematic for some patients. Adjustments of stimulation parameters may ameliorate this problem but this may also reduce the degree of tremor control.[19] Bilateral Vim stimulation is associated with more common side effects than unilateral procedures. Disequilibrium or even frank ataxia can be observed with the spread of current to the inferior border of the Vim into the posterior subthalamic region affecting the DRTT.[42] The most common adverse effects of stimulation are paresthesias, caused by the spread of current into the nucleus ventralis caudalis. Low-threshold paresthesias are seen in the posteriorly placed leads and reposition of the implanted lead may be necessary. However, most adverse effects from stimulation are induced by the current and disappear when the stimulation is off. Although the benefits of Vim DBS in patients with essential tremor tend to last for years to decades, the degree of tremor control tends to diminish compared with the peak efficacy and many patients show a reduction of tremor control of around 50% after several years.[43] A recent study of patients with essential tremor showed that the mean improvement decreased from 66% at 1 year to 48% at 10 years after surgery, although the patients still reported significant benefits for their activities of daily living.[36] The loss of efficacy may be caused by the development of brain tolerance, which may be offset by stimulation holiday. However, disease progression seems to be the more common explanation because tremor scores in these patients are worse when DBS is off than at their presurgical baseline.[43] Furthermore, frequency of arm tremor tends to decrease and the amplitude of tremor increases with longer disease duration, making it more difficult to control with electrical stimulation.[44] Worsening of tremor under these circumstances often requires adjustment of stimulation parameters with increased amplitude and/or increased pulse width. However, a higher

Table 2
Tremor improvement as evaluated by the Fahn-Tolosa-Marin scale in unilateral and bilateral tremor cases

	Unilateral Vim (%)	Bilateral Vim (%)	Number of Patients	Type
Dallapiazza et al,[9] 2018	53–63	66–78	1093	Meta-analysis
Wharen et al,[45] 2017	60	—	127	Controlled trial

Data from Dallapiazza RF, Lee DJ, De Vloo P, et al. Outcomes from stereotactic surgery for essential tremor. J Neurol Neurosurg Psychiatry 2018. [Epub ahead of print]; and Wharen RE Jr, Okun MS, Guthrie BL, et al. Thalamic DBS with a constant-current device in essential tremor: a controlled clinical trial. Parkinsonism Relat Disord 2017;40:18–26.

Table 3
Complication rate obtained from large meta-analyses of deep brain stimulation patients and the complication rate obtained in a recent controlled trial

	Hemorrhage (%)	Infection (%)	Lead Revision for Stimulation Side Effects (%)	Total Patients Studied (N)
Fenoy and Simpson,[35] 2014	5	1.9	2.6	728
Wharen et al,[45] 2017	2.3	2.3	3.1	127

Data from Fenoy AJ, Simpson RK Jr. Risks of common complications in deep brain stimulation surgery: management and avoidance. J Neurosurg 2014;120(1):132–9; and Wharen RE Jr, Okun MS, Guthrie BL, et al. Thalamic DBS with a constant-current device in essential tremor: a controlled clinical trial. Parkinsonism Relat Disord 2017;40:18–26.

DBS output is commonly associated with more pronounced adverse effects of stimulation, resulting in dysarthria, paresthesias, tonic motor contractures, and ataxia.

This article presents 2 tables summarizing Vim DBS outcomes from recent studies. Described are the tremor outcomes using the common FTM scale. **Table 2** provides tremor outcomes from a recently published large cohort of patients and from a recently published controlled trial.[9,45] **Table 3** lists complication rates from recent publications. These complication rates are consistent with rates describe in historical articles.

Although DBS provides impressive sustained improvement in medically refractory tremor, potential complications must be considered. **Table 3** provides the complication rate obtained from large meta-analyses of DBS patients and the complication rate obtained in a recent controlled trial. Of note, the meta-analysis pooled patients undergoing DBS for a variety of diagnoses, not just tremor.[35,45]

Most studies evaluating DBS outcomes for tremor have focused on appendicular tremor but substantial improvements can also be seen in axial tremor. In one recent study, a ~50% improvement in axial tremor symptoms, such as voice and head tremor, was noted with unilateral lead implantation, and with placement of a second lead the symptoms improved by another ~10%.[46]

FUTURE DIRECTIONS

DBS for tremor has resulted in dramatic quality-of-life improvements for numerous patients but there is room for refinement and improvement of this therapy. Some recent advancements in technology hold promise for the development of stimulation therapies that may have potential for improving battery life and or reducing stimulation-related side effects.

Directional leads are purported to allow more precise shaping of the therapeutic electrical field and may result in an incremental benefit in therapy. Ability to closely control the shape the electrical field surrounding the DBS lead could lead to reduced stimulation side effects such as dysarthria or paresthesias. It may also allow a lower energy usage.[47]

Closed-loop stimulation is also a technique being explored for DBS treatment of tremor. This strategy could be especially useful in action tremor such as essential tremor because stimulation could be activated at the time of movement and then turned off or turned down during rest. Sensing methods to which stimulation may respond include local field potentials at the lead as well as electrocorticography and other biomarkers.[48]

SUMMARY

Tremor is the most common movement disorder. Tremor can be classified as either action or resting tremor. Essential tremor is the most common type of action tremor. Initial treatment of action tremor is with medication. Patients with medically refractory tremor may be offered surgical intervention with neuromodulation therapies such as DBS of the thalamus. DBS is an effective treatment of medically refractory tremor symptoms. Neuromodulation with thalamic DBS is currently the most common treatment of tremor. Classic essential tremor is the action tremor that, in most cases, responds best to thalamic DBS. Although DBS has shown satisfactory results, practitioners continue to seek improvement in therapeutic outcome with newer technologies such as closed-loop stimulation and directional leads. Although the risks and side effect profile are favorable for this treatment, technological advances hold promise for improved treatment paradigms in the future.

REFERENCES

1. Bhatia KP, Bain P, Bajaj N, et al. Consensus statement on the classification of tremors. From the Task Force

on Tremor of the International Parkinson and Movement Disorder Society. Mov Disord 2018;33(1):75–87.
2. Benabid AL, Pollak P, Louveau A, et al. Combined (thalamotomy and stimulation) stereotactic surgery of the VIM thalamic nucleus for bilateral Parkinson disease. Appl Neurophysiol 1987; 50(1–6):344–6.
3. Benabid AL, Pollak P, Gao D, et al. Chronic electrical stimulation of the ventralis intermedius nucleus of the thalamus as a treatment of movement disorders. J Neurosurg 1996;84(2):203–14.
4. Benabid AL, Pollak P, Gervason C, et al. Long-term suppression of tremor by chronic stimulation of the ventral intermediate thalamic nucleus. Lancet 1991;337(8738):403–6.
5. Tasker RR. Deep brain stimulation is preferable to thalamotomy for tremor suppression. Surg Neurol 1998;49(2):145–53 [discussion: 153–4].
6. Blomstedt P, Hariz MI. Are complications less common in deep brain stimulation than in ablative procedures for movement disorders? Stereotact Funct Neurosurg 2006;84(2–3):72–81.
7. Matsumoto K, Asano T, Baba T, et al. Long-term follow-up results of bilateral thalamotomy for parkinsonism. Appl Neurophysiol 1976;39(3–4):257–60.
8. Nagaseki Y, Shibazaki T, Hirai T, et al. Long-term follow-up results of selective VIM-thalamotomy. J Neurosurg 1986;65(3):296–302.
9. Dallapiazza RF, Lee DJ, De Vloo P, et al. Outcomes from stereotactic surgery for essential tremor. J Neurol Neurosurg Psychiatry 2018. https://doi.org/10.1136/jnnp-2018-318240.
10. Jankovic J, Fahn S. Physiologic and pathologic tremors. Diagnosis, mechanism, and management. Ann Intern Med 1980;93(3):460–5.
11. Hallett M. Tremor: pathophysiology. Parkinsonism Relat Disord 2014;20(Suppl 1):S118–22.
12. Coenen VA, Allert N, Paus S, et al. Modulation of the cerebello-thalamo-cortical network in thalamic deep brain stimulation for tremor: a diffusion tensor imaging study. Neurosurgery 2014;75(6):657–69 [discussion: 669–70].
13. Fiechter M, Nowacki A, Oertel MF, et al. Deep brain stimulation for tremor: is there a common structure? Stereotact Funct Neurosurg 2017;95(4):243–50.
14. Wong JK, Cauraugh JH, Ho KWD, et al. STN vs GPi deep brain stimulation for tremor suppression in Parkinson disease: a systematic review and meta-analysis. Parkinsonism Relat Disord 2018. https://doi.org/10.1016/j.parkreldis.2018.08.017.
15. Artusi CA, Farooqi A, Romagnolo A, et al. Deep brain stimulation in uncommon tremor disorders: indications, targets, and programming. J Neurol 2018; 265(11):2473–93.
16. Albanese A, Asmus F, Bhatia KP, et al. EFNS guidelines on diagnosis and treatment of primary dystonias. Eur J Neurol 2011;18(1):5–18.
17. Ondo W, Hashem V, LeWitt PA, et al. Comparison of the Fahn-Tolosa-Marin clinical rating scale and the essential tremor rating assessment scale. Mov Disord Clin Pract 2018;5(1):60–5.
18. Samotus O, Lee J, Jog M. Long-term tremor therapy for Parkinson and essential tremor with sensor-guided botulinum toxin type A injections. PLoS One 2017;12(6):e0178670.
19. Baizabal-Carvallo JF, Kagnoff MN, Jimenez-Shahed J, et al. The safety and efficacy of thalamic deep brain stimulation in essential tremor: 10 years and beyond. J Neurol Neurosurg Psychiatry 2014; 85(5):567–72.
20. Ferrara JM, Kenney C, Davidson AL, et al. Efficacy and tolerability of pregabalin in essential tremor: a randomized, double-blind, placebo-controlled, crossover trial. J Neurol Sci 2009;285(1–2):195–7.
21. Higuchi M-A, Topiol DD, Ahmed B, et al. Impact of an interdisciplinary deep brain stimulation screening model on post-surgical complications in essential tremor patients. PLoS One 2015;10(12):e0145623.
22. Chen T, Mirzadeh Z, Chapple K, et al. "Asleep" deep brain stimulation for essential tremor. J Neurosurg 2016;124(6):1842–9.
23. Montgomery EB Jr. Microelectrode targeting of the subthalamic nucleus for deep brain stimulation surgery. Mov Disord 2012;27(11):1387–91.
24. Raz A, Eimerl D, Zaidel A, et al. Propofol decreases neuronal population spiking activity in the subthalamic nucleus of Parkinsonian patients. Anesth Analg 2010;111(5):1285–9.
25. Gross RE, Krack P, Rodriguez-Oroz MC, et al. Electrophysiological mapping for the implantation of deep brain stimulators for Parkinson's disease and tremor. Mov Disord 2006;21(Suppl 14):S259–83.
26. Starr PA, Martin AJ, Ostrem JL, et al. Subthalamic nucleus deep brain stimulator placement using high-field interventional magnetic resonance imaging and a skull-mounted aiming device: technique and application accuracy. J Neurosurg 2010; 112(3):479–90.
27. Burchiel KJ, McCartney S, Lee A, et al. Accuracy of deep brain stimulation electrode placement using intraoperative computed tomography without microelectrode recording. J Neurosurg 2013;119(2): 301–6.
28. Park CK, Jung NY, Kim M, et al. Analysis of delayed intracerebral hemorrhage associated with deep brain stimulation surgery. World Neurosurg 2017; 104:537–44.
29. Zrinzo L, Foltynie T, Limousin P, et al. Reducing hemorrhagic complications in functional neurosurgery: a large case series and systematic literature review. J Neurosurg 2012;116(1):84–94.
30. Saleh C, Dooms G, Berthold C, et al. Post-operative imaging in deep brain stimulation: a controversial issue. Neuroradiol J 2016;29(4):244–9.

31. Ramayya AG, Abdullah KG, Mallela AN, et al. Thirty-day readmission rates following deep brain stimulation surgery. Neurosurgery 2017;81(2):259–67.
32. Fenoy AJ, Villarreal SJ, Schiess MC. Acute and subacute presentations of cerebral edema following deep brain stimulation lead implantation. Stereotact Funct Neurosurg 2017;95(2):86–92.
33. Kluger BM, Foote KD, Jacobson CE, et al. Lessons learned from a large single center cohort of patients referred for DBS management. Parkinsonism Relat Disord 2011;17(4):236–9.
34. Almeida L, Rawal PV, Ditty B, et al. Deep brain stimulation battery longevity: comparison of monopolar versus bipolar stimulation modes. Mov Disord Clin Pract 2016;3(4):359–66.
35. Fenoy AJ, Simpson RK Jr. Risks of common complications in deep brain stimulation surgery: management and avoidance. J Neurosurg 2014;120(1):132–9.
36. Cury RG, Fraix V, Castrioto A, et al. Thalamic deep brain stimulation for tremor in Parkinson disease, essential tremor, and dystonia. Neurology 2017;89(13):1416–23.
37. Huss DS, Dallapiazza RF, Shah BB, et al. Functional assessment and quality of life in essential tremor with bilateral or unilateral DBS and focused ultrasound thalamotomy. Mov Disord 2015;30(14):1937–43.
38. Nazzaro JM, Pahwa R, Lyons KE. Long-term benefits in quality of life after unilateral thalamic deep brain stimulation for essential tremor. J Neurosurg 2012;117(1):156–61.
39. Flora ED, Perera CL, Cameron AL, et al. Deep brain stimulation for essential tremor: a systematic review. Mov Disord 2010;25(11):1550–9.
40. Hariz G-M, Blomstedt P, Koskinen L-OD. Long-term effect of deep brain stimulation for essential tremor on activities of daily living and health-related quality of life. Acta Neurol Scand 2008;118(6):387–94.
41. Tröster AI, Pahwa R, Fields JA, et al. Quality of life in Essential Tremor Questionnaire (QUEST): development and initial validation. Parkinsonism Relat Disord 2005;11(6):367–73.
42. Reich MM, Brumberg J, Pozzi NG, et al. Progressive gait ataxia following deep brain stimulation for essential tremor: adverse effect or lack of efficacy? Brain 2016;139(11):2948–56.
43. Favilla CG, Ullman D, Wagle Shukla A, et al. Worsening essential tremor following deep brain stimulation: disease progression versus tolerance. Brain 2012;135(Pt 5):1455–62.
44. Deuschl G, Wenzelburger R, Löffler K, et al. Essential tremor and cerebellar dysfunction clinical and kinematic analysis of intention tremor. Brain 2000;123(Pt 8):1568–80.
45. Wharen RE Jr, Okun MS, Guthrie BL, et al. Thalamic DBS with a constant-current device in essential tremor: a controlled clinical trial. Parkinsonism Relat Disord 2017;40:18–26.
46. Mitchell KT, Larson P, Starr PA, et al. Benefits and risks of unilateral and bilateral ventral intermediate nucleus deep brain stimulation for axial essential tremor symptoms. Parkinsonism Relat Disord 2018. https://doi.org/10.1016/j.parkreldis.2018.09.004.
47. Schüpbach WMM, Chabardes S, Matthies C, et al. Directional leads for deep brain stimulation: opportunities and challenges. Mov Disord 2017;32(10):1371–5.
48. Kuo C-H, White-Dzuro GA, Ko AL. Approaches to closed-loop deep brain stimulation for movement disorders. Neurosurg Focus 2018;45(2):E2.

Neuromodulation
Deep Brain Stimulation for Treatment of Dystonia

Nicholas Dietz, BS, Joseph Neimat, MD, MS*

KEYWORDS

• Neuromodulation • Dystonia • Deep brain stimulation • Neurosurgery

KEY POINTS

- Consensus guidelines regarding the classification of dystonia describe axis I and axis II defining relevant clinical features and etiology, respectively.
- Pathophysiology of dystonia involves the cortico-basal ganglia-thalamo-cortical loop with direct and indirect pathway models and the cerebello-thalamo-cortical pathway.
- Historically, peripheral denervation, rhizotomy, and ablative procedures, including thalamotomy and pallidotomy, were performed to improve dystonic features.
- Deep brain stimulation became widely incorporated in 1999 after several landmark studies and has been effectively used in targets of the thalamus, pallidum, and subthalamic nucleus.
- Improved understanding of neural pathways and pathophysiology and increased genetic analysis capabilities continue to guide precise surgical technique toward increasingly-effective treatment of dystonia.

INTRODUCTION

Dystonia is a heterogeneous, hyperkinetic movement disorder that can manifest as sustained or intermittent abnormal postures, hyperkinetic muscle contractions, or repetitive movements.[1] Although dystonic patterns vary significantly across clinical phenotype, causes are multifactorial and are attributed to genetic and environmental factors.[2,3] Medical treatment varies based on anatomic distribution and classification but may include oral pharmaceuticals for generalized dystonia, intramuscular injections of botulinum toxin (BTX) for focal dystonias, and finally surgery for either form. A subset of severe dystonias, focal or generalized, that is refractory to medical therapy may benefit from surgical intervention through deep brain stimulation (DBS). This article discusses the classification, diagnosis, pathogenesis, and treatment of dystonia and the evolution of surgical intervention from ablation to stereotactic DBS since its inception in the mid-twentieth century.

DISEASE OVERVIEW
Classification

Traditional classification of dystonia has focused on etiology, age of onset, and anatomic distribution.[4,5] Evolution of descriptions in recent decades has distinguished primary dystonia and secondary dystonia.[6] Primary dystonia refers to phenotypically isolated dystonia, in which it is a standalone or pure clinical manifestation.[7] In contrast, secondary dystonia covers a broader scope of dystonia stemming from syndromic neurologic conditions or environmental factors that contributed to dystonic features.[8] Additionally, fixed dystonia includes dystonic features that remain in hyperkinetic or abnormally postured states at

Disclosures: The authors have nothing to disclose.
Department of Neurosurgery, University of Louisville, School of Medicine, 200 Abraham Flexner Highway, Louisville, KY 40202, USA
* Corresponding author.
E-mail address: joseph.neimat@louisvilleneuroscience.com

Neurosurg Clin N Am 30 (2019) 161–168
https://doi.org/10.1016/j.nec.2018.12.001

rest. Fixed forms of dystonia have been associated with psychogenic etiology or complex regional pain syndrome.[9] In contrast, mobile dystonia arises with movement and may relieve in rest or neural positions. Sensory tricks, or gestes antagonistes, are a classic feature of primary dystonia in which a specific movement or internal stimulus alleviates the dystonic features.[10] Moreover, the sensory trick has traditionally represented a way to differentiate primary dystonia from essential tremor (ET), for example.[10] New classification proposals underscore the importance of a multitude of clinical characteristics and etiology under 2 axes.[8,11] The identification of genetic causes may begin to play an increasing role in the evolving nomenclature. This has been exemplified in the identification and classification of the DYT mutations.[12]

In 2013, Albanese and colleagues[8] presented a set of widely accepted consensus guidelines regarding the classification of dystonia. They describe the distinction of 2 axes, axis I and axis II, that aid in diagnosis of subtypes of dystonia in a clinically useful fashion. Axis I defines clinical features of the dystonia in a meaningful way to include description of the phenomenology and 5 other features: anatomic distribution, age of onset, temporal pattern, comorbid movement disorders, and additional neurologic manifestations.[8] Axis I criteria provide key information regarding expected therapy and prognosis of the subtype depicted from movement behavior and individual history of the disease. Importantly, clinicians may also begin to recognize syndromic dystonia from symptomatic patterns uncovered in axis I. Axis II underscores the etiology of the dystonia, with emphasis on acquired versus inherited forms and anatomic changes that may have induced dystonic symptoms. Imaging, such as brain MRI, laboratory values, or genetic testing, may inform axis II, providing evidence for structural neurologic abnormalities, gene mutations, or degeneration at gross or microscopic levels.

Anatomic Distribution

Distribution tends to inform prognostic evaluations and treatment options and can be separated into focal, segmental, multifocal, hemidystonia, or generalized.[8] Focal involves 1 isolated region of the body, whereas segmental involves multiple adjacent body regions. Focal dystonia includes well-described patterns, such as writer's cramp, blepharospasm, oromandibular, and cervical dystonia—the most common of focal dystonias, including abnormal horizontal head posturing (torticollis) and head tilting (laterocollis). Combinations of cranial muscle dystonia, such as blepharospasm and oromandibular dystonia, called Meige syndrome, may be classified as segmental. Multifocal dystonia involves 2 or more noncontiguous body regions and hemidystonia relates to a symptomatic distribution along 1 side of the body. Generalized dystonia involves the trunk and 2 other body regions, often the lower extremities.

Age of Onset

A bimodal distribution of dystonia onset has been observed with peaks at 9 years of age and 55 years of age.[13] Clinical features also segregate with age of onset, because those of younger age are more likely to have generalized dystonia, which is less commonly diagnosed in older cohorts.[13] Delineation of age cutoffs have been criticized for being arbitrary in their differentiation of childhood early onset from adulthood late onset, with some divisions at 20 years or 26 years, for example.

Ideal demarcations of age may aid in diagnosis of type or etiology to incorporate errors of metabolism, cerebral palsy, or neurotransmitter deficiency. Cervical dystonia, the most common type of dystonia, which includes torticollis and laterocollis, typically arises between the fourth and fifth decades of life, for example.[14] Recent discussions have been more precise in their grouping by age of onset. Albanese and colleagues[8] propose a new guideline for age groups to include infancy (birth to 2 years), childhood (3–12 years), adolescence (13–20 years), early adulthood (21–40 years), and late adulthood (>40 years).

Etiology

The etiologies of dystonia may be classified as inherited or acquired, according to Jinnah and Albanese.[1] Axis II classification schemes that incorporate etiology define 2 distinct subgroups: nervous system pathology and mechanism of acquisition.[11] Degenerative, structural changes or lesions and absence of degenerative or structural changes are categories of nervous system pathology whereas inherited, acquired, and idiopathic are categories of acquisition.[11] Certain distributions relate to secondary causes of dystonia, including hemidystonia, which is most commonly due to stroke, childhood trauma, or perinatal injury.[15]

Epidemiology

Combined analyses from several studies estimate the prevalence of primary dystonia, the most common form of dystonia, to be 16.4 per 100,000 individuals.[16] Incidence of primary cervical dystonia has been calculated to be 8 million to 12 per million, from a pooled analysis of studies based out of Rochester, Minnesota, and Northern California.[17] Defazio and colleagues[18] characterize prevalence of early-onset (<20 years old) primary dystonia as 50 per million and late-onset (>20 years old) primary dystonia as 30 cases to 7320 cases per million. This broad range suggests the uncertainty or failure to diagnose many cases.

NEURAL SUBSTRATES OF DYSTONIA

Pathophysiology

Basal ganglia

The cortico-basal ganglia-thalamo-cortical loop is understood to be responsible for the regulation of voluntary movement. The classic model of this motor circuitry is segregated in direct and indirect pathways that regulate motivational and inhibitory effects through the basal ganglia (**Fig. 1**). The direct pathway is composed of connections between the motor cortex and dorsal striatum (caudate and putamen). Inhibitory signals are then sent to the globus pallidus internus (GPi) and substantia nigra pars reticulata that tonically suppress the ventral lateral nucleus of the thalamus through γ-aminobutyric acid (GABA)-ergic signal. The subsequent inhibition of the GABAergic signals to the thalamus excite projections to the ventral anterior nucleus and activates the motor cortex, promoting movement. In contrast, the indirect pathway inhibits movement through the basal ganglia. The indirect pathway is responsible for disinhibiting the subthalamic nucleus (STN), which stimulates the GPi. The inhibitory signal of the GPi on the ventral lateral nucleus suppresses movement.

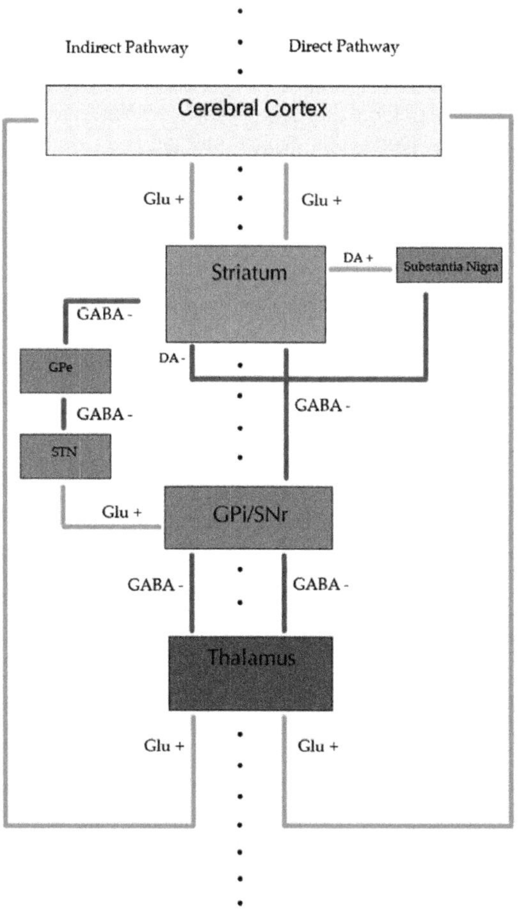

Fig. 1. Basal ganglia: direct and indirect pathways.

Some theories regarding the mechanism of dystonia posit that an imbalance exists between direct and indirect pathways in the cortico-basal ganglia-thalamo-cortical loop such that the indirect pathway may be dysfunctional. The constellation of symptoms resulting in muscle hypertonicity may be related to an uninhibited stimulation of the direct pathway. Furthermore, imaging studies using functional MRI and PET studies show abnormal activity of the basal ganglia in the absence of structural changes.[19,20]

Cerebellum

Evidence suggests that the cerebello-thalamo-cortical circuit also may play a role in dystonia. Hoover and Strick[21] describe cortical projections from the basal ganglia and cerebellum converging on overlapping regions of the motor cortex. A variety of pathologies, such as stroke, tumor, and other lesions, related to the cerebellum and its projections to the pathway have been linked to dystonic features. For example, it has been found that posterior fossa tumors and other pathology have led to secondary dystonia that have been improved with tumor excision.[22] Additionally, stroke has been found to result in cervical dystonia[23] and hemidystonia.[24]

Diagnosis and Work-up

Diagnosis

Variability in presentation and etiology traditionally challenges the streamlined diagnosis of dystonia. Several algorithms have been suggested, however, to identify subtype that guide work-up and specific diagnosis. Important first steps in diagnosis include history and physical examination to identify and separate dystonia from similar pathologies, such as myoclonus, tremor, or chorea.[5] Dystonic features are often stereotyped, unidirectional, and sustained and may involve torsion compared with other hyperkinetic pathologies. It is commonly cited that dystonia fundamentally involves the simultaneous activation of agonist and corresponding antagonist muscle groups.[25] Additionally, voluntary movement in the associated muscle group as well as emotional stress and fatigue tend to worsen patterned symptoms of dystonia.

Correct classification of the dystonia represents the next clinical step in narrowing the diagnosis that informs potential prognosis, work-up, and management options. A common starting point is to differentiate isolated from combined dystonia, with acknowledgment of predominant movement phenomenology and presence of additional neurologic or systemic symptoms.[26] Distinction of fixed versus mobile forms of dystonia, with presence of sensory trick or comorbid complex regional pain syndrome features, for example, also guides clinicians down management pathways. Classification schemes may involve axis I and axis II characteristics, such as body distribution, age of onset, temporality of symptoms, and etiology.

Work-up

Although clinical examination often may be sufficient to achieve diagnosis, especially in isolated forms of dystonia, a host of tests may be used to aid conclusions. Commonly implemented tools include electromyography to quantify hypertonicity of select muscle groups and differentiate from tremor and myoclonus; neuroimaging to determine structural abnormalities, such as mass lesion or metal or calcium deposits that may be higher yield for combined, hemidystonia, and generalized forms; and laboratory studies.

Routine studies include a levodopa trial, lysosomal enzyme assays, plasma and urine amino acids, serum copper, 24-hour urine copper, serum ceruloplasmin for suspicion of Wilson disease, iron studies, and peripheral blood smear to identify acanthocytes.[11] More-specific, disease-targeted analyses may be performed with genetic testing, cerebrospinal fluid analysis for dopaminergic analysis, or metabolic screenings for suspected syndromes. Several reports conclude that genetic testing is not recommended in adults with focal or segmental dystonia because results do not aid in management.[27]

Genetic Analysis

Recent genetic analyses have offered more precise description of pathogenesis and prognosis of primary dystonia. In 1997, DYT1-TOR1A was an autosomal dominant mutation identified to relate to isolated, early-onset dystonia patterns.[28] Since then, many more mutations, including autosomal recessive, X-linked, and mitochondrial, have been identified and linked to dystonic distribution, temporality, and prognosis. Clinical relevance, however, remains questionable because the odds of identifying a genetic correlation from sporadic onset isolated dystonia are estimated at less than 1%.[29] Dystonia that is of isolated form, early-onset temporality, or arising in the setting of positive family history for dystonia is an indication for which genetic testing is more likely to be helpful in clinical management.

MEDICAL THERAPY

A multitude of medical therapy options exist in the treatment of dystonia and vary based on etiology, age, and distribution of the pathology. Symptomatic management options for dystonia regardless of etiology include physical and occupational therapy to maintain range of motion and prevent contractures.[29,30] Braces and medical devices that maintain posture and prevent torsion also may be useful in localized dystonic manifestations. Also notable is the use of rehabilitation for maintenance and recovery from sensory loss or sensory cortical control for muscle movements. Training regimens have been described to facilitate recovery of sensory and motor discrimination.[31]

BTX injections into dystonic muscles have emerged as a standardized approach for symptomatic relief of focal and segmental dystonias in recent decades. Numerous clinical studies have demonstrated BTX efficacy in restoring posture and movement and improving pain from cervical dystonia for which it is a first-line treatment.[32] BTX causes a localized paralysis from chemical denervation that arrests presynaptic release of acetylcholine, providing safe symptomatic relief. Although standard guidelines do not specify dosing and frequency of administration, injections are often administered every 12 weeks or more for patients with persistent symptoms of cervical dystonia.[33]

Oral medications are typically reserved for generalized dystonia and may be used in combination treatment regimens. Commonly used anticholinergic therapies include trihexyphenidyl and benztropine. A landmark double-blind randomized controlled study in 1986 by Burke and colleagues[34] demonstrated that high-dose trihexyphenidyl up to 30 mg daily resulted in a clinically significant improvement of primary and secondary dystonia symptoms in 71% of the study cohort at 36 weeks, with 42% reporting lasting improvements at 2.4 years. After anticholinergic agents, baclofen is another oral medication useful in treatment of dystonic spasticity that interrupts neural transmission through GABA receptor agonist activity. Benzodiazepines, such as clonazepam, also may be used to supplement oral regimens.

SURGICAL INTERVENTION

Surgical ablation and stimulation techniques to treat dystonia generally target the cortico-basal ganglia-thalamo-cortical pathway and are reserved for severe, debilitating, generalized dystonia and hemidystonia refractory to medical therapy. Surgical candidates are those who have failed optimal medical treatments and experience significant disability. It is also important to intervene with surgical methods before progression of dystonia leads to contractures or fixed deformity.[35] Since the 1950s, ablative procedures, including thalamotomy and pallidotomy, were performed and showed improvements in dystonic features. Localized stimulation was observed, however, to have favorable outcomes in alleviating movement pathology in a reversible manner. Other neurosurgical interventions for the treatment of dystonia include peripheral denervation, myotomies, rhizotomies, and placement of intrathecal baclofen pumps.

Historical Procedures

Thalamotomies were performed to treat dystonia beginning in the 1950s because dystonic symptoms were found to diminish after procedures for Parkinson disease (PD). In 1976, Cooper[36] described the success of thalamotomy in a case series spanning 2 decades during which 226 patients with dystonia were treated, with 65% showing improvement. Later reports of stereotactic thalamotomy for generalized dystonia demonstrated improvement of more than 50% of function in 34% of the patients treated and at least 25% in another 23% of patients.[37] A variety of thalamic nuclei were targeted across procedures to include the ventralis oralis anterior (VOa), ventralis oralis posterior, ventralis intermedius (VIM), and centromedian nuclei, complicating the standardized evaluation of the procedures peformed.[36,38]

Postoperative complications, however, were noted more frequent in bilateral thalamotomies. In a case study of 55 patients undergoing thalamotomy procedures, dysarthria was observed in 56% of those with bilateral thalamotomies compared with 11% with unilateral thalamotomy.[38] To a lesser extent, pallidotomy was also performed in early pioneering functional procedures for dystonia,[39,40] with results more favorable for primary than for secondary dystonia.[41]

Until the 1980s, the selective dorsal rhizotomy was frequently used for a group of patients with early-onset diffuse spasticity, cerebral palsy, or torticollis, in which intradural cervical dorsal nerve roots were lesioned.[42] In those patients amenable to the procedure, sensory nerve roots were exposed and selectively targeted with electromyography to confirm spastic muscle innervations.[43] Those rootlets contributing to the spasticity were then sectioned to reduce spasticity. In 1982, Bertrand and colleagues[44] described a targeted peripheral denervation for treatment of torticollis. This technique was later demonstrated in 1988 on a sample of 111 patients with symptomatic torticollis, showing 87% success rate with resolution of symptoms and return of function.[45] The success of this procedure was replicated in 1993, when 260 patients with torticollis were treated, with 88% experiencing postoperative clinical improvement.[45,46] Newer surgical interventions like DBS offer increased safety, improved adverse effect profiles, and reversibility that have largely replaced lesional procedures, including, rhizotomy, thalamotomy, and pallidotomy.[47]

Deep Brain Stimulation

DBS represents an adjustable and reversible intervention, using electrical impulses that may alter neural signals in specific subcortical brain regions to reverse pathology. Electrode leads are implanted and connected to a pacemaker that is typically placed subcutaneously in the subclavicular region. DBS has eclipsed many of the previous lesional therapies that had been used more routinely in dystonia and offered the possibility of dramatic symptom reduction in some of the most severely disabled patients. It is considered safe and with low risk of readmission: 1.9% within 30 days for all DBS procedures.[48]

Although DBS is a modern procedure, arising in the past 30 years, there had been previous forays into targeted stimulation for similar medically refractory conditions. In 1978, Cooper described one of the first applications of DBS for hypertonicity via chronic cerebellar stimulation to elicit thalamic inhibition.[49] In late 1970s, Mundinger[50] describe stereotaxic thalamic stimulation for torticollis in 7 patients. The technique of stimulation remained quiescent until the mid-1980s and 1990s, when it was used by Alim Benabid and other investigators for the treatment of ET and PD. In 1999, a series of DBS studies, using unilateral pallidal stimulation attempted for focal cervical dystonia[51] and bilateral pallidal stimulation for generalized dystonia, were successful in relief of symptoms.[52,53] Stimulation techniques for dystonia were widely adopted thereafter. In 1998, DBS was approved for treatment of ET by the US Food and Drug Administration. Indications for DBS expanded soon after to include PD in 2002 and dystonia in 2003. Because it was believed that the number of patients who would require DBS for treatment of advanced dystonia was few, it was approved under a Humanitarian Device Exemption, presuming that fewer than 4000 per year would require the therapy.

Targets for Dystonia

Thalamus

In 1977, Mundinger[50] described a successful clinical outcome 8 months postoperatively with stereotaxic thalamic stimulation for torticollis in 7 patients.[50] Specific targets included Ventro-oralis Anterior (VOa)m Ventro-oralis Internus (VOi) and subthalamic regions. Despite this reported success, few publications followed regarding use of thalamic stimulation for treatment of dystonia except a small study with 2 patients with torticollis.[54] In 2001, however, Vercueil and collegues[55] described an analysis of 12 patients with generalized dystonia treated with DBS targeted in the ventrolateral thalamic nucleus. A total of 8 reported improved global function and 5 experienced some improvement in limb dystonia but did not show symptomatic improvement in Burke-Fahn-Marsden Dystonia Rating Scale (BFMDRS) movement or BFMDRS disability outcomes. Subsequently, Cury and colleagues[56] performed VIM DBS for 6 patients with dystonic tremor, with primary outcome of reduction of tremor after 1 year. A moderate reduction of dystonic tremor after 1 year described as a 41% improvement according to the BFMDRS was observed.

Pallidum

Historically, studies on DBS for dystonia have largely focused on the GPi target. The shift toward pallidal targets for DBS was likely a byproduct of the success seen from DBS for treatment of PD that saw a secondary reduction in dystonic symptoms. Although the pathophysiology of dystonia is not clearly defined, a subset of trials indicates that the globus pallidus plays a significant role in mechanism. A landmark study demonstrated that local field potentials in the GPi were seen in those with untreated dystonia that differed from those with treated dystonia.[57] The first randomized controlled trial on bilateral pallidal DBS found improvement in 54% BFMDRS movement and 41% BFMDRS disability scores in 22 patients with primary generalized dystonia after 12 months of stimulation.[58] In 2006, Kupsch and colleagues[59] conducted a blinded, randomized controlled trial of 40 patients with segmented or generalized dystonia who received either DBS or sham stimulation for 3 months. Movement scores improved by 15.8 points, with 39.3% reduction in symptoms, compared with 1.6-point improvement and 4.9% reduction in the sham control group.[59] A host of GPi targets for primary generalized dystonia shows clinical improvements, ranging from 34% to 92%.[60–63]

Subthalamic nucleus

Although the STN represents a primary DBS target for PD, its use for dystonia has not been as strongly considered. Yet, interest in its effectiveness for dystonia has shown that it may represent at least an appropriate alternative to the more commonly targeted GPi.[64,65] Ostrem and colleagues[65] report a significant improvement on the Toronto Western Spasmodic Torticollis Rating Scale (TWSTRS) for 9 patients with cervical dystonia who received bilateral STN DBS. A follow-up study with 20 patients having primary dystonia was later conducted to determine long-term treatment efficacy and showed sustained clinical improvement over 3 years in 14 of the patients with isolated dystonia, with 70% improvement in BFMDRS and 66.6% improvement in TWSTRS.[66]

SUMMARY

Given the heterogeneity of dystonia, it is important to recognize the nuanced diagnostic classification and evaluation of treatment. For those cases refractory to the various forms of medical management, DBS through GPi or thalamic nuclei may be targeted. As the pathophysiology of dystonia is further characterized, targets may be specified for different classifications that more appropriately treat abnormal regions in the cortico-basal ganglia-thalamo-cortical or cerebello-thalamo-cortical circuits. Although the GPi represents the premier site for dystonic stimulation, certain thalamic nuclei have emerged as more appropriate for particular pathologies, such as bilateral Ventro-oralis DBS for musicians' dystonia[67] or thalamic stimulation for dystonic tremor.[68]

Additionally, future directions in the treatment of dystonia may incorporate genetic analysis to redefine classification schemes and further individualize treatment approach. Certain genotypes, for example, are more inclined toward effective DBS or particular stimulation targets. Panov and colleagues[69] have shown that GPi DBS is especially effective for patients with DYT1-associated dystonia, whereas DYT6 patients were less successfully treated with GPi stimulation. As implementable sequencing techniques become increasingly incorporated into practice, indications of surgical options may broaden from precision of subcortical targets in DBS. Moreover, improved understanding of neural pathways, neuroanatomic subtleties in pathophysiology, and increased genetic analysis capabilities will guide precise surgical technique toward ever-safer and more effective treatment of dystonia.

REFERENCES

1. Jinnah HA, Albanese A. The new classification system for the dystonias: why was it needed and how was it developed? Mov Disord Clin Pract 2014;1(4):280–4.
2. Phukan J, Albanese A, Gasser T, et al. Primary dystonia and dystonia-plus syndromes: clinical characteristics, diagnosis, and pathogenesis. Lancet Neurol 2011;10(12):1074–85.
3. Fahn S, Bressman SB, Marsden CD. Classification of dystonia. Adv Neurol 1998;78:1–10.
4. Fahn S. Classification of movement disorders. Mov Disord 2011;26(6):947–57.
5. Geyer HL, Bressman SB. The diagnosis of dystonia. Lancet Neurol 2006;5(9):780–90.
6. Bressman SB. Dystonia genotypes, phenotypes, and classification. Adv Neurol 2004;94:101–7.
7. Fahn S, Eldridge R. Definition of dystonia and classification of the dystonic states. Adv Neurol 1976;14:1–5.
8. Albanese A, Bhatia K, Bressman SB, et al. Phenomenology and classification of dystonia: a consensus update. Mov Disord 2013;28(7):863–73.
9. LeDoux MS. Dystonia: phenomenology. Parkinsonism Relat Disord 2012;18(Suppl 1):S162–4.
10. Schrag A, Trimble M, Quinn N, et al. The syndrome of fixed dystonia: an evaluation of 103 patients. Brain 2004;127(Pt 10):2360–72.
11. De Pablo-Fernandez E, Warner TT. Dystonia. Br Med Bull 2017;123(1):91–102.
12. Muller U, Steinberger D, Nemeth AH. Clinical and molecular genetics of primary dystonias. Neurogenetics 1998;1(3):165–77.
13. Bressman SB, de Leon D, Brin MF, et al. Idiopathic dystonia among Ashkenazi Jews: evidence for autosomal dominant inheritance. Ann Neurol 1989;26(5):612–20.
14. Defazio G, Jankovic J, Giel JL, et al. Descriptive epidemiology of cervical dystonia. Tremor Other Hyperkinet Mov (N Y) 2013;3 [pii:tre-03-193-4374-2].
15. Pettigrew LC, Jankovic J. Hemidystonia: a report of 22 patients and a review of the literature. J Neurol Neurosurg Psychiatry 1985;48(7):650–7.
16. Steeves TD, Day L, Dykeman J, et al. The prevalence of primary dystonia: a systematic review and meta-analysis. Mov Disord 2012;27(14):1789–96.
17. Marras C, Van den Eeden SK, Fross RD, et al. Minimum incidence of primary cervical dystonia in a multiethnic health care population. Neurology 2007;69(7):676–80.
18. Defazio G, Abbruzzese G, Livrea P, et al. Epidemiology of primary dystonia. Lancet Neurol 2004;3(11):673–8.
19. Asanuma K, Carbon-Correll M, Eidelberg D. Neuroimaging in human dystonia. J Med Invest 2005;52(Suppl):272–9.
20. Kerrison JB, Lancaster JL, Zamarripa FE, et al. Positron emission tomography scanning in essential blepharospasm. Am J Ophthalmol 2003;136(5):846–52.
21. Hoover JE, Strick PL. The organization of cerebellar and basal ganglia outputs to primary motor cortex as revealed by retrograde transneuronal transport of herpes simplex virus type 1. J Neurosci 1999;19(4):1446–63.
22. Krauss JK, Seeger W, Jankovic J. Cervical dystonia associated with tumors of the posterior fossa. Mov Disord 1997;12(3):443–7.
23. Zadro I, Brinar VV, Barun B, et al. Cervical dystonia due to cerebellar stroke. Mov Disord 2008;23(6):919–20.
24. Rumbach L, Barth P, Costaz A, et al. Hemidystonia consequent upon ipsilateral vertebral artery occlusion and cerebellar infarction. Mov Disord 1995;10(4):522–5.
25. Yanagisawa N, Goto A. Dystonia musculorum deformans. Analysis with electromyography. J Neurol Sci 1971;13(1):39–65.
26. Fung VS, Jinnah HA, Bhatia K, et al. Assessment of patients with isolated or combined dystonia: an update on dystonia syndromes. Mov Disord 2013;28(7):889–98.
27. Jinnah HA, Berardelli A, Comella C, et al. The focal dystonias: current views and challenges for future research. Mov Disord 2013;28(7):926–43.
28. Ozelius LJ, Hewett JW, Page CE, et al. The early-onset torsion dystonia gene (DYT1) encodes an ATP-binding protein. Nat Genet 1997;17(1):40–8.
29. Jinnah HA, Factor SA. Diagnosis and treatment of dystonia. Neurol Clin 2015;33(1):77–100.
30. Jankovic J. Medical treatment of dystonia. Mov Disord 2013;28(7):1001–12.
31. Byl NN, Nagajaran S, McKenzie AL. Effect of sensory discrimination training on structure and function in patients with focal hand dystonia: a case series. Arch Phys Med Rehabil 2003;84(10):1505–14.
32. Jankovic J. Botulinum toxin therapy for cervical dystonia. Neurotox Res 2006;9(2–3):145–8.
33. Evidente VG, Pappert EJ. Botulinum toxin therapy for cervical dystonia: the science of dosing. Tremor Other Hyperkinet Mov (N Y) 2014;4:273.
34. Burke RE, Fahn S, Marsden CD. Torsion dystonia: a double-blind, prospective trial of high-dosage trihexyphenidyl. Neurology 1986;36(2):160–4.
35. Cloud LJ, Jinnah HA. Treatment strategies for dystonia. Expert Opin Pharmacother 2010;11(1):5–15.
36. Cooper IS. 20-year followup study of the neurosurgical treatment of dystonia musculorum deformans. Adv Neurol 1976;14:423–52.
37. Tasker RR, Doorly T, Yamashiro K. Thalamotomy in generalized dystonia. Adv Neurol 1988;50:615–31.

38. Andrew J, Fowler CJ, Harrison MJ. Stereotaxic thalamotomy in 55 cases of dystonia. Brain 1983;106(Pt 4):981–1000.
39. Burzaco J. Stereotactic pallidotomy in extrapyramidal disorders. Appl Neurophysiol 1985;48(1–6): 283–7.
40. Lozano AM, Kumar R, Gross RE, et al. Globus pallidus internus pallidotomy for generalized dystonia. Mov Disord 1997;12(6):865–70.
41. Alkhani A, Khan F, Lang AE, et al. 716 the response to pallidal surgery for dystonia is dependent on the etiology. Neurosurgery 2000;47(2):504.
42. Taira T, Hori T. Selective peripheral neurotomy and selective dorsal rhizotomy. Brain Nerve 2008; 60(12):1427–36 [in Japanese].
43. Engsberg JR, Ross SA, Collins DR, et al. Effect of selective dorsal rhizotomy in the treatment of children with cerebral palsy. J Neurosurg 2006; 105(1 Suppl):8–15.
44. Bertrand C, Molina Negro P, Martinez SN. Technical aspects of selective peripheral denervation for spasmodic torticollis. Appl Neurophysiol 1982;45(3): 326–30.
45. Bertrand CM, Molina-Negro P. Selective peripheral denervation in 111 cases of spasmodic torticollis: rationale and results. Adv Neurol 1988;50:637–43.
46. Bertrand CM. Selective peripheral denervation for spasmodic torticollis: surgical technique, results, and observations in 260 cases. Surg Neurol 1993; 40(2):96–103.
47. Ostrem JL, Starr PA. Treatment of dystonia with deep brain stimulation. Neurotherapeutics 2008;5(2): 320–30.
48. Rumalla K, Smith KA, Follett KA, et al. Rates, causes, risk factors, and outcomes of readmission following deep brain stimulation for movement disorders: analysis of the U.S. Nationwide Readmissions Database. Clin Neurol Neurosurg 2018;171:129–34.
49. Cooper IS, Upton AR. Use of chronic cerebellar stimulation for disorders of disinhibition. Lancet 1978;1(8064):595–600.
50. Mundinger F. New stereotactic treatment of spasmodic torticollis with a brain stimulation system (author's transl). Med Klin 1977;72(46):1982–6 [in German].
51. Islekel S, Zileli M, Zileli B. Unilateral pallidal stimulation in cervical dystonia. Stereotact Funct Neurosurg 1999;72(2–4):248–52.
52. Kumar R, Dagher A, Hutchison WD, et al. Globus pallidus deep brain stimulation for generalized dystonia: clinical and PET investigation. Neurology 1999;53(4):871–4.
53. Coubes P, Echenne B, Roubertie A, et al. Treatment of early-onset generalized dystonia by chronic bilateral stimulation of the internal globus pallidus. Apropos of a case. Neurochirurgie 1999;45(2): 139–44 [in French].
54. Andy OJ. Thalamic stimulation for control of movement disorders. Appl Neurophysiol 1983;46(1–4): 107–11.
55. Vercueil L, Pollak P, Fraix V, et al. Deep brain stimulation in the treatment of severe dystonia. J Neurol 2001;248(8):695–700.
56. Cury RG, Fraix V, Castrioto A, et al. Thalamic deep brain stimulation for tremor in Parkinson disease, essential tremor, and dystonia. Neurology 2017; 89(13):1416–23.
57. Silberstein P, Kuhn AA, Kupsch A, et al. Patterning of globus pallidus local field potentials differs between Parkinson's disease and dystonia. Brain 2003;126(Pt 12):2597–608.
58. Vidailhet M, Vercueil L, Houeto JL, et al. Bilateral deep-brain stimulation of the globus pallidus in primary generalized dystonia. N Engl J Med 2005; 352(5):459–67.
59. Kupsch A, Benecke R, Muller J, et al. Pallidal deep-brain stimulation in primary generalized or segmental dystonia. N Engl J Med 2006;355(19): 1978–90.
60. Katayama Y, Fukaya C, Kobayashi K, et al. Chronic stimulation of the globus pallidus internus for control of primary generalized dystonia. Acta Neurochir Suppl 2003;87:125–8.
61. Cersosimo MG, Raina GB, Piedimonte F, et al. Pallidal surgery for the treatment of primary generalized dystonia: long-term follow-up. Clin Neurol Neurosurg 2008;110(2):145–50.
62. Pinsker MO, Volkmann J, Falk D, et al. Deep brain stimulation of the internal globus pallidus in dystonia: target localisation under general anaesthesia. Acta Neurochir (Wien) 2009;151(7):751–8.
63. Alterman RL, Miravite J, Weisz D, et al. Sixty hertz pallidal deep brain stimulation for primary torsion dystonia. Neurology 2007;69(7):681–8.
64. Chou KL, Hurtig HI, Jaggi JL, et al. Bilateral subthalamic nucleus deep brain stimulation in a patient with cervical dystonia and essential tremor. Mov Disord 2005;20(3):377–80.
65. Ostrem JL, Racine CA, Glass GA, et al. Subthalamic nucleus deep brain stimulation in primary cervical dystonia. Neurology 2011;76(10):870–8.
66. Ostrem JL, San Luciano M, Dodenhoff KA, et al. Subthalamic nucleus deep brain stimulation in isolated dystonia: a 3-year follow-up study. Neurology 2017;88(1):25–35.
67. Horisawa S, Goto S, Nakajima T, et al. Bilateral stereotactic thalamotomy for bilateral musician's hand dystonia. World Neurosurg 2016;92:585.e21-25.
68. Fasano A, Bove F, Lang AE. The treatment of dystonic tremor: a systematic review. J Neurol Neurosurg Psychiatry 2014;85(7):759–69.
69. Panov F, Tagliati M, Ozelius LJ, et al. Pallidal deep brain stimulation for DYT6 dystonia. J Neurol Neurosurg Psychiatry 2012;83(2):182–7.

Spinal Cord Stimulation

Andrew K. Rock, MD, MHS[a], Huy Truong, MD[a], Yunseo Linda Park[b], Julie G. Pilitsis, MD, PhD[a,b,*]

KEYWORDS

• Spinal cord stimulation • Neuromodulation • Failed back surgery syndrome
• Complex regional pain syndromes • Pain • Review

KEY POINTS

- Randomized clinical trials for failed back surgery syndrome (FBSS), complex regional pain syndrome (CRPS), and refractory angina pectoris (RAP) suggest that SCS has successful outcomes.
- Psychological screening is paramount when determining who should be eligible for treatment with SCS.
- The patient's response to a trial period of SCS is essential for predicting outcomes and identifying who should undergo permanent SCS implantation.
- Several decisions including the type of lead, anesthesia, and waveform programming need to be considered for each patient.
- SCS has been shown to have long-term cost-effectiveness for the treatment of chronic pain when compared with alternative treatment modalities.

INTRODUCTION

Spinal cord stimulation (SCS) of the dorsal columns was first used by Shealy and colleagues[1] at Case Western Reserve University for the treatment of chronic intractable cancer pain in 1967. Premised around Melzack and Wall's gate control theory of pain, it was initially hypothesized that electrical stimulation of Aβ fiber projections within the dorsal horn would inhibit nociceptive signals conducted by small Aδ and C fibers.[2,3] This mechanism of action has been supported through observations that stimulating paresthesia coverage that overlaps with painful regions provides therapeutic relief.[4,5] However, recent investigations have established nonconventional stimulation patterns that challenge this traditional paradigm and believed mechanism of action.[6,7] Nonetheless, SCS has been well established as a safe and effective treatment of pain derived from a wide variety of etiologies. In this review, we discuss the common indications for SCS, patient selection criteria, and pertinent outcomes from randomized clinical trials (RCT) related to common indications treated with SCS.

INDICATIONS

Currently, the Food and Drug Administration has approved several SCS systems for the use in the management of chronic intractable pain of the trunk and limbs, including unilateral or bilateral pain associated with failed back surgery syndrome (FBSS), intractable low back and leg pain, complex regional pain syndrome (CRPS) type I and II, and neuropathic pain. Several governing bodies have published recommendations and guidelines pertaining to the use of SCS.[8–15] These recommendations are summarized in **Table 1**. For a wide variety of indications, there remains a paucity

Disclosure Statement: Dr J.G. Pilitsis is a consultant for Medtronic, Boston Scientific, Nevro, Jazz Pharmaceuticals, Neurobridge Therapeutics, and Abbott; receives grant support from Medtronic, Boston Scientific, Abbott, Nevro, Jazz Pharmaceuticals, GE Global Research, and NIH 1R01CA166379; and is medical advisor for Centauri and Karuna and has stock equity.
[a] Department of Neurosurgery, Albany Medical College, 43 New Scotland Avenue, Albany, NY 12208, USA; [b] Department of Neuroscience and Experimental Therapeutics, Albany Medical College, 43 New Scotland Avenue, Albany, NY 12208, USA
* Corresponding author. Albany Medical College Neurosurgery Group, 47 New Scotland Avenue, MC 10, Physicians Pavilion, 1st Floor, Albany, NY 12208.
E-mail address: jpilitsis@yahoo.com

Neurosurg Clin N Am 30 (2019) 169–194
https://doi.org/10.1016/j.nec.2018.12.003

Table 1
Summary of published guidelines on common indications for spinal cord stimulation

	FBSS	CRPS-I	CRPS-II	RAP
NICE[8]	Recommended for adults who continue to experience chronic pain (≥50 mm on 0–100 Visual Analog Scale) for ≥6 mo despite conventional medical management, and have a successful SCS trial	Recommended for adults who continue to experience chronic pain (≥50 mm on 0–100 Visual Analog Scale) for ≥6 mo despite conventional medical management, and have a successful SCS trial	Recommended for adults who continue to experience chronic pain (≥50 mm on 0–100 Visual Analog Scale) for ≥6 mo despite conventional medical management, and have a successful SCS trial	
BPS[9]	Clinical evidence supports SCS in pain from FBSS	Clinical evidence supports SCS in pain from CRPS-I	Clinical evidence supports SCS in pain from CRPS-II	
Dutch Society of Rehabilitation Specialists and Anaesthesiologists[10]		Level 3; SCS administered to CRPS-I patients who are carefully selected and undergo successful trial stimulation causes long-term pain reduction and improves quality of life, but does not improve function		
NeuPSIG[11]	Evidence quality, good; certainty, moderate; strength of recommendation, grade B	Evidence quality, good; certainty, moderate; strength of recommendation, grade B	Evidence quality, good; certainty, moderate; strength of recommendation, grade B	
NeuPSIG[12]	Evidence quality, moderate; strength of recommendation, weak; comments, seems better than reoperation and conventional medical management based on two RCTs, but low response rate and high complication rate	Evidence quality, moderate; strength of recommendation, weak; comments, long-term benefit demonstrated, 5-y reoperation rate for complications (42%), but 95% of patients would undergo implantation again for same result		

NACC[13]		Recommends SCS for the treatment of CRPS-I and CRPS-II with pain $\geq$3-mo duration or severe, rapidly progressing disease not responding to more conservative measures, but only after informed consent, psychological evaluation, and a successful trial have been performed	SCS recommended as evidence level 2a, degree of recommendation A Based on accumulated evidence, SCS for angina is accepted in the European Society of Cardiology and American Heart Association/ American College of Cardiology guidelines
Netherlands Society of Anaesthesiologists and Rehabilitation Specialists[14]		Level 3; there is evidence that spinal cord stimulation administered to CRPS-I patients who are carefully selected and undergo successful trial stimulation causes long-term pain reduction and improves quality of life, but does not improve function	
EFNS[15]	Weak recommendation as an alternative to reoperation, low or moderate quality of evidence	Weak recommendation as an addition to conventional medical management vs conventional management alone	

Evidence-based guidelines and recommendations on indications for SCS over the past 10 years.
Abbreviations: BPS, British Pain Society; EFNS, European Federation of Neurologic Societies; NACC, Neurostimulation Appropriateness Consensus Committee; NeuSIG, Canadian Pain Society Special Interest Group on Neuropathic Pain; NICE, National Institute for Health and Care Excellence; RAP, refractory angina pectoris.

of quality evidence to support or refute the utility of SCS as an adjunct or alternative to conventional medical management (CMM) strategies. Most evidence supports the use of SCS for the treatment of FBSS, CRPS, and refractory angina pectoris (RAP). Therefore, these indications are the primary focus for discussion in this review.

Failed Back Surgery Syndrome

Table 2 summarizes studies related to SCS treatment of FBSS. FBSS is a condition where patients experience recurring low back pain following prior spinal surgery. Approximately 10% to 30% of patients experience postoperative low back pain, and SCS has been found to successfully treat this pain with a low morbidity rate compared with reoperation.[16] In a case series with long-term follow-up, North and colleagues[17] reported promising results of SCS therapy for FBSS patients, with success rates of 53% to 60% at 2.2 years and 47% to 54% at 5 years. The results were later replicated by LeDoux and Langford[18] within a series of 32 patients with FBSS, in which 82% and 74% patients had good results at 6-month and 2-year time points, respectively. These results prompted more definitive studies. In a RCT, North and colleagues[16,19] randomized 51 FBSS patients to SCS or reoperation. Clinical improvement and treatment satisfaction, indicated by the desire to crossover to the other randomized treatment, were reported and analyzed. The initial results at 6-month follow-up[19] and later on with 3-year average follow-up[16] both confirmed SCS to be more satisfactory than reoperation in terms of self-reported pain relief and the crossover rate. In a multicenter RCT for patients with FBSS (n = 100), Kumar and colleagues[20] demonstrated SCS to be more effective than conservative medical management (CMM) at improving pain relief, quality of life (QoL), and functional capacity at 1-year follow-up. These benefits were sustained at 2-year follow-up.[21] QoL also seemed to markedly improve when patients were randomized to SCS as compared with CMM.[22]

In recent years, new waveforms, including burst and high-frequency stimulation, have been introduced. Burst stimulation, which delivers five spikes at 500 Hz 40 times per second, has been found to suppress pain and tonic stimulation, but without evoking paresthesia. Initial results in 48 patients who were on tonic stimulation and switched to burst stimulation showed improved pain relief with minimal to no paresthesias in 60% of patients.[23] The SUNBURST trial compared burst stimulation and traditional tonic stimulation in a randomized crossover trial.[24] Patients had greater improvement on Visual Analog Scale (VAS) for pain with burst SCS when compared to tonic SCS; with most patients preferring burst SCS (70.8%). This preference was maintained at 1-year follow-up. Similarly, 10-kHz high-frequency (HF10) therapy has shown promise. In the SENZA-RCT, 171 SCS-naive patients were randomized to tonic versus HF10 stimulation therapy. There were significantly more responders (defined as 50% pain relief) in the HF10 group as compared with tonic SCS.[25] The benefit was maintained at 2-year follow-up.[26]

Complex Regional Pain Syndrome

Table 3 summarizes studies related to SCS treatment of CRPS. CRPS is a form of chronic pain, usually affecting a single limb, which typically arises after sustaining injury or having surgery. Patients with CRPS experience extreme burning pain with greater sensitivity to acute pain. According to the Budapest classification, patients with CRPS exhibit lower thresholds for pain perception in response to hot and/or cold stimuli. Other diagnostic criteria include: hyperesthesia, allodynia, temperature asymmetry, skin color changes, edema, decreased range of motion, and trophic changes.[27] After early case series showed positive benefits of SCS for CRPS,[28] Kemler and colleagues[29] provided level I evidence on the topic with a well-designed single-center RCT comparing SCS plus physical therapy (PT) with PT alone for patients with CRPS who were unresponsive to at least 6 months of conventional treatment. At 6-month follow-up, SCS was successful in 56% of patients, with a 3.6-point improvement in VAS and improvement in QoL. The benefits were sustained at 2 years with an average VAS improvement of three points compared with no change in the group receiving PT alone. Furthermore, 63% of the SCS group reported "much improvement" as compared with only 6% within the group with PT alone. Complications were reported in 38% of patients, which included lead and generator pocket revision, lead replacement, generator replacement, and explantation.[30] Despite the risk of complications, 95% of patients stated they would repeat the procedure again for the same outcome when asked at 5-year follow-up.[31]

Refractory Angina Pectoris

Table 4 summarizes studies related to SCS treatment of RAP. RAP is anginal pain commonly caused by coronary artery disease that does not respond to antianginal medications. Patients tend to experience episodes of heavy, pressure-like chest pain. SCS has been proposed as a treatment of anginal pain when it becomes refractory to

Table 2
Level of evidence of studies related to spinal cord stimulation treatment of failed back surgery syndrome

First Author, Year	Study Design	Exposures	Primary Outcomes	Key Findings	Level of Evidence
Schu et al,[79] 2014	Double-blinded, crossover RCT; n = 20	Tonic vs burst vs placebo	Pain intensity	Burst stimulation had significantly lower pain scores compared with tonic and placebo stimulation	I
North et al,[19] 1994	Prospective RCT; n = 27	SCS vs reoperation	Frequency of crossover	6-mo crossover point showed significant advantage for SCS over reoperation	I
North et al,[16] 2005	Prospective RCT; n = 45	SCS vs reoperation	Frequency of crossover	SCS was more successful than reoperation with patients initially randomized to SCS less likely to crossover	I
Manca et al,[22] 2008	RCT; n = 100	SCS plus CMM vs CMM alone	Health resource utilization; QoL; costs; clinical outcomes	SCS had significantly higher costs and greater improvement in QoL when compared with CMM alone	I
Kumar et al,[20] 2007	RCT; n = 100	SCS plus CMM vs CMM alone	50% pain relief	Compared with CMM alone, SCS improved pain relief, QoL, functional capacity, and patient satisfaction in a greater number of patients than CMM alone	I
Kumar et al,[21] 2008	RCT; n = 100	SCS plus CMM vs CMM alone	Pain relief; functional capacity; QoL; satisfaction	At 24 mo, SCS had significantly higher pain relief, functional capacity, QoL, and satisfaction than CMM alone	I
van Gorp et al,[81] 2016	RCT; n = 97	SCS plus subcutaneous stimulation vs SCS alone	VAS scores	Percentage of patients with pain relief were significantly higher when subcutaneous stimulation was added on in addition to SCS	I
Kinfe et al,[88] 2014	Nonrandomized, single-center trial; n = 100	Paddle vs cylindrical SCS leads	VAS scores; ODI	Similar pain relief (69%) was observed for both groups, but there was higher dislocation and infection rate in the cylindrical group	II-1

(*continued on next page*)

Table 2
(continued)

First Author, Year	Study Design	Exposures	Primary Outcomes	Key Findings	Level of Evidence
Sweet et al,[89] 2016	Randomized crossover trial; n = 15	Conventional vs subthreshold high-density vs sham	50% pain relief	Subthreshold SCS had significantly greater improvement in pain relief compared with conventional SCS, but not sham	II-1
Turner et al,[93] 2010	Prospective, population-based controlled cohort study; n = 168	SCS vs pain clinic vs CMM	Pain; function; medication use; work status	SCS group did not differ in outcomes at 12 or 24 mo compared with other intervention groups	II-1
Choi et al,[83] 2017	Case control observational study; n = 21	3-column vs 5-column stimulation	VAS score; pain relief; CT assessment of T9 canal area	No difference in paresthesia area, trial success rate, clinical outcomes, or percent pain relief between the two groups; contact area was greater for 5-column stimulation	II-2
Zucco et al,[80] 2015	Observational, multicenter, longitudinal ambispective study; n = 80	Pre- vs post-SCS	Pain status; QoL; direct and indirect costs	SCS improved clinical outcomes and QoL; societal costs increased from €6600 to €13,200 per patient per year; SCS would be cost-effective in 80%–85% of cases	II-3
Rigoard et al,[82] 2015	Prospective, nonrandomized observational study; n = 76	Multicolumn stimulation	Paresthesia coverage; VAS scores	At 6 mo, 75.4% and 42.1% of patients had at least a 30% and 50% improvement of VAS scores, respectively	III
Remacle et al,[84] 2017	Prospective observational study; n = 29	Multicolumn SCS	VAS scores; ADLs	Multicolumn SCS had greater improvement in pain relief, quality of sleep, and decreased analgesic medication use during the follow-up period	III
Paul et al,[85] 2017	Prospective observational study; n = 48	SCS	ODI; BDI; McGill pain score; VAS scores	Minimal clinically important difference for SCS placement could be calculated using each of the different outcome measures	III

North et al,[17] 1991	Retrospective study; n = 50	SCS	50% pain relief; ADL	53% and 47% of patients had successful pain relief at 2.2 and 5.0 y, respectively	III
Logé et al,[86] 2013	Prospective observational study; n = 21	Small profile plate-type SCS electrode	VAS scores	With mean follow-up of 40.8 mo, a significant mean reduction was seen at follow-up visits	III
Avellanal et al,[87] 2014	Prospective observational study; n = 133	Algorithm including surgical management for severe FBSS	50% pain relief	The proposed algorithm was effective with 9.84% of patients receiving palliative SCS	III
Vonhogen et al,[90] 2011	Retrospective review; n = 20	Percutaneous plate SCS electrodes	VAS scores	Significant reduction of 55% and 45.7% in leg and back pain, respectively	III
Tomycz et al,[91] 2010	Retrospective; n = 11	Nonsimultaneous surgical implantation of intrathecal opioid pump and SCS	QoL; pain control; ADL	All patients (100%) believed that the dual placement had improved their QoL and continued use for pain control	III
Reverberi et al,[92] 2013	Prospective observational study; n = 8	SCS plus peripheral nerve stimulation	VAS scores; BDI; McGill score; ODI; QoL	At 1-y follow-up, all outcomes of interest showed significant improvement	III
LeDoux and Langford,[18] 1993	Prospective observational study; n = 32	SCS	50% pain relief	67% of patients at 1 y and 74% at 2 y had 50% or better pain relief	III
Devulder et al,[94] 1997	Cross-sectional study; n = 69	SCS	Long-term results and cost-effectiveness	26 patients stopped SCS, whereas 43 patients continued SCS with good relief; SCS cost on average $3660 per patient per year	III
Lad et al,[95] 2014	Retrospective review; n = 16,455	SCS vs reoperation	Health care resource use	2.4% of patients underwent SCS; complications, hospital stay, and associated charges were significantly lower for SCS compared with reoperation	III

Summary of key findings on studies related to spinal cord stimulation for the treatment of failed back surgery syndrome.

Abbreviations: ADL, activities of daily living; BDI, Beck Depression Inventory; CT, computed tomography; ODI, Oswestry Disability Index; QoL, quality of life; VAS, Visual Analog Scale for pain.

Table 3
Level of evidence of studies related to spinal cord stimulation for treatment of complex regional pain syndrome

First Author, Year	Study Design	Exposures	Primary Outcomes	Key Findings	Level of Evidence
Kriek et al,[96] 2015	Double-blind crossover RCT; n = 0	Five SCS frequencies: 40 Hz, 500 Hz, 1200 Hz, burst, placebo	Pain relief; satisfaction	No data reported yet	N/A
Deer et al,[97] 2017	Prospective, multicenter, randomized comparative effectiveness trial; n = 152	DRG stimulation vs SCS	Composite safety and efficacy	DRG had greater improvement in pain relief, QoL, and psychological disposition when compared with SCS	I
Kemler et al,[31] 2008	RCT; n = 36	SCS plus PT vs PT alone	Pain intensity; global perceived effect; satisfaction; QoL	At 5-y follow-up, SCS plus PT had similar results for pain relief and all other measured variables compared with PT alone	I
Kemler et al,[98] 2001	RCT; n = 54	SCS plus PT vs PT alone	Temperature and pain detection thresholds	SCS showed no effect on detection thresholds after 3 mo	I
Kemler et al,[29] 2000	RCT; n = 54	SCS plus PT vs PT alone	Pain intensity; global perceived effect; satisfaction; QoL	SCS plus PT had significantly higher improvement in pain reduction and QoL at 6 mo compared with PT alone	I
Kemler et al,[30] 2004	RCT; n = 54	SCS plus PT vs PT alone	Pain intensity; global perceived effect; satisfaction; QoL	SCS plus PT had significantly higher improvement in pain intensity, global perceived effect, and QoL at 24 mo compared with PT alone	I
Geurts et al,[101] 2013	Prospective cohort study; n = 84	SCS	VAS score; Patients Global Impressions of Change Scale	During 11 y, 41% of patients had 30% pain reduction During 12 y, 63% of patients still used their devices Pain relief of 50% at 1 wk predicted long-term success	II-2
van Eijs et al,[102] 2012	Prospective study; n = 74	SCS	Pain; QoL; function	Mean pain relief at 1 y was 35% with improvements on mental, but not physical or functional QoL	II-2
Sears et al,[99] 2011	Cross-sectional study; n = 35	SCS	Pain relief; satisfaction	More than 50% of patients with CRPS reported >50% pain relief at 4.4 y of follow-up, but 77.8% reported they would undergo the procedure again	III

Goto et al,[100] 2013	Retrospective review; n = 5	SCS plus intrathecal baclofen	VAS scores	Combined SCS plus baclofen neuromodulation decreased pain intensity in refractory CRPS and improves abnormal dystonic posture, movement disorders, and pain fluctuations	III
Forouzanfar et al,[103] 2004	Prospective observational study; n = 36	SCS	Pain intensity; Global Perceived Effect; QoL	Pain relief was reduced at 6 mo, 1 and 2 y, but 42% of cervical and 47% of lumbar patients reported "much improvement"; complications occurred in 64% of patients	III
Harke et al,[104] 2005	Prospective trial; n = 29	SCS	Deep pain; allodynia; functional disability	SCS permanently relieved deep pain and allodynia and restored ADLs	III
Kumar et al,[105] 2011	Retrospective review; n = 25	SCS	VAS scores; ODI; BDI; QoL	At 88-mo follow-up, there were ongoing improvements in all outcomes of interest when compared with baseline	III
Kumar et al,[106] 1997	Retrospective review; n = 12	SCS	Case review	At 41 mo, all patients used their stimulators regularly and only 2 received adjunctive minor pain medication	III
Barolat et al,[28] 1989	Prospective observational study; n = 18	SCS	Clinical outcomes	In the implanted group, pain relief was absent in 3 patients, minimal in 1, moderate in 5, and good in 6	III

Summary of key findings on studies related to spinal cord stimulation for the treatment of complex regional pain syndrome.

Abbreviations: ADL, activities of daily living; BDI, Beck Depression Inventory; DRG, dorsal root ganglia; N/A, not applicable; ODI, Oswestry Disability Index; PT, physical therapy.

Table 4
Level of evidence for studies related to spinal cord stimulation for the treatment of angina pectoris

First Author, Year	Study Design	Exposures	Primary Outcomes	Key Findings	Level of Evidence
McNab et al,[107] 2006	Open-label, single-center RCT; n = 68	SCS vs percutaneous myocardial laser revascularization	Exercise treadmill time; CCS class; QoL	No difference in angina-free exercise capacity, CCS class, and quality of life between treatments	I
Lanza et al,[108] 2005	Randomized crossover trial; n = 10	Continued vs withdrawal of SCS	Angina symptoms; QoL; VAS scores; 24-h Holter monitoring; dobutamine stress echocardiography	SCS reduced number, duration, and severity of angina episodes, nitrate consumption, improved QoL and VAS scores; and decreased number of ST-segment depressions and time to angina	I
DeJongste et al,[34] 1994	Prospective RCT; n = 17	SCS within 2 wk vs delayed SCS at 8 wk for intractable angina	Treadmill exercise testing; QoL; angina attacks	Spinal cord stimulation significantly improves exercise capacity and QoL by increasing exercise capacity and rate-pressure product	I
Mannheimer et al,[36] 1998	RCT; n = 104	SCS vs CABG	Symptoms; exercise capacity; ECG changes; mortality; cardiovascular morbidity	CABG had increased exercise capacity, less ST-segment depression, comparable workloads, and increased rate-pressure product; both groups had adequate symptom relief; mortality rate was lower in the SCS group	I
Lanza et al,[109] 2011	Multicenter, single-blind RCT; n = 25	SCS: paresthesia vs subliminal vs sham	Angina episodes; nitrate use; angina class; QoL	Paresthesia, but not subliminal SCS, was superior to sham SCS for improving outcomes	I
DeJongste et al,[34] 1994	RCT; n = 25	SCS vs control	Exercise capacity; angina attacks; nitrate use; QoL	Compared with control subjects, exercise duration and time to angina increased, angina attacks and nitrate use decreased, and ischemic episodes and ST-segment depression decreased when treated with SCS	I

Zipes et al,[110] 2012	Multicenter, single-blind RCT; n = 68	SCS: high vs low stimulation vs baseline	Anginal attacks; major cardiac events	Early termination based on futility analysis; high stimulation was not significantly different from low stimulation at 6 mo	I
Eddicks et al,[111] 2007	Placebo-controlled RCT; n = 12	SCS: 3 × 2-h conventional vs 24-h conventional vs 3 × 2-h subthreshold vs 24-h 0.1-V output	Functional status; QoL; CCS class; nitrate use	Improvement in functional status and symptoms was revealed in phases with conventional or subthreshold stimulation when compared with low-output placebo stimulation	I
Bondesson et al,[112] 2008	Nonrandomized clinical trial; n = 153	EECP vs SCS vs CMM	Glyceryl trinitrate use, CCS classification	EECP and SCS reduce angina in patients with RAP; EECP was slightly more effective than SCS	II-1
Anselmino et al,[113] 2009	Randomized self-controlled crossover trial; n = 8	SCS: paresthesia (on) vs subliminal vs off	30-min heart rate variability recordings	Stimulation resulted in a median 52% (33%–65%) reduction of the sympathetic activity compared when not stimulated; no difference between on and subliminal responses	II-2
Andrell et al,[114] 2010	Prospective study; n = 121	SCS vs CMM	Angina symptoms; QoL; cardiac events; mortality	SCS is associated with symptom relief and improved QoL	II-2
Sgueglia et al,[115] 2007	Prospective controlled trial; n = 30	SCS vs CMM	Angina symptoms; QoL; cardiac stress testing	SCS had long-term efficacy for angina symptoms, QoL and stress test performance	II-2
Di Pede et al,[116] 2003	Prospective registry; n = 104	SCS	Angina attacks; nitrate use; CCS class	SCS is performed safely and is associated with a sustained improvement in symptoms of angina	II-3
Lapenna et al,[117] 2006	Prospective observational study; n = 51	SCS	Angina symptoms; QoL; CCS class; mortality	SCS improved angina symptoms (82%), QoL, CCS class, number of angina attacks, and 3-y survival rate in RAP	II-3

(*continued on next page*)

Table 4
(*continued*)

First Author, Year	Study Design	Exposures	Primary Outcomes	Key Findings	Level of Evidence
TenVaarwerk et al,[118] 1999	Retrospective series	SCS	Cardiovascular mortality and function	Clinical outcomes of patients with intractable angina is not adversely affected by the chronic use of neurostimulation	III
Andersen et al,[119] 1994	Prospective observational study; n = 50	SCS	Necropsy findings; symptoms; serum enzymes; ECG changes	There was no evidence that SCS concealed acute myocardial infarction	III
Hautvast et al,[120] 1998	Prospective observational study; n = 19	SCS	Heart rate variability	No significant changes in heart rate variability were detected with SCS	III
Hautvast et al,[121] 1996	Prospective observational study; n = 9	SCS	Regional myocardial blood flow; frequency of attacks; nitrate use	Despite clinical improvement at 6 wk, there was no significant change in coronary blood flow from SCS	III
Saraste et al,[122] 2015	Prospective observational study; n = 18	SCS	Dobutamine stress echocardiography	Short-term SCS improved myocardial ischemia tolerance, absolute MPR, and endothelium-mediated vasomotor function in RAP	III
Mannheimer et al,[32] 1993	Prospective observational study; n = 20	SCS	Response to atrial pacing	SCS had antianginal and anti-ischemic effects on severe CAD caused by decreased myocardial oxygen consumption	III
DeJongste et al,[123] 1994	Prospective self-controlled trial; n = 10	SCS	Ambulatory ECG	SCS reduced symptoms and signs of myocardial ischemia on ECG	III
Ekre et al,[124] 2003	Prospective observation study; n = 18	SCS in cardiac permanent pacemaker use	Continuous ECG monitoring; serious events	SCS is safely combined with cardiac permanent pacemakers for RAP	III
Bagger et al,[125] 1998	Prospective observational study; n = 10	SCS	Atrial pacing	Long-term clinical benefits were seen in 57% of patients	III

Jitta et al,[126] 2011	Retrospective study; n = 127	SCS	Predictors of QoL	Female gender, COPD, DM, and obesity adversely influence the effect of SCS on RAP	III
Eliasson et al,[33] 1994	Prospective observational study; n = 19	SCS	Repeated long-term ECG recordings	SCS did not increase the frequency or severity of myocardial ischemia in severe CAD	III
Jessurun et al,[127] 1997	Retrospective study; n = 57	SCS	Efficacy; adverse events; mortality	Mortality of patients with SCS is similar to that of patients with CAD and stable angina pectoris	III
Sestito et al,[128] 2008	Randomized crossover trial; n = 16	SCS: on vs off	Laser evoked potentials	SCS re-establishes normal habituation to cutaneous painful stimuli in cardiac syndrome X	III
Murray et al,[129] 1999	Retrospective case review; n = 19	Baseline vs revascularization vs SCS time periods	Readmission rate	Annual admission rate was 0.97/patient/y after revascularization and 0.27/patient/y after SCS; SCS is effective without masking ischemic symptoms	III
De Vries et al,[130] 2007	Prospective trial; n = 36	Baseline vs TENS vs SCS	QoL; antianginal effects	Neurostimulation with TENS or SCS had widespread value for treating RAP	III
Chua and Keogh,[131] 2005	Prospective observational study; n = 11	SCS	Subjective symptoms	Spinal cord stimulation improves 6-min-walk distance, exercise duration, New York Heart Association functional class, Likert score, and number of angina-free days per wk for at least 1 y over 2 y of follow-up	III

Summary of key findings on studies related to spinal cord stimulation for the treatment of angina pectoris.

Abbreviations: CABG, coronary artery bypass surgery; CAD, coronary artery disease; CCS, Canadian Cardiovascular Society classification; COPD, chronic obstructive pulmonary disease; DM, diabetes mellitus; ECG, electrocardiography; EECP, enhanced external counterpulsation; MPR, myocardial perfusion reserve; TENS, transcutaneous electrical nerve stimulation.

medical therapy. Initial concerns arose that SCS may mask the signs of myocardial ischemia, but early case series demonstrated antianginal effects without an increased risk for ischemia.[32,33] Notably, a small RCT (n = 17) demonstrated improved performance on cardiac treadmill stress testing and reduced nitrate intake among those treated with SCS.[34] Similar results were observed in other RCTs and case series that followed.[35] In a larger scale RCT (n = 100) by Mannheimer and colleagues,[36] SCS was compared with coronary artery bypass surgery for the treatment of RAP. Patients who received coronary artery bypass surgery performed significantly better on exercise tolerance testing, but both groups experienced adequate symptom relief with no significant difference between the two cohorts.

Table 5 summarizes studies related to SCS treatment of peripheral vascular disease and critical limb ischemia. The use of SCS for the treatment of critical limb ischemia has mixed evidence within the literature. Case series and case control studies report promising clinical outcomes with pain relief and the promotion of wound healing when SCS was added to the standard medical treatment.[37–43] However, RCTs have had less robust results with only one out of three RCTs suggesting improved pain relief with SCS.[44–46]

PATIENT SELECTION

Patient selection is critical for promoting positive outcomes following SCS. Other treatment modalities, such as medication, steroid injections, and/or PT, should be pursued before proposing the possibility of SCS. Then, several factors need to be considered before pursuing SCS, including: psychiatric comorbidities, MRI eligibility, preoperative surgical risk, and expected response to a trial of SCS. If patients are ineligible to receive MRI, they need to be followed with computed tomography or computed tomography myelography. From a surgical perspective, general contraindications include uncontrolled bleeding disorders, sepsis, cognitive impairments, unresolved psychological disorders, and/or substance use disorders. In particular, tobacco use has been associated with early SCS failure.[47] The importance of tobacco use cessation should be emphasized with each patient and urine drug and ethanol screening should be performed to better optimize other comorbidities preoperatively.

Evaluation and treatment of comorbid mental health conditions is an important step before a trial of SCS, because chronic pain can severely affect each patients' QoL, interpersonal relationships, and activities of daily living. Establishing effective coping skills helps improve outcomes following SCS surgery.[48] For emphasis, patients should expect an upfront goal not to relieve all pain, but to decrease it by 50%. Thorough preoperative psychiatric evaluations can help identify underlying untreated depression, anxiety, personality, substance use, or post traumatic stress disorders that may need further clinical management. Prior studies have demonstrated that 63% and 23% of patients may exhibit symptoms of depression or anxiety, respectively.[49] These rates are higher than the general population, indicating the importance of pre-SCS psychological screening. Instruments that have demonstrated efficacy in the diagnosis and treatment of comorbid mental health conditions in SCS include the Beck Depression Inventory, Pain Catastrophizing Scale, and the Minnesota Multiphasic Personality Inventory.[50,51]

TRIALING

One of the benefits of SCS is the opportunity for patients to pursue a trial period with a temporary device before permanent implantation. This allows the clinician and patient to gauge the potential benefits that may be achieved on permanent implantation. Typically, a 5- to 7-day trial period is recommended for all patients, during which clinicians follow-up closely. If initial pain relief is limited, patients should follow-up in the outpatient setting for a radiographic evaluation and/or potential device reprogramming. At the end of the trial, patients decide whether their pain, QoL, and/or functionality improved by at least 50% and whether they want to pursue permanent implantation. Common instruments to assess the response to SCS trials include the VAS, McGill Pain Questionnaire, and Oswestry Disability Index. These subjective and objective instruments help patients in making a decisive decision about their long-term management with SCS. If they remain indecisive, the trial period is extended or programming parameters adjusted for more informed decision-making.

During a trial, it is important to obtain radiographic imaging of lead placement as a way to guide permanent implantation. Imaging should extend from the bottommost rib and have clear identification of each vertebral body and the laterality clearly designated. It is then necessary to obtain data on the location of stimulation on each lead in reference to these landmarks and areas of perceived clinical benefit. For instance, if the "sweet spot" of the lead is at the top of the lead, the lead is placed higher during permanent placement than in the trial so that the "sweet spot" is in the middle (**Fig. 1**). Optimal lead positioning plays a crucial role in postoperative pain relief. Lead

Table 5
Level of evidence of studies related to spinal cord stimulation treatment of peripheral vascular disease and critical limb ischemia

First Author, Year	Study Design	Exposures	Primary Outcomes	Key Findings	Level of Evidence
Jivegard et al,[44] 1995	Prospective RCT; n = 51	SCS	Limb salvage and amount of tissue loss at 18 mo; pain relief	SCS provided long-term pain relief but limb not salvage at 18 mo	I
Ubbink et al,[45] 1999	Multicenter RCT; n = 120	SCS plus CMM vs CMM alone	Measures of microcirculation	For intermediate skin microcirculation amputation, frequency was twice as low for SCS plus CMM when compared with CMM alone	I
Spincemaille et al,[46] 2000	Multicenter RCT; n = 120	SCS plus CMM vs CMM alone	VAS scores; McGill pain score; analgesic use; QoL	Pain relief was considerable for both groups; SCS had fewer nonnarcotic and narcotic drug use	I
Klomp et al,[132] 1999	RCT; n = 120	SCS plus CMM vs CMM alone	Mortality; amputation	No significant difference between groups for all outcomes	I
Amann et al,[135] 2003	Prospective, controlled, multicenter study; n = 112	SCS vs SCS-no-match vs non-SCS	$TcPo_2$; limb survival	Cumulative limb survival of patients treated with SCS was significantly better than that of patients not treated with SCS	II-1
Kumar et al,[42] 1997	Prospective study; n = 46	SCS	Macrocirculation and microcirculation	SCS was successful in 77% of patients with significantly higher foot $TcPo_2$ and pulse volume recording	II-2
Tshomba et al,[134] 2014	Retrospective review; n = 101	SCS	Predictors of treatment success	Reduced delay between the onset of ulcer and SCS was associated with improved QoL and walking distance	II-3
Robaina et al,[39] 1989	Retrospective review; n = 11	SCS	VAS scores	Good or excellent results were reported in 90.9% cases	II-3

(*continued on next page*)

Table 5
(*continued*)

First Author, Year	Study Design	Exposures	Primary Outcomes	Key Findings	Level of Evidence
Mingoli et al,[41] 1993	Retrospective review; n = 76	SCS	Pain control; walking distance; lesion healing	Overall limb salvage rate was 42%; pain control was obtained in 80% of patients at the 1-y and 75% at the 2-y follow-up	III
Augustinsson,[37] 1987	Case series; n = 34	SCS	Pain relief; lesion healing	32/34 patients experienced some pain relief and 12/24 patients showed healing of ischemic ulcers	III
Claeys,[133] 1997	Retrospective review; n = 169	SCS	Microcirculatory blood flow	At 31.2 mo, major pain relief was noticed in patients who retained their limbs; clinical improvement was confirmed with increased $TcPo_2$	III
Bracale et al,[38] 1989	Case series	SCS	Pain relief; lesion healing	Pain relief in more than 70% and healing of ischemic lesions in 32%	III
Sampere et al,[40] 1989	Case series	SCS	Pain relief; lesion healing	SCS was beneficial in 70.6% of cases	III
Broseta et al,[43] 1986	Case series	SCS	Pain, walking distance; blood flow; lesion changes	Pain relief was obtained in 73%; 15/33 improved claudication; 12/23 and 13/23 improve on Doppler and skin temperature, respectively	III
De Caridi et al,[136] 2016	Case series	SCS	Lesion healing; $TcPo_2$	$TcPo_2$ and wound healing were improved with SCS	III
Colini et al,[137] 2011	Prospective observational study; n = 40	SCS	Change in $TcPo_2$ and $TcPco_2$	After 1 mo of SCS, there was improvement in metabolic parameters and greater percentage of open capillaries	III

Summary of studies related to spinal cord stimulation treatment of peripheral vascular disease and critical limb ischemia.

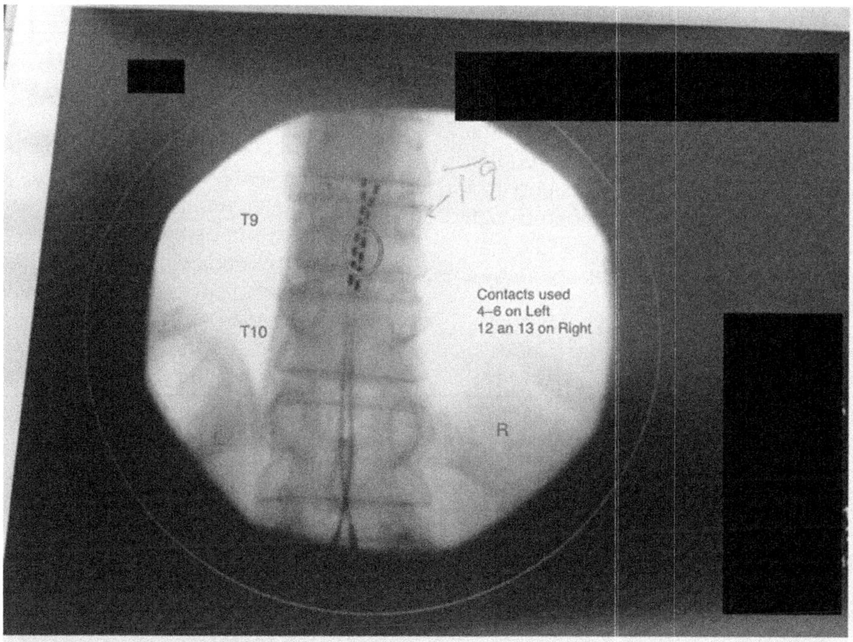

Fig. 1. If the "sweet spot" of the lead is at the top of the lead, the lead is placed higher during permanent placement than in the trial so that the "sweet spot" is in the middle.

location for back and leg coverage varies among devices and varying waveforms, thus trial periods are a good way to ascertain vital information on expected efficacy. In the case of HF10, the leads should always be placed for coverage over the T9-10 regions. For arm and neck pain, we typically place cervical leads either with a retrograde paddle from occiput to C3 or one/two leads depending on symptoms in a "blooming flower" configuration up to C1-2. Details on these procedures have been previously described by Haider and colleagues.[52] Lastly, leads for managing RAP should typically cover the T4-6 region.

TECHNICAL CONSIDERATIONS

Once a patient undergoes a successful SCS trial, several decisions must be made: (1) should patients undergo percutaneous or paddle implantation, (2) are there any technical nuances that must be considered, (3) should the procedure be performed asleep or awake, and (4) what waveform should be used? The patients' trial data, their overall health, surgeon comfort, and local expertise or resources are factors that play a role in making these decisions. However, there is often not a single "right or wrong" decision to be made.

Lead Type

Experiences with percutaneous and paddle implants are well documented in the literature. Although both are excellent options, the choice of one type of lead over another depends on the expertise, work flow, and practical issues. Percutaneous leads involve a less invasive procedure and are less likely to result in postoperative complications (2.2% compared with 3.4% in patients with paddle leads).[53] For patients with multiple comorbidities, percutaneous leads may be a better choice. Although paddle leads require a more invasive surgery through hemilaminotomy, satisfaction and pain relief may be higher.[54] Similar rates of lead migration have been described for each type of lead, but migration tends to be less extreme for paddle implants.[55] Lastly, the contacts of paddle implants all face the epidural space, which allows for more effective energy delivery.[56] A recent study suggested that minimally invasive surgery techniques is feasible for placement of SCS with possible advantage.[57]

Asleep Versus Awake

Although trial implants are generally performed under local anesthesia, permanent implants may either be performed awake or asleep with intraoperative neuromonitoring. The decision usually depends on the type of lead being implanted and the workflow of the surgeon and their team. Both modalities involve direct feedback from the patient, electromyography, and/or somatosensory evoked potentials with intraoperative neuromonitoring.

Difficulties for awake implantation may arise when paddle leads are being implanted or when the patient is anxious, obese, or has a history of obstructive sleep apnea.[58] In some cases, waking up the patient intraoperatively places extra stress on the surgeon and/or anesthesiologist. Reports suggest that placement while the patient is asleep has similar or superior outcomes as compared with awake placement.[58–62] Occasionally, paddle lead placement may also be offered under epidural or spinal anesthesia.[63,64]

Waveforms

Results from major RCTs related to types of waveform patterns used for SCS are presented in **Table 6**. Over the past 10 years, alternative waveforms have become the most dynamic part in SCS. Traditional systems deliver continuous stimulation at low frequency around 50 Hz and provide pain relief together with paresthesia. Successful stimulation was explained by gate control theory of pain and guided practice toward stimulation-induced paresthesia that overlaps with the painful region.

Table 6
Results from randomized controlled trials of various waveforms for spinal cord stimulation

First Author, Year	Exposures	Diagnosis	Main Findings
Yearwood et al,[138] 2010	Wide range (50–1000 μs); n = 19	Neuropathy/ radiculopathy; CRPS	7/19 patients selected new pulse width programming and achieved significantly increased paresthesia-pain overlap
Perruchoud et al,[139] 2013	High vs sham; n = 33	Chronic low back pain	High frequency was equivalent to sham for improvement of pain and QoL outcomes
Washburn et al,[140] 2014	Constant current vs constant voltage; n = 30	FBSS; radiculopathies; CRPS	More patients preferred constant voltage, which produced larger decrease in pain scores
Van Havenbergh et al,[141] 2015	500 Hz vs 1000 Hz; n = 15	FBSS; radiculopathies; CRPS	No significant difference between two modes of stimulation
North et al,[6] 2016	Supraperception vs subperception; n = 22	Chronic pain	Subperception provided greater pain relief than paresthesia-based SCS at lower frequencies, suggesting that 1-kHz subperception stimulation is an effective alternative
Kapural et al,[26] 2016	HF10 therapy vs traditional low-frequency; n = 179	Chronic intractable pain of the trunk or limbs	HF10 therapy exhibits a long-term superiority to traditional SCS in treating back and leg pain
Tjepkema-Cloostermans et al,[142] 2016	Burst vs tonic; n = 40	Neuropathic pain in lower limbs	Burst stimulation was more effective than tonic, but therapeutic range of amplitudes requires individual assessment
Kriek et al,[143] 2017	Standard 40 Hz vs 500 Hz vs 1200 Hz vs burst vs placebo; n = 29	CRPS	Pain reduction was found in all settings compared with placebo but the 4 settings did not differ from each other
Kinfe et al,[144] 2016	Burst vs HF10; n = 16	FBSS	6/8 HF10 and 8/8 burst patients experienced significant back pain reduction; both were safe and effective in treating intractable FBSS patients
Deer et al,[24] 2018	Tonic vs burst; n = 100	FBSS; radiculopathies	70.8% of the subjects preferred burst over tonic; burst provided superior pain relief compared with tonic

Summary of results from randomized clinical trials that compared differing waveforms for spinal cord stimulation.

Table 7
Level of evidence for studies related to adjuvant therapies to spinal cord stimulation

First Author, Year	Study Design	Exposures	Primary Outcomes	Key Findings	Level of Evidence
Lind et al,[70] 2004	Nonrandomized trial	SCS with baclofen vs SCS alone	Pain rating; ADL improvement; global satisfaction	Intrathecal baclofen enhances and prolongs the pain-reducing capacity of SCS Trials of SCS with baclofen should be considered for patients who do not respond to SCS alone	II-3
Schechtmann et al,[71] 2010	Double-blind, placebo-controlled RCT; n = 10	Intrathecal clonidine vs baclofen vs saline	VAS scores	Clonidine may be an alternative to baclofen as an adjunct to SCS A trial with clonidine and baclofen combined with SCS may be warranted in patients who do not respond to SCS alone	I

Summary of key findings from studies on adjuvant therapies in addition to spinal cord stimulation for pain relief.
Abbreviation: ADL, activities of daily living.

In 2010, the notion of "paresthesia-free pain suppression," was introduced,[65] which has substantially changed SCS. The mechanism of action remains unclear. Arle and coworkers[66] suggest that (1) high frequency preferentially blocks large-diameter fibers, (2) large diameter fibers convey vibratory sensation, which is associated with paresthesia; and (3) high-frequency stimulation, while blocking action potentials of large fibers, recruits medium-diameter fibers, which produce the pain relief effect. Others implicate involvement of wide dynamic range neurons and/or modulation of the dorsal horn.

HF10 has been shown to have equivalent or superior outcomes to tonic SCS in patients with chronic back and leg pain, with response rates of 76.5% for HF10 SCS and 49.3% for tonic SCS.[26] Burst stimulation also offers promise in RCT.[24] Additional value may result from high-density programming, which provides stimulation at higher frequencies and delivery of higher charges per second.[67] Algorithmic programming, which uses patient-specific, three-dimensional model-based neural targeting, demonstrates sustained relief of back pain at 24 months.[55] Most recently, efficacy of closed-loop SCS systems using evoked compound action potentials can maintain desired levels of stimulation. Profound responses of 80% overall pain relief in 64.3% of patients at 6 months have been reported.[68] The impact of new waveforms on increasing numbers of patients that benefit from SCS and prevention from habituation are currently under study.

Adjuncts

A summary of results from studies evaluating adjuncts to SCS therapy are presented in **Table 7**. The standard goal for SCS is to reduce each patients' pain by 50%. This is obtained through a multimodal approach. First, SCS programming should be performed as an iterative process because pain symptoms change over time and regularly scheduled visits allow for ongoing fine-tuned adjustments of care.[69] One feared complication of SCS is habituation, where patients become accustomed to the effects of stimulation. Theoretically, this is minimized by varying the signal and its focal point, which creates alternating waveforms. Whether habituation occurs with ongoing changes in waveforms of stimulation has not been truly elucidated. Medications may also be used concurrently with SCS to optimize pain relief. Specifically, baclofen in addition to SCS has been shown to produce greater pain relief than SCS alone.[70,71] Intrathecal clonidine and oral duloxetine have each independently shown similar adjunctive benefits.[71,72] With the growing recognition of the ongoing opioid epidemic, it should be heavily emphasized that patients on opioids at time of implantation who continue opioid use at similar doses tend to have poorer long-term outcomes.[73]

ECONOMIC EVALUATION

Despite the high cost of SCS, several studies have demonstrated long-term cost-effectiveness of SCS when compared with CMM alone.[74] A RCT using crossover design with SCS versus reoperation for FBSS showed that the cost per patient for long-term success with SCS and reoperation were $48,357 and $105,928, respectively. SCS was most cost-effective when patients did not attempt reoperation before SCS, and reoperation did not succeed in relieving pain in any patient where SCS was previously unsuccessful.[75] A review of 128 patients who underwent SCS or peripheral nerve stimulation found that on average $93,685 was saved over 3.1 years of implantation as compared with health care expenditures before device implantation.[76] Among patients with CRPS, the costs of treatment with SCS within the first year were $4000 more than control subjects, but lifetime analysis demonstrated a savings of $60,000.[77] In 2017, comparisons across commercial, Medicaid, and Medicare cohorts demonstrated cost-effectiveness in all groups for periods from 2 to 9 years of follow-up following implantation.[78]

SUMMARY

SCS is commonly used for the treatment of FBSS, CRPS, and neuropathic pain. There is level 1 evidence to support its use in FBSS and CRPS. Careful patient selection including a rigorous trial period and psychological evaluation are essential. When patients proceed to permanent implantation, various considerations should be made, such as the type of lead, type of anesthesia, and waveform. This decision-making process is multifactorial and must take into account characteristics unique to each patient and workflow of each operative team. New waveforms hold promise for improving pain relief, but their mechanisms of action still need to be elucidated. Finally, the evidence to date suggests SCS is cost-effective when compared with CMM and this should be emphasized when patients and insurers face the upfront economic costs.

REFERENCES

1. Shealy CN, Mortimer JT, Reswick JB. Electrical inhibition of pain by stimulation of the dorsal columns: preliminary clinical report. Anesth Analg 1967;46(4):489–91.

2. Melzack R, Wall PD. Pain mechanisms: a new theory. Science 1965;150(3699):971–9.
3. Vallejo R, Bradley K, Kapural L. Spinal cord stimulation in chronic pain: mode of action. Spine (Phila Pa 1976) 2017;42 Suppl 14:S53–60.
4. Barolat G, Massaro F, He J, et al. Mapping of sensory responses to epidural stimulation of the intraspinal neural structures in man. J Neurosurg 1993;78(2):233–9.
5. Gordon AT, Zou SP, Kim Y, et al. Challenges to setting spinal cord stimulator parameters during intraoperative testing: factors affecting coverage of low back and leg pain. Neuromodulation 2007; 10(2):133–41.
6. North JM, Hong KJ, Cho PY. Clinical outcomes of 1 kHz subperception spinal cord stimulation in implanted patients with failed paresthesia-based stimulation: results of a prospective randomized controlled trial. Neuromodulation 2016;19(7):731–7.
7. De Ridder D, Lenders MW, De Vos CC, et al. A 2-center comparative study on tonic versus burst spinal cord stimulation: amount of responders and amount of pain suppression. Clin J pain 2015; 31(5):433–7.
8. NICE. Technology Appraisal Guidelines 159-spinal cord stimulation for chronic pain of neuropathic or ischaemic origin 2008. Available at: https://www.nice.org.uk/guidance/ta159. Accessed July 31, 2018.
9. Pain SA, Raff M, Raff M, et al. Spinal cord stimulation for the management of pain: recommendations for best clinical practice. S Afr Med J 2013;103(6 Pt 2):423–30.
10. Perez RS, Zollinger PE, Dijkstra PU, et al. Evidence based guidelines for complex regional pain syndrome type 1. BMC Neurol 2010;10:20.
11. Mailis A, Taenzer P. Evidence-based guideline for neuropathic pain interventional treatments: spinal cord stimulation, intravenous infusions, epidural injections and nerve blocks. Pain Res Manag 2012; 17(3):150–8.
12. Dworkin RH, O'Connor AB, Kent J, et al. Interventional management of neuropathic pain: NeuPSIG recommendations. Pain 2013;154(11):2249–61.
13. Deer TR, Krames E, Mekhail N, et al. The appropriate use of neurostimulation: new and evolving neurostimulation therapies and applicable treatment for chronic pain and selected disease states. Neuromodulation Appropriateness Consensus Committee. Neuromodulation 2014;17(6):599–615 [discussion: 615].
14. Netherlands Society of Rehabilitation Specialists, Netherlands Society of Anaesthesiologists. Updated guiddelines complex regional pain syndrome type 1. Available at: http://pdver.atcomputing.nl/pdf/Executive_summary_guideline_CRPS_I_2014_docx.pdf. Accessed July 31, 2018
15. Cruccu G, Garcia-Larrea L, Hansson P, et al. EAN guidelines on central neurostimulation therapy in chronic pain conditions. Eur J Neurol 2016; 23(10):1489–99.
16. North RB, Kidd DH, Farrokhi F, et al. Spinal cord stimulation versus repeated lumbosacral spine surgery for chronic pain: a randomized, controlled trial. Neurosurgery 2005;56(1):98–106 [discussion: 106–7].
17. North RB, Ewend MG, Lawton MT, et al. Failed back surgery syndrome: 5-year follow-up after spinal cord stimulator implantation. Neurosurgery 1991;28(5):692–9.
18. LeDoux MS, Langford KH. Spinal cord stimulation for the failed back syndrome. Spine 1993;18(2):191–4.
19. North RB, Kidd DH, Lee MS, et al. A prospective, randomized study of spinal cord stimulation versus reoperation for failed back surgery syndrome: initial results. Stereotact Funct Neurosurg 1994; 62(1–4):267–72.
20. Kumar K, Taylor RS, Jacques L, et al. Spinal cord stimulation versus conventional medical management for neuropathic pain: a multicentre randomised controlled trial in patients with failed back surgery syndrome. Pain 2007;132(1–2): 179–88.
21. Kumar K, Taylor RS, Jacques L, et al. The effects of spinal cord stimulation in neuropathic pain are sustained: a 24-month follow-up of the prospective randomized controlled multicenter trial of the effectiveness of spinal cord stimulation. Neurosurgery 2008;63(4):762–70 [discussion: 770].
22. Manca A, Kumar K, Taylor RS, et al. Quality of life, resource consumption and costs of spinal cord stimulation versus conventional medical management in neuropathic pain patients with failed back surgery syndrome (PROCESS trial). Eur J Pain 2008;12(8):1047–58.
23. De Ridder D, Vancamp T, Lenders MW, et al. Is preoperative pain duration important in spinal cord stimulation? A comparison between tonic and burst stimulation. Neuromodulation 2015;18(1):13–7 [discussion: 17].
24. Deer T, Slavin KV, Amirdelfan K, et al. Success using neuromodulation with BURST (SUNBURST) study: results from a prospective, randomized controlled trial using a novel burst waveform. Neuromodulation 2018;21(1):56–66.
25. Kapural L, Yu C, Doust MW, et al. Novel 10-kHz high-frequency therapy (HF10 therapy) Is superior to traditional low-frequency spinal cord stimulation for the treatment of chronic back and leg pain: the SENZA-RCT randomized controlled trial. Anesthesiology 2015;123(4):851–60.
26. Kapural L, Yu C, Doust MW, et al. Comparison of 10-kHz high-frequency and traditional low-frequency spinal cord stimulation for the treatment of chronic back and leg pain: 24-month results

from a multicenter, randomized, controlled pivotal trial. Neurosurgery 2016;79(5):667–77.
27. Harden RN, Bruehl S, Perez RS, et al. Validation of proposed diagnostic criteria (the "Budapest Criteria") for complex regional pain syndrome. Pain 2010;150(2):268–74.
28. Barolat G, Schwartzman R, Woo R. Epidural spinal cord stimulation in the management of reflex sympathetic dystrophy. Stereotact Funct Neurosurg 1989;53(1):29–39.
29. Kemler MA, Barendse GA, van Kleef M, et al. Spinal cord stimulation in patients with chronic reflex sympathetic dystrophy. N Engl J Med 2000; 343(9):618–24.
30. Kemler MA, De Vet HC, Barendse GA, et al. The effect of spinal cord stimulation in patients with chronic reflex sympathetic dystrophy: two years' follow-up of the randomized controlled trial. Ann Neurol 2004;55(1):13–8.
31. Kemler MA, de Vet HC, Barendse GA, et al. Effect of spinal cord stimulation for chronic complex regional pain syndrome type I: five-year final follow-up of patients in a randomized controlled trial. J Neurosurg 2008;108(2): 292–8.
32. Mannheimer C, Eliasson T, Andersson B, et al. Effects of spinal cord stimulation in angina pectoris induced by pacing and possible mechanisms of action. BMJ 1993;307(6902):477–80.
33. Eliasson T, Jern S, Augustinsson LE, et al. Safety aspects of spinal cord stimulation in severe angina pectoris. Coron Artery Dis 1994;5(10):845–50.
34. de Jongste MJ, Hautvast RW, Hillege HL, et al. Efficacy of spinal cord stimulation as adjuvant therapy for intractable angina pectoris: a prospective, randomized clinical study. Working Group on Neurocardiology. J Am Coll Cardiol 1994;23(7):1592–7.
35. Hautvast RW, DeJongste MJ, Staal MJ, et al. Spinal cord stimulation in chronic intractable angina pectoris: a randomized, controlled efficacy study. Am Heart J 1998;136(6):1114–20.
36. Mannheimer C, Eliasson T, Augustinsson LE, et al. Electrical stimulation versus coronary artery bypass surgery in severe angina pectoris: the ESBY study. Circulation 1998;97(12):1157–63.
37. Augustinsson LE. Epidural spinal electrical stimulation in peripheral vascular disease. Pacing Clin Electrophysiol 1987;10(1 Pt 2):205–6.
38. Bracale GC, Selvetella L, Mirabile F. Our experience with spinal cord stimulation (SCS) in peripheral vascular disease. Pacing Clin Electrophysiol 1989;12(4 Pt 2):695–7.
39. Robaina FJ, Dominguez M, Diaz M, et al. Spinal cord stimulation for relief of chronic pain in vasospastic disorders of the upper limbs. Neurosurgery 1989;24(1):63–7.
40. Sampere CT, Guasch JA, Paladino CM, et al. Spinal cord stimulation for severely ischemic limbs. Pacing Clin Electrophysiol 1989;12(2): 273–9.
41. Mingoli A, Sciacca V, Tamorri M, et al. Clinical results of epidural spinal cord electrical stimulation in patients affected with limb-threatening chronic arterial obstructive disease. Angiology 1993; 44(1):21–5.
42. Kumar K, Toth C, Nath RK, et al. Improvement of limb circulation in peripheral vascular disease using epidural spinal cord stimulation: a prospective study. J Neurosurg 1997;86(4):662–9.
43. Broseta J, Barbera J, de Vera JA, et al. Spinal cord stimulation in peripheral arterial disease. A cooperative study. J Neurosurg 1986;64(1):71–80.
44. Jivegard LE, Augustinsson LE, Holm J, et al. Effects of spinal cord stimulation (SCS) in patients with inoperable severe lower limb ischaemia: a prospective randomised controlled study. Eur J Vasc Endovasc Surg 1995;9(4):421–5.
45. Ubbink DT, Spincemaille GH, Prins MH, et al. Microcirculatory investigations to determine the effect of spinal cord stimulation for critical leg ischemia: the Dutch multicenter randomized controlled trial. J Vasc Surg 1999;30(2):236–44.
46. Spincemaille GH, Klomp HM, Steyerberg EW, et al. Pain and quality of life in patients with critical limb ischaemia: results of a randomized controlled multicentre study on the effect of spinal cord stimulation. ESES study group. Eur J Pain 2000;4(2): 173–84.
47. De La Cruz P, Fama C, Roth S, et al. Predictors of spinal cord stimulation success. Neuromodulation 2015;18(7):599–602 [discussion: 602].
48. Celestin J, Edwards RR, Jamison RN. Pretreatment psychosocial variables as predictors of outcomes following lumbar surgery and spinal cord stimulation: a systematic review and literature synthesis. Pain Med 2009;10(4):639–53.
49. Shamji MF, Westwick HJ, Heary RF. Complications related to the use of spinal cord stimulation for managing persistent postoperative neuropathic pain after lumbar spinal surgery. Neurosurg Focus 2015;39(4):E15.
50. Fama CA, Chen N, Prusik J, et al. The use of preoperative psychological evaluations to predict spinal cord stimulation success: our experience and a review of the literature. Neuromodulation 2016;19(4): 429–36.
51. Block AR, Marek RJ, Ben-Porath YS, et al. Associations between pre-implant psychosocial factors and spinal cord stimulation outcome: evaluation using the MMPI-2-RF. Assessment 2017;24(1): 60–70.
52. Haider S, Owusu-Sarpong S, Peris Celda M, et al. A single center prospective observational study

of outcomes with tonic cervical spinal cord stimulation. Neuromodulation 2017;20(3):263–8.
53. Babu R, Hazzard MA, Huang KT, et al. Outcomes of percutaneous and paddle lead implantation for spinal cord stimulation: a comparative analysis of complications, reoperation rates, and health-care costs. Neuromodulation 2013;16(5):418–26 [discussion: 426–7].
54. North RB, Kidd DH, Petrucci L, et al. Spinal cord stimulation electrode design: a prospective, randomized, controlled trial comparing percutaneous with laminectomy electrodes: part II-clinical outcomes. Neurosurgery 2005;57(5):990–6 [discussion: 990–6].
55. Veizi E, Hayek SM, North J, et al. Spinal cord stimulation (SCS) with anatomically guided (3D) neural targeting shows superior chronic axial low back pain relief compared to traditional SCS-LUMINA study. Pain Med 2017;18(8):1534–48.
56. North RB, Kidd DH, Olin JC, et al. Spinal cord stimulation electrode design: prospective, randomized, controlled trial comparing percutaneous and laminectomy electrodes-part I: technical outcomes. Neurosurgery 2002;51(2):381–9 [discussion: 389–90].
57. Rigoard P, Luong AT, Delmotte A, et al. Multicolumn spinal cord stimulation lead implantation using an optic transligamentar minimally invasive technique. Neurosurgery 2013;73(3):550–3.
58. Roth SG, Lange S, Haller J, et al. A prospective study of the intra- and postoperative efficacy of intraoperative neuromonitoring in spinal cord stimulation. Stereotact Funct Neurosurg 2015;93(5):348–54.
59. Shils JL, Arle JE. Intraoperative neurophysiologic methods for spinal cord stimulator placement under general anesthesia. Neuromodulation 2012; 15(6):560–71 [discussion: 571–2].
60. Falowski SM, Celii A, Sestokas AK, et al. Awake vs. asleep placement of spinal cord stimulators: a cohort analysis of complications associated with placement. Neuromodulation 2011;14(2):130–4 [discussion: 134–5].
61. Tamkus AA, Scott AF, Khan FR. Neurophysiological monitoring during spinal cord stimulator placement surgery. Neuromodulation 2015;18(6):460–4 [discussion: 464].
62. Schoen N, Chieng LO, Madhavan K, et al. The use of intraoperative electromyogram during spinal cord stimulator placement surgery: a case series. World Neurosurg 2017;100:74–84.
63. Zhang K, Bhatia S, Oh M, et al. Epidural anesthesia for placement of spinal cord stimulators with paddle-type electrodes. Stereotact Funct Neurosurg 2009;87(5):292–6.
64. Sarubbo S, Latini F, Tugnoli V, et al. Spinal anesthesia and minimal invasive laminotomy for paddle electrode placement in spinal cord stimulation: technical report and clinical results at long-term followup. ScientificWorldJournal 2012;2012:201053.
65. De Ridder D, Vanneste S, Plazier M, et al. Burst spinal cord stimulation: toward paresthesia-free pain suppression. Neurosurgery 2010;66(5):986–90.
66. Arle JE, Mei L, Carlson KW, et al. High-frequency stimulation of dorsal column axons: potential underlying mechanism of paresthesia-free neuropathic pain relief. Neuromodulation 2016;19(4): 385–97.
67. Provenzano DA, Rebman J, Kuhel C, et al. The efficacy of high-density spinal cord stimulation among trial, implant, and conversion patients: a retrospective case series. Neuromodulation 2017; 20(7):654–60.
68. Russo M, Cousins MJ, Brooker C, et al. Effective relief of pain and associated symptoms with closed-loop spinal cord stimulation system: preliminary results of the avalon study. Neuromodulation 2018;21(1):38–47.
69. Health Quality O. Spinal cord stimulation for neuropathic pain: an evidence-based analysis. Ont Health Technol Assess Ser 2005;5(4):1–78.
70. Lind G, Meyerson BA, Winter J, et al. Intrathecal baclofen as adjuvant therapy to enhance the effect of spinal cord stimulation in neuropathic pain: a pilot study. Eur J Pain 2004;8(4):377–83.
71. Schechtmann G, Lind G, Winter J, et al. Intrathecal clonidine and baclofen enhance the pain-relieving effect of spinal cord stimulation: a comparative placebo-controlled, randomized trial. Neurosurgery 2010;67(1):173–81.
72. Prabhala T, Sabourin S, DiMarzio M, et al. Duloxetine improves spinal cord stimulation outcomes for chronic pain. Neuromodulation 2018. [Epub ahead of print].
73. Gee L, Smith HC, Ghulam-Jelani Z, et al. Spinal cord stimulation for the treatment of chronic pain reduces opioid use and results in superior clinical outcomes when used without opioids. Neurosurgery 2018;84(1):217–26.
74. Kumar K, Rizvi S. Cost-effectiveness of spinal cord stimulation therapy in management of chronic pain. Pain Med 2013;14(11):1631–49.
75. North RB, Kidd D, Shipley J, et al. Spinal cord stimulation versus reoperation for failed back surgery syndrome: a cost effectiveness and cost utility analysis based on a randomized, controlled trial. Neurosurgery 2007;61(2):361–8 [discussion: 368–9].
76. Mekhail NA, Aeschbach A, Stanton-Hicks M. Cost benefit analysis of neurostimulation for chronic pain. Clin J pain 2004;20(6):462–8.
77. Kemler MA, Furnee CA. Economic evaluation of spinal cord stimulation for chronic reflex sympathetic dystrophy. Neurology 2002;59(8):1203–9.

78. Elsamadicy AA, Farber SH, Yang S, et al. Impact of insurance provider on overall costs in failed back surgery syndrome: a cost study of 122,827 patients. Neuromodulation 2017;20(4):354–60.
79. Schu S, Slotty PJ, Bara G, et al. A prospective, randomised, double-blind, placebo-controlled study to examine the effectiveness of burst spinal cord stimulation patterns for the treatment of failed back surgery syndrome. Neuromodulation 2014; 17(5):443–50.
80. Zucco F, Ciampichini R, Lavano A, et al. Cost-effectiveness and cost-utility analysis of spinal cord stimulation in patients with failed back surgery syndrome: results from the PRECISE study. Neuromodulation 2015;18(4):266–76 [discussion: 276].
81. van Gorp EJ, Teernstra OP, Gultuna I, et al. Subcutaneous stimulation as ADD-ON therapy to spinal cord stimulation is effective in treating low back pain in patients with failed back surgery syndrome: a multicenter randomized controlled trial. Neuromodulation 2016;19(2):171–8.
82. Rigoard P, Jacques L, Delmotte A, et al. An algorithmic programming approach for back pain symptoms in failed back surgery syndrome using spinal cord stimulation with a multicolumn surgically implanted epidural lead: a multicenter international prospective study. Pain Pract 2015;15(3):195–207.
83. Choi JG, Ha SW, Son BC. Comparison of clinical efficacy and computed tomographic analysis of lead position between three-column and five-column paddle leads spinal cord stimulation for failed back surgery syndrome. World Neurosurg 2017; 97:292–303.
84. Remacle TY, Bonhomme VL, Renwart HP, et al. Effect of multicolumn lead spinal cord stimulation on low back pain in failed back surgery patients: a three-year follow-up. Neuromodulation 2017;20(7):668–74.
85. Paul AR, Kumar V, Roth S, et al. Establishing minimal clinically important difference of spinal cord stimulation therapy in post-laminectomy syndrome. Neurosurgery 2017;81(6):1011–5.
86. Loge D, Vanneste S, Vancamp T, et al. Long-term outcomes of spinal cord stimulation with percutaneously introduced paddle leads in the treatment of failed back surgery syndrome and lumboischialgia. Neuromodulation 2013;16(6):537–45 [discussion: 545].
87. Avellanal M, Diaz-Reganon G, Orts A, et al. One-year results of an algorithmic approach to managing failed back surgery syndrome. Pain Res Manag 2014;19(6):313–6.
88. Kinfe TM, Quack F, Wille C, et al. Paddle versus cylindrical leads for percutaneous implantation in spinal cord stimulation for failed back surgery syndrome: a single-center trial. J Neurol Surg A Cent Eur Neurosurg 2014;75(6):467–73.
89. Sweet J, Badjatiya A, Tan D, et al. Paresthesia-free high-density spinal cord stimulation for postlaminectomy syndrome in a prescreened population: a prospective case series. Neuromodulation 2016;19(3):260–7.
90. Vonhogen LH, Vancamp T, Vanneste S, et al. Percutaneously implanted plates in failed back surgery syndrome (FBSS). Neuromodulation 2011; 14(4):319–24 [discussion: 324–5].
91. Tomycz ND, Ortiz V, Moossy JJ. Simultaneous intrathecal opioid pump and spinal cord stimulation for pain management: analysis of 11 patients with failed back surgery syndrome. J Pain Palliat Care Pharmacother 2010;24(4):374–83.
92. Reverberi C, Dario A, Barolat G. Spinal cord stimulation (SCS) in conjunction with peripheral nerve field stimulation (PNfS) for the treatment of complex pain in failed back surgery syndrome (FBSS). Neuromodulation 2013;16(1):78–82 [discussion: 83].
93. Turner JA, Hollingworth W, Comstock BA, et al. Spinal cord stimulation for failed back surgery syndrome: outcomes in a workers' compensation setting. Pain 2010;148(1):14–25.
94. Devulder J, De Laat M, Van Bastelaere M, et al. Spinal cord stimulation: a valuable treatment for chronic failed back surgery patients. J Pain Symptom Manage 1997;13(5):296–301.
95. Lad SP, Babu R, Bagley JH, et al. Utilization of spinal cord stimulation in patients with failed back surgery syndrome. Spine 2014;39(12):E719–27.
96. Kriek N, Groeneweg JG, Stronks DL, et al. Comparison of tonic spinal cord stimulation, high-frequency and burst stimulation in patients with complex regional pain syndrome: a double-blind, randomised placebo controlled trial. BMC Musculoskelet Disord 2015;16:222.
97. Deer TR, Levy RM, Kramer J, et al. Dorsal root ganglion stimulation yielded higher treatment success rate for complex regional pain syndrome and causalgia at 3 and 12 months: a randomized comparative trial. Pain 2017;158(4):669–81.
98. Kemler MA, Reulen JP, Barendse GA, et al. Impact of spinal cord stimulation on sensory characteristics in complex regional pain syndrome type I: a randomized trial. Anesthesiology 2001;95(1): 72–80.
99. Sears NC, Machado AG, Nagel SJ, et al. Long-term outcomes of spinal cord stimulation with paddle leads in the treatment of complex regional pain syndrome and failed back surgery syndrome. Neuromodulation 2011;14(4):312–8 [discussion: 318].
100. Goto S, Taira T, Horisawa S, et al. Spinal cord stimulation and intrathecal baclofen therapy: combined neuromodulation for treatment of advanced complex regional pain syndrome. Stereotact Funct Neurosurg 2013;91(6):386–91.
101. Geurts JW, Smits H, Kemler MA, et al. Spinal cord stimulation for complex regional pain syndrome

type I: a prospective cohort study with long-term follow-up. Neuromodulation 2013;16(6):523–9 [discussion: 529].
102. van Eijs F, Geurts JW, Van Zundert J, et al. Spinal cord stimulation in complex regional pain syndrome type I of less than 12-month duration. Neuromodulation 2012;15(2):144–50 [discussion: 150].
103. Forouzanfar T, Kemler MA, Weber WE, et al. Spinal cord stimulation in complex regional pain syndrome: cervical and lumbar devices are comparably effective. Br J Anaesth 2004;92(3):348–53.
104. Harke H, Gretenkort P, Ladleif HU, et al. Spinal cord stimulation in sympathetically maintained complex regional pain syndrome type I with severe disability. A prospective clinical study. Eur J Pain 2005;9(4):363–73.
105. Kumar K, Rizvi S, Bnurs SB. Spinal cord stimulation is effective in management of complex regional pain syndrome I: fact or fiction. Neurosurgery 2011;69(3):566–78 [discussion: 578–80].
106. Kumar K, Nath RK, Toth C. Spinal cord stimulation is effective in the management of reflex sympathetic dystrophy. Neurosurgery 1997;40(3):503–8 [discussion: 508–9].
107. McNab D, Khan SN, Sharples LD, et al. An open label, single-centre, randomized trial of spinal cord stimulation vs. percutaneous myocardial laser revascularization in patients with refractory angina pectoris: the SPiRiT trial. Eur Heart J 2006;27(9): 1048–53.
108. Lanza GA, Sestito A, Sgueglia GA, et al. Effect of spinal cord stimulation on spontaneous and stress-induced angina and 'ischemia-like' ST-segment depression in patients with cardiac syndrome X. Eur Heart J 2005;26(10):983–9.
109. Lanza GA, Grimaldi R, Greco S, et al. Spinal cord stimulation for the treatment of refractory angina pectoris: a multicenter randomized single-blind study (the SCS-ITA trial). Pain 2011;152(1):45–52.
110. Zipes DP, Svorkdal N, Berman D, et al. Spinal cord stimulation therapy for patients with refractory angina who are not candidates for revascularization. Neuromodulation 2012;15(6):550–8 [discussion: 558–9].
111. Eddicks S, Maier-Hauff K, Schenk M, et al. Thoracic spinal cord stimulation improves functional status and relieves symptoms in patients with refractory angina pectoris: the first placebo-controlled randomised study. Heart 2007;93(5): 585–90.
112. Bondesson S, Pettersson T, Erdling A, et al. Comparison of patients undergoing enhanced external counterpulsation and spinal cord stimulation for refractory angina pectoris. Coron Artery Dis 2008; 19(8):627–34.
113. Anselmino M, Ravera L, De Luca A, et al. Spinal cord stimulation and 30-minute heart rate variability in refractory angina patients. Pacing Clin Electrophysiol 2009;32(1):37–42.
114. Andrell P, Yu W, Gersbach P, et al. Long-term effects of spinal cord stimulation on angina symptoms and quality of life in patients with refractory angina pectoris: results from the European Angina Registry Link Study (EARL). Heart 2010;96(14): 1132–6.
115. Sgueglia GA, Sestito A, Spinelli A, et al. Long-term follow-up of patients with cardiac syndrome X treated by spinal cord stimulation. Heart 2007; 93(5):591–7.
116. Di Pede F, Lanza GA, Zuin G, et al. Immediate and long-term clinical outcome after spinal cord stimulation for refractory stable angina pectoris. Am J Cardiol 2003;91(8):951–5.
117. Lapenna E, Rapati D, Cardano P, et al. Spinal cord stimulation for patients with refractory angina and previous coronary surgery. Ann Thorac Surg 2006;82(5):1704–8.
118. TenVaarwerk IA, Jessurun GA, DeJongste MJ, et al. Clinical outcome of patients treated with spinal cord stimulation for therapeutically refractory angina pectoris. The Working Group on Neurocardiology. Heart 1999;82(1):82–8.
119. Andersen C, Hole P, Oxhoj H. Does pain relief with spinal cord stimulation for angina conceal myocardial infarction? Br Heart J 1994;71(5):419–21.
120. Hautvast RW, Brouwer J, DeJongste MJ, et al. Effect of spinal cord stimulation on heart rate variability and myocardial ischemia in patients with chronic intractable angina pectoris–a prospective ambulatory electrocardiographic study. Clin Cardiol 1998;21(1):33–8.
121. Hautvast RW, Blanksma PK, DeJongste MJ, et al. Effect of spinal cord stimulation on myocardial blood flow assessed by positron emission tomography in patients with refractory angina pectoris. Am J Cardiol 1996;77(7):462–7.
122. Saraste A, Ukkonen H, Varis A, et al. Effect of spinal cord stimulation on myocardial perfusion reserve in patients with refractory angina pectoris. Eur Heart J Cardiovasc Imaging 2015;16(4): 449–55.
123. de Jongste MJ, Haaksma J, Hautvast RW, et al. Effects of spinal cord stimulation on myocardial ischaemia during daily life in patients with severe coronary artery disease. A prospective ambulatory electrocardiographic study. Br Heart J 1994;71(5): 413–8.
124. Ekre O, Borjesson M, Edvardsson N, et al. Feasibility of spinal cord stimulation in angina pectoris in patients with chronic pacemaker treatment for cardiac arrhythmias. Pacing Clin Electrophysiol 2003;26(11):2134–41.
125. Bagger JP, Jensen BS, Johannsen G. Long-term outcome of spinal cord electrical stimulation in

patients with refractory chest pain. Clin Cardiol 1998;21(4):286–8.
126. Jitta DJ, DeJongste MJ, Kliphuis CM, et al. Multimorbidity, the predominant predictor of quality-of-life, following successful spinal cord stimulation for angina pectoris. Neuromodulation 2011;14(1):13–8 [discussion: 18–9].
127. Jessurun GA, Ten Vaarwerk IA, DeJongste MJ, et al. Sequelae of spinal cord stimulation for refractory angina pectoris. Reliability and safety profile of long-term clinical application. Coron Artery Dis 1997;8(1):33–8.
128. Sestito A, Lanza GA, Le Pera D, et al. Spinal cord stimulation normalizes abnormal cortical pain processing in patients with cardiac syndrome X. Pain 2008;139(1):82–9.
129. Murray S, Carson KG, Ewings PD, et al. Spinal cord stimulation significantly decreases the need for acute hospital admission for chest pain in patients with refractory angina pectoris. Heart 1999;82(1):89–92.
130. de Vries J, Dejongste MJ, Durenkamp A, et al. The sustained benefits of long-term neurostimulation in patients with refractory chest pain and normal coronary arteries. Eur J Pain 2007;11(3):360–5.
131. Chua R, Keogh A. Spinal cord stimulation significantly improves refractory angina pectoris-a local experience spinal cord stimulation in refractory angina. Heart Lung Circ 2005;14(1):3–7.
132. Klomp HM, Spincemaille GH, Steyerberg EW, et al. Spinal-cord stimulation in critical limb ischaemia: a randomised trial. ESES Study Group. Lancet 1999;353(9158):1040–4.
133. Claeys LG. Improvement of microcirculatory blood flow under epidural spinal cord stimulation in patients with nonreconstructible peripheral arterial occlusive disease. Artif Organs 1997;21(3):201–6.
134. Tshomba Y, Psacharopulo D, Frezza S, et al. Predictors of improved quality of life and claudication in patients undergoing spinal cord stimulation for critical lower limb ischemia. Ann Vasc Surg 2014;28(3):628–32.
135. Amann W, Berg P, Gersbach P, et al. Spinal cord stimulation in the treatment of non-reconstructable stable critical leg ischaemia: results of the European Peripheral Vascular Disease Outcome Study (SCS-EPOS). Eur J Vasc Endovasc Surg 2003;26(3):280–6.
136. De Caridi G, Massara M, David A, et al. Spinal cord stimulation to achieve wound healing in a primary lower limb critical ischaemia referral centre. Int Wound J 2016;13(2):220–5.
137. Colini Baldeschi G, Carlizza A. Spinal cord stimulation: predictive parameters of outcome in patients suffering from critical lower limb ischemia. A preliminary study. Neuromodulation 2011;14(6):530–2 [discussion: 533].
138. Yearwood TL, Hershey B, Bradley K, et al. Pulse width programming in spinal cord stimulation: a clinical study. Pain Physician 2010;13(4):321–35.
139. Perruchoud C, Eldabe S, Batterham AM, et al. Analgesic efficacy of high-frequency spinal cord stimulation: a randomized double-blind placebo-controlled study. Neuromodulation 2013;16(4):363–9 [discussion: 369].
140. Washburn S, Catlin R, Bethel K, et al. Patient-perceived differences between constant current and constant voltage spinal cord stimulation systems. Neuromodulation 2014;17(1):28–35 [discussion: 35–6].
141. Van Havenbergh T, Vancamp T, Van Looy P, et al. Spinal cord stimulation for the treatment of chronic back pain patients: 500-Hz vs. 1000-Hz burst stimulation. Neuromodulation 2015;18(1):9–12 [discussion: 12].
142. Tjepkema-Cloostermans MC, de Vos CC, Wolters R, et al. Effect of burst stimulation evaluated in patients familiar with spinal cord stimulation. Neuromodulation 2016;19(5):492–7.
143. Kriek N, Groeneweg JG, Stronks DL, et al. Preferred frequencies and waveforms for spinal cord stimulation in patients with complex regional pain syndrome: A multicentre, double-blind, randomized and placebo-controlled crossover trial. Eur J Pain 2017;21(3):507–19.
144. Kinfe TM, Pintea B, Link C, et al. High frequency (10 kHz) or burst spinal cord stimulation in failed back surgery syndrome patients with predominant back pain: preliminary data from a prospective observational study. Neuromodulation 2016;19(3):268–75.

Intrathecal Pain Therapy for the Management of Chronic Noncancer Pain

Vishad V. Sukul, MD

KEYWORDS

• Intrathecal drug delivery • Intrathecal pain therapy • Intrathecal pumps • Morphine • Ziconotide • Chronic pain • Neuropathic pain • Review

KEY POINTS

- Randomized controlled trials, prospective and retrospective series, and clinical consensus guidelines have established successful outcomes for patients treated with intrathecal pain therapy (ITPT).
- Intrathecal drug delivery/ITPT should be considered early after failure of more conservative treatment options, and not as a salvage therapy alone.
- Two medication options approved by the Food and Drug Administration exist for IDD: intrathecal morphine and intrathecal ziconotide. Choice of medication to use is dependent on indication for therapy, but ziconotide is recommended as first-line monotherapy when possible.
- Patient selection, psychological screening, and intrathecal medical trial are integral to the success of the therapy.
- Technical considerations and management of adverse events are both important to avoid complications and ensure longevity of therapy and good patient response.

INTRODUCTION

Intrathecal pain therapies first began to emerge in the late 1970s with the World Health Organization's call for a focus on the management of chronic malignant cancer pain. Interest in the use of intraspinal analgesics increased after clinical demonstration of efficacy of intrathecal morphine.[1] The first reported use of an implanted pump for the delivery of intrathecal medication was described by Onofrio and colleagues[2] in 1981, followed by several case reports and outcomes studies including epidural infusion systems as well as the advent of programmable pumps.[1,3] The therapy was quickly used for the management of both intractable cancer and noncancer pain. Several expert and evidence-based guidelines have been published over the years to help clinicians navigate the complexities of intrathecal pain management.[4,5]

INDICATIONS

Not unlike other types of neuromodulation (ie, spinal cord stimulation [SCS]), the indications for the use of intrathecal pain therapy (ITPT) in the noncancer, nonpalliative setting has broadened considerably. ITPT is officially labeled by the Food and Drug Administration (FDA) for both moderate and severe trunk/limb pain, as well as intractable pain in the setting of the failure of other conservative therapies. Like SCS, it can be considered in the setting of failed back surgery/post-laminectomy syndrome,[6] chronic axial/limb/visceral or neuropathic pain syndromes,[7,8] and to a degree chronic regional pain syndrome.[9]

There continues to be some debate as to when ITPT should be considered in the management of chronic pain; however, the 2017 Polyanalgesic Consensus Conference (PACC) guidelines suggest its use within the same line as SCS and other

Disclosure: Dr V.V. Sukul is a consultant for Medtronic.

AMC Department of Neurosurgery, 47 New Scotland Avenue, MC10, Albany, NY 12208, USA
E-mail address: sukulv@amc.edu

Neurosurg Clin N Am 30 (2019) 195–201
https://doi.org/10.1016/j.nec.2018.12.010
1042-3680/19/

neurostimulation strategies in the treatment of chronic noncancer pain is warranted (level C recommendation), while noting that there is strong evidence to support the use of intrathecal ziconotide in chronic noncancer pain and moderate evidence to support the use of intrathecal opioid therapy. They deemed insufficient evidence to formally recommend it as a second-line neuromodulation option after the failure of SCS, and clinical judgment should be applied on a case-by-case basis.[4] At present, the suggestion is to consider neurostimulation if it will be able to adequately treat the affected pain region, and to consider ITPT if the painful region would not be adequately treated by a neurostimulation option. Most importantly however, neuromodulation (including SCS and ITPT) should be considered before the escalation of long-term oral opioid therapy.[4]

PATIENT SELECTION

As noted previously, ITPT should be considered in the setting of chronic, intractable pain (neuropathic, nociceptive, or mechanical) unable to be managed via typical conservative and interventional therapies. Importantly, patients should have a clear diagnosis and source for their pain before the initiation of ITPT.[4] If neurostimulation, such as SCS, is a viable option for patients with neuropathic pain, this should be considered first. ITPT should be considered if the pain pattern is diffuse, difficult to treat with (or failed) neurostimulation, or if anatomic factors predispose to pump placement. In addition, anatomic factors should be taken into consideration (ie, ability to safely place an intrathecal catheter) when deciding on long-term ITPT. As with SCS, consensus guidelines suggest value in performing a pretrial psychological screening and assessment. Aspects of a patient's psychiatric history can influence the choice of intrathecal medication (ie, ziconotide) as well as the decision to trial.

CHOICE OF INTRATHECAL THERAPY

There are a number of choices for ITPT. Two FDA-approved medication options are available: intrathecal ziconotide and intrathecal morphine. Formulations of other opioids (ie, hydromorphone, fentanyl) and other anesthetics (ie, bupivacaine) can be used; however, they are considered off label and should not be considered first-line therapy.

Morphine

Intrathecal opioids have been for many practitioners a drug of choice for intrathecal pain management since the 1970s.[1] Morphine (preservative-free) was one of the original drugs used in the early intrathecal pumps,[2] and there is some familiarity with the pharmacokinetics of this medication. Intrathecal administration of morphine acts locally, affecting mu opioid receptors in an agonist fashion. By also acting as on indirect calcium channels and causing resulting hyperpolarization of postsynaptic receptors/neurons, it is able to produce a gestalt effect resulting in decreased pain signaling.[10] However, due to the widespread prevalence of opioid receptors and the longevity of the medication in the central nervous system, it is important to remember that adverse effects (eg, respiratory depression, somnolence) can occur at higher doses.

Intrathecal opioid therapy has been well studied in both cancer-related and non–cancer-related severe chronic pain. Smith and colleagues[11] showed in a randomized clinical trial of ITPT versus conventional medical management (CMM) that 84.5% of ITPT patients versus 70.8% of CMM patients achieved clinical success (>20% reduction in visual analog scale [VAS] scores or >20% reduction in toxicity with equal VAS scores). They demonstrated the longevity of therapy to both 4 and 12 weeks in surviving patients.[12] A retrospective survey–based multicenter study of 429 patients collected from 35 physicians suggested a mean pain relief of 61%, with patients with noncancer pain showing greater pain relief and a more gradual dose increase over time to maintenance therapy.[13] Adverse drug events were uncommon, but system malfunctions did occur over time in approximately 21% of patients, most of which were catheter related. Several single-center studies have shown persistent improvements in chronic pain with ITPT in the long term, including 2 prospective studies evaluating ITPT over a 36-month[14] and 49-month period,[15] and a randomized double-blind study of 24 patients (median VAS change of 30.5 vs 11).[16] An open-label evaluation of a newer pump technology delivering intrathecal morphine again reported decreases in pain at approximately 70% of patient visits, with indications of sustained benefit over 6 to 12 months.[17] Overall, localized pain appears to be better treated with ITPT than global pain.[4] More recently, microdose or low-dose intrathecal opioid therapy regimens have been discussed, allowing for successful chronic pain management on morphine monotherapy with minimal side-effect profile.[18]

Respiratory depression is the most severe medication-related adverse event from intrathecal opioid therapy, and can be fatal if not appropriately treated. High dosing, rapid titration, and higher catheter placements in the spine may predispose to this complication. As such, 12 to 24 hours of monitoring is recommended for patients undergoing trials, priming boluses,[10] and significant dose escalations. In contrast, ziconotide has not been shown to cause respiratory depression, even at maximum reported doses. Peripheral edema, endocrine dysfunction, urinary retention, and immunosuppression may be observed in long-term treatment with intrathecal opioid therapy; and it has been suggested that patients with known peripheral edema should be considered for alternative therapies if possible, but this is not specifically delineated in the most recent clinical guidelines.[19] Sudden interruption of therapy may precipitate opioid withdrawal, and should be treated rapidly.

Intrathecal granuloma formation is a rare but serious complication of intrathecal opioid therapy. An inflammatory mass forms at the intrathecal catheter tip and can affect medication delivery and cause spinal cord compression. It has been described in up to 8% of patients, and is associated with higher doses and concentrations of intrathecal morphine.[20] As such, lower doses/concentrations of intrathecal morphine are recommended.[19] Symptoms of cord compression, such as weakness, worsening pain, sensory loss, and myelopathic clinical findings, in the absence of other obvious disease process should precipitate a granuloma workup, including MRI with and without contrast or computed tomography myelogram. Many granulomas resolve with cessation of intrathecal morphine therapy or lowering the morphine concentration and increasing the volume infused through the catheter. Surgical management may be necessary if there is evidence of spinal cord compression and significant neurologic symptoms.

Ziconotide

Ziconotide is a complex synthetic peptide approved by the FDA in 2004 for the management of severe chronic pain, which generates its effect through reversible binding of calcium channels (N-type voltage gated) in the spinal cord. It is the synthetic version of a peptide naturally found in the venom of the marine cone snail.[21] It has a slow diffusivity, and as such remains in the cerebrospinal fluid (CSF) longer and disperses much less supraspinally, but still has the potential to cause adverse effects with rapid dose titration.[10,22]

Ziconotide has good clinical evidence supporting efficacy. One double-blind placebo-controlled study demonstrated statistical significance of efficacy of ziconotide (via visual analog pain scores) in the management of chronic pain (14.7% vs 7.0%).[23] A long-term, multicenter, open-label study with stable dosing of the drug through the study showed a visual analog pain score reduction of 10% to 30%.[24] A single-center, 15-patient study found 53% of patients to be effectively treated (>30% improvement in numeric rating scale) with a low-dose ziconotide (1.1–2.8 mcg/d) protocol at approximately 70 days after initiation of therapy.[25] Another single-institution study found a 91% reduction in opioid consumption (morphine equivalents) in patients treated with ziconotide.[22]

Adverse events varied through these studies. Commonly described adverse events associated with short-term and long-term ziconotide therapy typically occur at higher doses. Adverse events typically are mild, but more severe alterations in mood, changes in mental status, and psychiatric symptoms (up to 12% of patients in early trials) can be observed with rapid titration or high doses of the drug. As such, a history of psychiatric disease can be a strong relative contraindication to intrathecal ziconotide therapy. Elevations in serum creatine kinase (CK) were seen in as many as 40% of patients in a review of clinical studies, and as such, CK screening may be indicated on a routine basis within the first 2 to 3 months of therapy or if patients experience muscle weakness or related symptoms.[19,21] Of note, only 1 case report of rhabdomyolysis has been described in the literature.[26]

It is important to remember that although ziconotide is very effective, it has a narrow therapeutic window and should be titrated slowly and carefully to achieve maximal effect without adverse events.

TRIALING

It is strongly recommended that a trial of intrathecal therapy should always be performed before considering a permanent implant.[27] The goal of the trial is to ascertain whether patients have adequate pain relief and improvement in function with the proposed medication, and to ensure that they have no acute side effects. Typically, the goal of therapy is a 50% or greater improvement in pain with the trial. This is similar to and was extrapolated from the SCS literature and guidelines.

The 2017 PACC guidelines consensus recommend that in the setting of noncancer chronic pain of neuropathic or somatic origin, an FDA approved intrathecal opioid (morphine) or ziconotide should be considered as a first-line drugs in most patients unless contraindicated, prior to trialing other opioids or adjuvant medications.[4]

Many physicians will attempt to wean patients off oral opioid therapy before performing an intrathecal trial. Some have described weaning patients to 50% of their chronic maintenance dose before trial,[28] with others taking patients entirely off medication by the time of implant. Consensus guidelines suggest reducing to less than 100 morphine equivalents per day, as higher chronic doses have been associated with failure of intrathecal monotherapy.[4]

Anticoagulation therapies should be discontinued 5 to 10 days before a trial procedure or implant and resumed at a minimum of 24 hours after the procedure.[4]

The trial can be performed in the outpatient setting as a single bolus trial. In this setting, a lumbar puncture is done under sterile conditions. A small amount of CSF is removed, and the appropriate dose of medication for the trial bolus is injected. It is important to ensure that the medication has been formulated for intrathecal use, as serious complications can arise otherwise. Following the injection, patients are observed in a monitored setting for several hours to ensure no side effects or complications (ie, respiratory depression) before discharge home. With a bolus dose trial, it is expected that patients should have some degree of relief within a few hours that should last for a short duration postprocedure. For ziconotide, the recommended bolus dose is 1 to 2 μg. For intrathecal morphine, the recommended bolus dose is no greater than 0.15 mg for the opioid naive patient, with 0.1mg felt to be a safe dose.[19]

Continuous infusion trials also are performed. In this setting, a lumbar intrathecal catheter or lumbar epidural catheter is placed, and a continuous infusion of medication is performed while the patient is monitored for several days. Again, 50% pain improvement is sought. The patient is typically kept in a monitored, inpatient setting for the duration of the trial. Infusions should be started at low doses, taking care to observe for side effects as the dosing is advanced slowly to a therapeutic level. With regard to ziconotide, trial infusions should be advanced slowly to avoid adverse events and side effects.

There appears to be some variability in which type of trial is performed. The 2017 PACC guidelines reference several survey-based studies showing a greater prevalence of continuous infusion trials compared with single bolus. Kim and colleagues[6] discussed that there was little consensus in the literature as to the type of trialing process that should be performed, only some degree of consensus on the ultimate goal of the trial. At their institution, intrathecal catheter trials were performed. Hamza and colleagues[28] in 2015 performed a randomized double-blind study that found no statistically significant difference between the method of a successful trial and long-term outcome with the implanted pump for patients undergoing a trial of intrathecal opioid medication. In the setting of an intrathecal ziconotide trial, Bäckryd and colleagues[8] and Mohammed and colleagues[29] found an intrathecal bolus trial to be feasible, with reasonable trial response rates; however, they cautioned that it was difficult to ascertain the predictive potential of an intrathecal bolus trial for long-term therapy efficacy. This is a contrast to the typical correlation of successful trial to permanent implant seen with neurostimulation devices.[22] McDowell and Pope,[30] in a review of the ziconotide literature, again revisited these findings, but noted that analysis of the ongoing PRIZM trial[31] suggested a shift toward intrathecal bolus trialing. Indeed, our institution and others perform bolus dose trialing with reasonable results.[22,25]

Ultimately, due to the lack of clear literature and consensus, either trialing method when used appropriately can be recommended in the setting of treating chronic, noncancer, non–end-of-life pain.

PERMANENT IMPLANT

Implant

Permanent implant of intrathecal pumps is a well-defined technique established for patients requiring intrathecal baclofen or pain medication therapy. Currently, there are 2 commonly used FDA-approved programmable intrathecal pumps. With regard to pain, one is indicated for both morphine and ziconotide (Synchromed II; Medtronic, Dublin, Ireland), and the other for morphine only (Prometra; Flowonix, Mount Olive, NJ). Before implantation, it is recommended that patients undergo a spinal imaging workup (typically MRI of the thoracolumbar spine) to better understand complex spinal anatomy or rule out pathology that may impact intrathecal catheter placement.[32,33]

Pump implantation is typically performed in a surgical setting under sterile conditions. There are many variances in technique, but typically an intrathecal catheter is placed and tunneled to a subcutaneously implanted pump in the abdominal region.[34,35] Fluoroscopic guidance[32] or other image guidance[35] is advised for placement of the intrathecal catheter, and a mid-lumbar entry (L2/3, L3/4) is recommended to avoid injury to the conus.[33] There is no clear consensus on the target spinal level for intrathecal catheter placement. Some physicians will try to target spinal levels near to or associated with the location of a patient's chronic pain, whereas others will place the catheters at a predefined level. Use of best clinical judgment is advised.[4] Anchoring of the catheter in the lumbar fascia is also recommended, to prevent catheter dislodgement, migration, and CSF leak. Catheters are then tunneled laterally to a pocket in the anterior abdominal wall, typically made in an epifascial plane. Subfascial approaches and pump placement in other regions (ie, thigh) have been described.[36,37]

Dosing, Initial Fill, and Medication-Induced Adverse Events

Depending on the abilities of the facility where the pump is being implanted, medication can be placed in the pump at the time of surgery or later on (once healing is completed) in the outpatient setting. In either scenario, is important to start with a low dosing and titrate up slowly in a controlled fashion over time to establish pain relief without systemic or local side effects. There are many options for dosing, including continuous dosing, bolus dosing, and other combinations. In most scenarios, continuous dosing is recommended as to avoid dosing-related complications.

Ziconotide

With intrathecal ziconotide, most recent protocols recommend initiating long-term therapy at a low dose. Prusik and colleagues[25] describe therapy initiation at 1.2 mcg/d escalating slowly in 0.2-mcg increments every 3 weeks as required for pain control with minimal side effects and reasonable efficacy. Other studies describe dose initiation at 0.5 to 2.0 mcg/d with slightly faster titration schedules.[21,22,27,30,38] Mean long-term dosing varies,[31] with some studies showing 2 to 3 mcg/d[22] and ranging to as high as 6 to 7 mcg/d.[23] Because side effects and adverse events with intrathecal ziconotide therapy are more likely to occur at doses >3 to 4 mcg, low dosage and slow titration are recommended.

Morphine

Intrathecal morphine dosing has been traditionally started at low to moderate doses and advanced at a slow titration to pain control. Newer "microdose" or low-dose strategies have indicated weaning patients entirely off oral opioid therapy before implantation, and starting at less than 400 μg/d[39,40] and titrating to no greater than 1 to 2 mg/d of therapy for pain relief. These strategies have proven effective, with some studies entirely eliminating systemic opioids in 51% of patients by 1 year.[41] This method of morphine and intrathecal opioid dosing is likely to be the norm in the future, and is included in the recommendations of the latest consensus guidelines.[27] Discussion of the nuances of long-term dose adjustment with or without microdosing/low-dose opioid therapy, compounded medications, and other nuances are beyond the scope of this review, but have been discussed to a great degree in the available literature.

Maintenance

Intrathecal pumps require physician maintenance. Pumps must be refilled in a timely fashion to avoid medication withdrawal. Refills are performed percutaneously. The reservoir is accessed with a syringe and needle, and all old medication is removed and measured to ensure that it corresponds with what is expected in the pump. New medication at the appropriate concentration and volume is then placed into the pump via sterile technique percutaneously, and the device is restarted/reprogrammed appropriately. Ultrasound guidance may be used to aid in refills and may decrease risk of inadvertent medication pocket fill.[42]

Complications and Concerns

As with any implanted device, complications can be a concern. With intrathecal therapy, this can manifest as either a medication-related adverse event, a malfunction/complication of the device itself, an iatrogenic complication, or some combination thereof.

Device-related complications, such as pump failure, catheter failure, and fractures, should be evaluated for and identified quickly and treated to reduce the risk of withdrawal events. Interrogation and electronic analysis of the device may help to identify hardware problems such as a motor stall. Catheter malfunction is typically the most common hardware-related malfunction described with intrathecal therapy.[43] Radiographic imaging to evaluate for catheter breaks and catheter-dye studies (injection of contrast medium through the catheter access port of a pump under live fluoroscopy) can be very beneficial to identify a catheter malfunction. Sudden withdrawal symptoms or escalating intrathecal doses without pain relief may indicate a catheter failure, and should be investigated. Pocket fill is an iatrogenic complication that providers should be on guard against, wherein some or all of the medication intended for a pump refill is accidentally injected into the subcutaneous pocket surrounding the pump. It can have considerable consequences, including under/overdosing or systemic complications, such as respiratory depression from the sudden bolus of medication.[10,19,33,44] Similarly, errors in the routine programming of intrathecal pumps can lead to overdose scenarios. In the setting of intrathecal morphine, if a pocket fill or medication programming error is suspected, one should monitor and manage following guidelines for opioid-induced respiratory depression.[10]

Infection is a significant complication and should be managed aggressively when suspected. If possible, in the setting of intrathecal opioid therapy, transition to oral opioids should be rapidly initiated to minimize withdrawal risk and the infected device removed. Medication transitions are less of a concern with intrathecal ziconotide, and oral opioid or other analgesic medication may be introduced at the discretion of the clinician for patient comfort/long-term pain management.

SUMMARY

ITPT is a well-established and effective therapy for the management of chronic refractory axial, extremity, and neuropathic pain. It should be considered in the setting of the failure of conservative management and when electrical neuromodulation is not a viable therapeutic option. Careful patient selection, psychological evaluation, systemic medication weaning, and a successful medication trial period are essential to long-term success of the therapy. Advances in patient care continue with the introduction of new low-dose protocols for intrathecal opioid therapy and with greater understanding of the clinical effects and therapeutic window of intrathecal ziconotide.

REFERENCES

1. Bottros MM, Christo PJ. Current perspectives on intrathecal drug delivery. J Pain Res 2014;7:615–26.
2. Onofrio BM, Yaksh TL, Arnold PG. Continuous low-dose intrathecal morphine administration in the treatment of chronic pain of malignant origin. Mayo Clin Proc 1981;56(8):516–20.
3. Penn RD, Paice JA, Gottschalk W, et al. Cancer pain relief using chronic morphine infusion. Early experience with a programmable implanted drug pump. J Neurosurg 1984;61(2):302–6.
4. Deer TR, Pope JE, Hayek SM, et al. The polyanalgesic consensus conference (PACC): recommendations on intrathecal drug infusion systems best practices and guidelines. Neuromodulation 2017; 20(2):96–132.
5. Deer TR, Prager J, Levy R, et al. Polyanalgesic Consensus Conference 2012: recommendations for the management of pain by intrathecal (intraspinal) drug delivery: report of an interdisciplinary expert panel. Neuromodulation 2012;15(5):436–64 [discussion: 464–6].
6. Kim D, Saidov A, Mandhare V, et al. Role of pretrial systemic opioid requirements, intrathecal trial dose, and non-psychological factors as predictors of outcome for intrathecal pump therapy: one clinician's experience with lumbar postlaminectomy pain. Neuromodulation 2011;14(2):165–75 [discussion: 175].
7. Smith TJ, Coyne PJ, Smith WR, et al. Use of an implantable drug delivery system for refractory chronic sickle cell pain. Am J Hematol 2005;78(2): 153–4.
8. Bäckryd E, Sörensen J, Gerdle B. Ziconotide trialing by intrathecal bolus injections: an open-label non-randomized clinical trial in postoperative/posttraumatic neuropathic pain patients refractory to conventional treatment. Neuromodulation 2015;18(5): 404–13.
9. Herring EZ, Frizon LA, Hogue O, et al. Long-term outcomes using intrathecal drug delivery systems in complex regional pain syndrome. Pain Med 2018. https://doi.org/10.1093/pm/pny104.
10. Webster LR. The relationship between the mechanisms of action and safety profiles of intrathecal morphine and ziconotide: a review of the literature. Pain Med 2015;16(7):1265–77.
11. Smith TJ, Staats PS, Deer T, et al. Randomized clinical trial of an implantable drug delivery system compared with comprehensive medical management for refractory cancer pain: impact on pain, drug-related toxicity, and survival. J Clin Oncol 2002;20(19):4040–9.
12. Smith TJ, Coyne PJ, Staats PS, et al. An implantable drug delivery system (IDDS) for refractory cancer pain provides sustained pain control, less drug-related toxicity, and possibly better survival compared with comprehensive medical management (CMM). Ann Oncol 2005;16(5):825–33.
13. Paice JA, Penn RD, Shott S. Intraspinal morphine for chronic pain: a retrospective, multicenter study. J Pain Symptom Manage 1996;11(2):71–80.
14. Thimineur MA, Kravitz E, Vodapally MS. Intrathecal opioid treatment for chronic non-malignant pain: a 3-year prospective study. Pain 2004;109(3): 242–9.
15. Kumar K, Kelly M, Pirlot T. Continuous intrathecal morphine treatment for chronic pain of nonmalignant etiology: long-term benefits and efficacy. Surg Neurol 2001;55(2):79–86 [discussion: 86–8].
16. Raphael JH, Duarte RV, Southall JL, et al. Randomised, double-blind controlled trial by dose reduction of implanted intrathecal morphine delivery in chronic non-cancer pain. BMJ Open 2013;3(7). https://doi.org/10.1136/bmjopen-2013-003061.
17. Rauck R, Deer T, Rosen S, et al. Accuracy and efficacy of intrathecal administration of morphine sulfate for treatment of intractable pain using the Prometra(®) Programmable Pump. Neuromodulation 2010;13(2):102–8.

18. Wilkes DM, Orillosa SJ, Hustak EC, et al. Efficacy, safety, and feasibility of the morphine microdose method in community-based clinics. Pain Med 2017. https://doi.org/10.1093/pm/pnx132.
19. Deer TR, Pope JE, Hayek SM, et al. The Polyanalgesic Consensus Conference (PACC): recommendations for intrathecal drug delivery: guidance for improving safety and mitigating risks. Neuromodulation 2017;20(2):155–76.
20. Kratzsch T, Stienen MN, Reck T, et al. Catheter-tip granulomas associated with intrathecal drug delivery–a two-center experience identifying 13 cases. Pain Physician 2015;18(5):E831–40.
21. Smith HS, Deer TR. Safety and efficacy of intrathecal ziconotide in the management of severe chronic pain. Ther Clin Risk Manag 2009;5(3):521–34.
22. Pope JE, Deer TR. Intrathecal pharmacology update: novel dosing strategy for intrathecal monotherapy ziconotide on efficacy and sustainability. Neuromodulation 2015;18(5):414–20.
23. Rauck RL, Wallace MS, Leong MS, et al. A randomized, double-blind, placebo-controlled study of intrathecal ziconotide in adults with severe chronic pain. J Pain Symptom Manage 2006;31(5):393–406.
24. Webster LR, Fisher R, Charapata S, et al. Long-term intrathecal ziconotide for chronic pain: an open-label study. J Pain Symptom Manage 2009;37(3):363–72.
25. Prusik J, Argoff C, Peng S, et al. Use of low dose ziconotide as first-line intrathecal monotherapy. Neuromodulation 2017;20(4):386–91.
26. Horazeck C, Huh AS, Huh BK. Acute rhabdomyolysis in a patient with long-term exposure to intrathecal ziconotide: a case report. Pain Pract 2015;15(3): E34–9.
27. Deer TR, Hayek SM, Pope JE, et al. The Polyanalgesic Consensus Conference (PACC): recommendations for trialing of intrathecal drug delivery infusion therapy. Neuromodulation 2017;20(2):133–54.
28. Hamza M, Doleys DM, Saleh IA, et al. A prospective, randomized, single-blinded, head-to-head long-term outcome study, comparing intrathecal (IT) boluses with continuous infusion trialing techniques prior to implantation of drug delivery systems (DDS) for the treatment of severe intractable chronic nonmalignant pain. Neuromodulation 2015;18(7): 636–48 [discussion: 649].
29. Mohammed SI, Eldabe S, Simpson KH, et al. Bolus intrathecal injection of ziconotide (Prialt®) to evaluate the option of continuous administration via an implanted intrathecal drug delivery (ITDD) system: a pilot study. Neuromodulation 2013;16(6):576–81 [discussion: 582].
30. McDowell GC 2nd, Pope JE. Intrathecal ziconotide: dosing and administration strategies in patients with refractory chronic pain. Neuromodulation 2016;19(5):522–32.
31. Deer T, Rauck RL, Kim P, et al. Effectiveness and safety of intrathecal ziconotide: interim analysis of the patient registry of intrathecal ziconotide management (PRIZM). Pain Pract 2018;18(2):230–8.
32. Prager J, Deer T, Levy R, et al. Best practices for intrathecal drug delivery for pain. Neuromodulation 2014;17(4):354–72 [discussion: 372].
33. Follett KA, Burchiel K, Deer T, et al. Prevention of intrathecal drug delivery catheter-related complications. Neuromodulation 2003;6(1):32–41.
34. Albright AL, Turner M, Pattisapu JV. Best-practice surgical techniques for intrathecal baclofen therapy. J Neurosurg 2006;104(4 Suppl):233–9.
35. Robinson S, Robertson FC, Dasenbrock HH, et al. Image-guided intrathecal baclofen pump catheter implantation: a technical note and case series. J Neurosurg Spine 2017;26(5):621–7.
36. Devine O, Harborne A, Lo WB, et al. Unusual placement of intrathecal baclofen pumps: report of two cases. Acta Neurochir 2016;158(1):167–70.
37. Narang S, Srinivasan SK, Zinboonyahgoon N, et al. Upper antero-medial thigh as an alternative site for implantation of intrathecal pumps: a case series. Neuromodulation 2016;19(6):655–63.
38. Raffaeli W, Sarti D, Demartini L, et al, Italian Ziconotide Group. Italian registry on long-term intrathecal ziconotide treatment. Pain Physician 2011;14(1): 15–24.
39. Grider JS, Etscheidt MA, Harned ME, et al. Trialing and maintenance dosing using a low-dose intrathecal opioid method for chronic nonmalignant pain: a prospective 36-month study. Neuromodulation 2016;19(2):206–19.
40. Caraway D, Walker V, Becker L, et al. Successful discontinuation of systemic opioids after implantation of an intrathecal drug delivery system. Neuromodulation 2015;18(6):508–15 [discussion: 515–6].
41. Hatheway JA, Caraway D, David G, et al. Systemic opioid elimination after implantation of an intrathecal drug delivery system significantly reduced health-care expenditures. Neuromodulation 2015;18(3): 207–13 [discussion: 213].
42. Gofeld M, McQueen CK. Ultrasound-guided intrathecal pump access and prevention of the pocket fill. Pain Med 2011;12(4):607–11.
43. Konrad PE, Huffman JM, Stearns LM, et al. Intrathecal drug delivery systems (IDDS): the implantable systems performance registry (ISPR). Neuromodulation 2016;19(8):848–56.
44. Maino P, Perez RSGM, Koetsier E. Intrathecal pump refills, pocket fills, and symptoms of drug overdose: a prospective, observational study comparing the injected drug volume vs. the drug volume effectively measured inside the pump. Neuromodulation 2017; 20(7):733–9.

Intrathecal Baclofen Infusion for the Treatment of Movement Disorders

Wendell Lake, MD[a,*], Hamid Shah, MD[b]

KEYWORDS

- Spasticity • Generalized dystonia • Secondary generalized dystonia • Baclofen
- Intrathecal infusion

KEY POINTS

- Intrathecal baclofen infusion is an accepted treatment for spasticity of cerebral or spinal origin that cannot be managed in a satisfactory fashion with oral medications.
- Evidence supports the use of intrathecal baclofen for the treatment of non-DYT1 generalized dystonias.
- A trial of treatment with oral baclofen is often recommended before intrathecal therapy and, in some cases, a single intrathecal injection for trial of baclofen therapy may provide useful information.
- Intrathecal baclofen therapy has a relatively high complication rate and practitioners offering this therapy need to be versed in the treatment of infection, system malfunction, withdrawal, overdose, and other expected complications.

INTRODUCTION: NATURE OF THE PROBLEM

Movement disorders owing to spinal or cerebral dysfunction are common in adult and pediatric patients. The first-line therapy for the treatment of these conditions often involves oral agents including baclofen, benzodiazepines, and other antispasmodics.[1] Intramuscular injection of botulinum toxin can also be useful in reducing spasticity of select muscle groups. Despite this broad armamentarium of therapies, many patients struggle to obtain satisfactory control of their spasticity and/or dystonia. This leads to complications, including pressure injury, pain, difficulty sitting in a wheelchair, bladder problems, difficulty performing basic hygiene, and overall degradations in quality of life. Some patients obtain significant relief from oral medications, but are unable to tolerate the side effects at the required dosage, such as sedation.[2,3]

Baclofen is a medication commonly administered orally to patients suffering from spasticity or secondary dystonia. The medication is an agonist of GABA type B receptors. Baclofen inhibits reflexive muscle contraction by blocking the release of excitatory neurotransmitters via interference with voltage gated calcium channels. Despite these positive attributes, the bioavailability of the drug at its site of action, the central nervous system is poor because of the blood central nervous system barrier.[4,5]

Owing to the marked number of problems associated with the oral treatment of spasticity and secondary dystonia, there was strong incentive to find new therapeutic options. In the 1980s, practitioners began to explore intrathecal baclofen infusion to achieve a high drug concentration at the site of action with relatively little systemic

Disclosure Statement: The authors have nothing to disclose.
[a] Department of Neurosurgery, University of Wisconsin-Madison, 600 Highland Avenue Box 8660, Madison, WI 53792, USA; [b] Department of Neurosurgery, Vanderbilt University, 1500 21st Avenue South, The Village at Vanderbilt, Suite 1506, Nashville, TN 37212, USA
* Corresponding author.
E-mail address: lake@neurosurgery.wisc.edu

Neurosurg Clin N Am 30 (2019) 203–209
https://doi.org/10.1016/j.nec.2018.12.002

toxicity.[6] Intrathecal infusion techniques are used with other medications such as morphine but are especially useful for baclofen because it does not easily cross the blood–central nervous system barrier.[6,7] Concentrations of baclofen in the central nervous system achievable by intrathecal infusion are 2 to 3 orders of magnitude greater than those achieved with systemic therapy.[8] With time, evidence has emerged that intrathecal baclofen infusion is an acceptable treatment for spasticity. Intrathecal baclofen therapy is also used for the treatment of secondary generalized dystonia, but less evidence is available supporting this application.[9,10]

At many centers, intrathecal baclofen infusion for spasticity and secondary generalized dystonia represents an important technique for managing symptoms and the therapy is used as part of a multimodal treatment approach. Frequently, the treatment teams include specialists in neurology, neurosurgery, and rehabilitation medicine. Treatments that may augment the use of intrathecal baclofen therapy include botulinum toxin injections, oral medications, neurectomies, physical therapy, and orthopedic procedures. This multidisciplinary approach often allows for the optimal treatment of these complex patients.[11]

INDICATIONS AND CONTRAINDICATIONS

The most common indications for baclofen therapy include spasticity and secondary dystonia. Spasticity can be of a cerebral or spinal origin. Common causes of spasticity of spinal origin include spinal cord injury, multiple sclerosis, and hereditary spastic paraparesis. Common cerebral causes of spasticity include cerebral palsy/perinatal brain injury, anoxic brain injury, and traumatic brain injury. Most cases of secondary generalized dystonia treated with intrathecal baclofen infusion are related to brain injury and, in some cases, patients may suffer from secondary dystonia and spasticity, both of a cerebral origin. If a patient exhibits signs of generalized dystonia, particularly with onset at a young age, and is being considered for treatment with intrathecal baclofen it is incumbent on the practitioner to rule out primary generalized dystonias.[9,11] This process may involve consulting a neurologist with movement disorders expertise and/or ordering specialized laboratory tests such as genetic testing for DYT1. If the patient suffers from an early-onset primary generalized dystonia, then treatment with deep brain stimulation of the globus pallidus interna is the preferred treatment strategy. Primary segmental dystonias (such as torticollis) are also generally managed with botulinum toxin injections as a first-line treatment and deep brain stimulation of the globus pallidus if this treatment method is insufficient. **Table 1** provides a list of common indications for intrathecal baclofen treatment, along with potential catheter locations and outcomes.[8,12,13]

Contraindications to intrathecal baclofen therapy include allergic reaction to baclofen, poor health precluding general anesthesia, and an inability to attend the necessary follow-up appointments for refills. Although absolute contraindications to baclofen therapy are relatively few, there are numerous considerations that practitioner must evaluate when deciding whether or not intrathecal baclofen is a useful treatment for a given patient. For example, the practitioner must evaluate the social situation and determine if the patient can either attend follow-up appointments for programming and refills under their own power or if they need significant logistical support.[13] If the patient is debilitated to the degree that they need help with transport and care, one must ensure that they have that support in place before embarking on this treatment. Another consideration is occult hydrocephalus. Many patients treated with intrathecal baclofen have cerebral palsy and may be at higher risk for subclinical hydrocephalus. If the patient has an increased intracranial pressure, this finding could significantly increase the risk of cerebrospinal fluid leak, infection, and other complications. Finally, many patients who require intrathecal baclofen have significant comorbidities that increase the risk of complications. These include underweight or overweight status, pressure wounds, and urinary tract infections. If possible, patients must be optimized medically to decrease the perioperative risks, including the risk of infection. At our center, we ensure that the patient has no open wounds or ongoing infectious processes before the implantation of a new baclofen pump system is undertaken.[6,11]

SURGICAL TECHNIQUE AND PROCEDURE

Preoperative Planning

- Most patients are evaluated in a multidisciplinary rehabilitation setting and deemed to be appropriate candidates based on failure to achieve adequate dystonia or spasticity management with oral medication, botulinum toxin injections, or both.
- A trial of intrathecal baclofen is considered for patients who are borderline ambulatory and may be using excess tone to assist in ambulation or transfers.
- A preoperative MRI of the spine is obtained in the prospective area of catheter implantation

Table 1
Common indications for intrathecal baclofen and potential catheter locations and outcomes

Standard Diagnoses for Which Intrathecal Baclofen Infusion is Administered	Treatment Strategy	Level of Evidence
Spasticity, quadriplegia in cerebral palsy	Pump with catheter tip placement at low cervical or high thoracic	Level I muscle tone lower extremeties,[15] Level II overall tone[16]
Spasticity, paraplegia of spinal origin	Pump with catheter tip at the midthoracic or lower thoracic level	Level I, rigidity and spasm severity,[17] Level III, functional improvement[18]
Hereditary spastic paraparesis	Pump with catheter tip at the midthoracic or lower thoracic level	Level IV, decreased spasticity, but possible decrease in muscle strength as well[19,20]
Secondary generalized dystonia	Pump with catheter tip placement at low cervical, high thoracic or intraventricular	Level IV[13,21]
Diagnoses where intrathecal baclofen is contraindicated or not preferred		
Primary generalized dystonia	Consider first line treatment with deep brain stimulation of the pallidum[8,12]	
Baclofen induced anaphylaxis	Consider botulinum toxin injection and management with oral medications other than baclofen[22]	

- Ensure that the patient does not have any underlying infections, either systemic or localized.
- Consider cervical laminotomy for catheter introduction in patients with an extensive history of spinal fusion surgery (ie, prior scoliosis surgery with fusion).

Patient Preparation and Positioning

- The patient is positioned under general anesthesia in the lateral decubitus position with the operative side up (usually right side up unless there is a contraindication; **Fig. 1**).[14]
- Fluoroscopy is brought in to localize the paramedian incision site. Usually the incision is centered over the L4 to L5 level in preparation for a catheter entry at the L2 to L3 or L1 to L2 level.
- A subcostal abdominal incision slightly rostral to the midpoint between the iliac crest and costal margin is marked out for implantation of the pump.
- The abdomen, flank, and back in the regions of the marked out incisions are prepped with chlorhexidine.
- A radiolucent table is used to facilitate fluoroscopy.
- Intrathecal baclofen is verified to be present in the room. Usually a concentration of 500 μg/mL is selected for new pump implantation.

Surgical Approach and Surgical Procedure

- Initially, a subcutaneous pocket is created at the abdominal site. In exceptionally thin patients, one may choose to make a subfascial pocket.
- Next, the paramedian incision is opened at the spine.
- Under fluoroscopic guidance, a Touhy needle is inserted into the intrathecal space and rotated such that the bevel faces rostrally. A brisk flow of cerebrospinal fluid is verified. **Fig. 2.**[14]
- Under fluoroscopy, the catheter with the stylet in place is advanced to the desired spinal level.
- A purse string stitch is placed but not tied with the Touhy needle in place.
- The stylet is removed from the catheter and cerebrospinal fluid flow from the catheter is verified.
- The Touhy needle is removed and the catheter level is again verified with fluoroscopy.

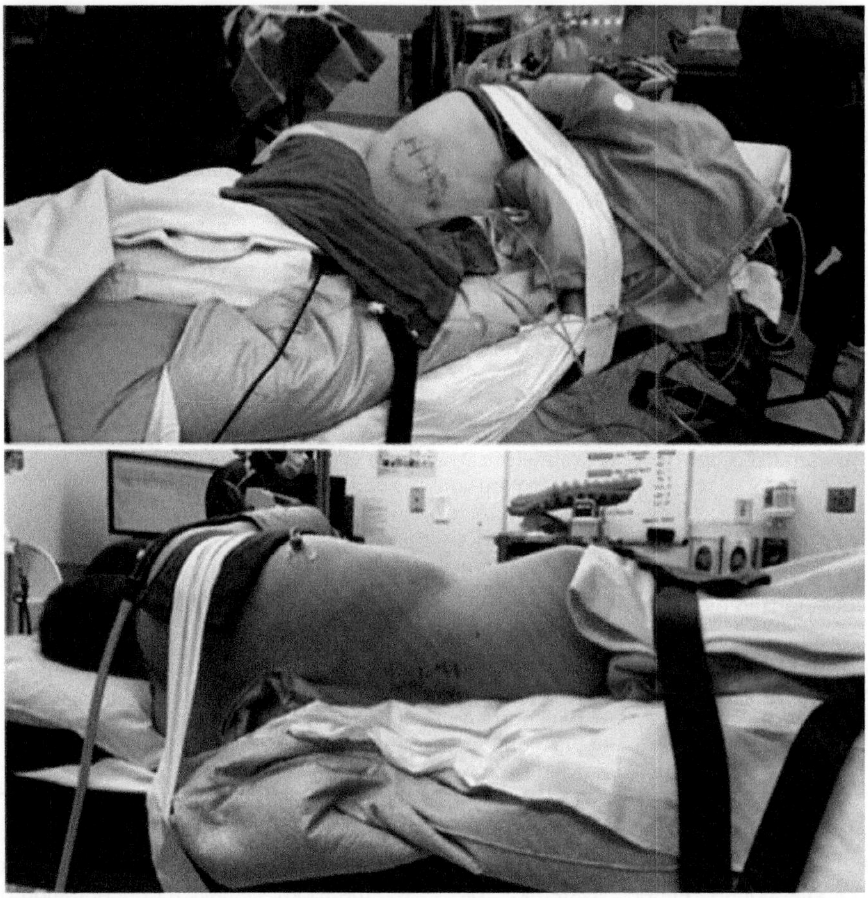

Fig. 1. Lateral decubitus positioning for baclofen pump and spinal catheter placement. (*From* Lake WB. Intrathecal baclofen infusion: a treatment for spasticity and secondary generalized dystonia. Contemp Neurosurg 2018;40(14):6; with permission.)

- A purse string stitch is tied and the catheter is anchored in place with the anchoring device.
- The catheter is tunneled from the back to the abdomen and connected to the pump.
- The pump is sutured down to the fascia and a side port tap is performed to verify good cerebrospinal fluid flow from the pump.
- Both wounds are copiously irrigated and vancomycin powder is placed in the wounds.
- Closure is performed in layers.

COMPLICATIONS AND THEIR MANAGEMENT

- If high risk (ie, cerebral palsy), assess the patient preoperatively for elevated intracranial pressure. This can be done, in some cases, with cranial imaging. If a trial intrathecal injection of baclofen is to be performed, one can measure the pressure of the cerebrospinal fluid with a manometer. Occult high intracranial pressure increases the risk for a cerebrospinal fluid leak.
- To further mitigate cerebrospinal fluid leak risk, place a purse string at the catheter entry site in the fascia.
- If the patient complains of positional headache postoperatively, they may be experiencing symptoms of intracranial hypotension. It may be reasonable to consider bed rest, an abdominal binder, or resort to an epidural blood patch under fluoroscopic guidance.
- Cerebrospinal fluid leak management may require all of or any combination of the following: epidural blood patch, exploration of the lumbar wound, system removal, or cerebrospinal fluid diversion with ventriculostomy
- Minimize the risk of infection. Ensure that the hemoglobin A1c is 7.5 or less. Inspect the patient for any ongoing infectious sources (urinalysis, inspect skin for cellulitis or breakdown, evaluate for poor dentition, evaluate nutritional where indicated). Use a standard preoperative scrub with chlorhexidine.

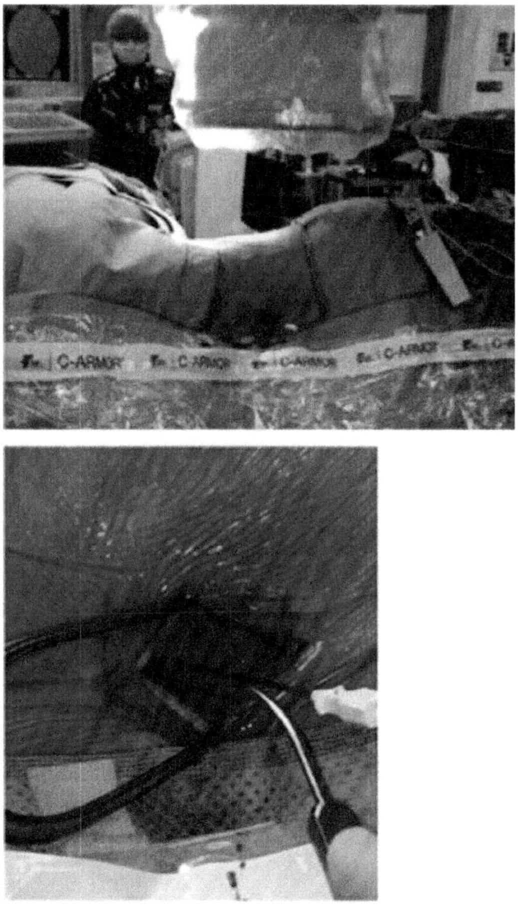

Fig. 2. Fluoroscopy position for spinal needle insertion during intrathecal catheter insertion. (*From* Lake WB. Intrathecal baclofen infusion: a treatment for spasticity and secondary generalized dystonia. Contemp Neurosurg 2018;40(14):6; with permission.)

- Use preoperative antibiotics and consider intraoperative topical antibiotics.
- Infection generally requires the removal of all hardware related to intrathecal baclofen infusion and treatment with intravenous antibiotics
- Avoid catheter fracture or dislocation. Firmly anchor the catheter to the fascia with a suture. Use a paramedian puncture site through the fascia to lower risk of catheter fracture or dislocation.
- Securely anchor the pump to the fascia with a suture and consider the perioperative use of an abdominal binder to decrease the risk of the pump flipping.
- Patients who are borderline ambulatory may be considered for an intrathecal trial so they can evaluate how a lowered tone effects their ambulation.
- If a patient with a baclofen pump is exhibiting signs of withdrawal (pruritis, irritability, hypertension, myoclonus), they should be admitted for workup of pump malfunction. This workup may consist of laboratory testing, urinalysis, pump interrogation, pump side port tap, test bolus through the pump, and reservoir aspiration to verify amount of medication in the pump.
- Patients with baclofen pump malfunction are generally admitted to an inpatient unit for cardiorespiratory monitoring and symptomatic treatment with benzodiazepines and oral baclofen.
- If a patient presents with withdrawal shortly after a refill appointment, consider the possibility of pocket fill.
- Baclofen overdose may present with respiratory depression and somnolence. Consider causes such as inaccurate pump programming or an inappropriate medication concentration placed in the reservoir if the symptoms occur shortly after a fill
- In cases with abnormal response to intrathecal baclofen infusion but normal side port tap, consider pump myelogram to rule septations of the intrathecal space and poor distribution of the drug into the intrathecal space.

Table 2 reviews the complication rates for intrathecal baclofen therapy from various papers.

POSTOPERATIVE CARE

- Start patients with new pumps at a low initial dosage of intrathecal baclofen.
- If a patient is undergoing a pump or catheter revision for a pump that has been malfunctioning for an unknown period of time, start at a low dosage and then titrate up as rapidly as the patient tolerates.
- For patients with new pumps or patients undergoing catheter revision, an overnight stay in an inpatient unit should be considered to observe for signs of overdose or withdrawal.
- Perform postoperative radiographs to note a baseline position of the pump and catheter tip. This step can assist in the refill process and pump trouble shooting (looking for flipped pumps or disconnection).
- Clearly document the pump low reservoir date after any pump programming or dosage change.
- Ensure that all patients are discharged with a supply of oral baclofen in case they need baclofen dosing for rescue during a pump malfunction.

Table 2
Complication rates for intrathecal baclofen therapy

Complication	Rate (%)	Intervention in Response
Infection	3,[23] 9.3[11]	Remove hardware and perform washout. Manage withdrawal following removal as an inpatient. Consider using vancomycin power in the wound bed when placing baclofen pumps in an attempt to prevent infection.
Cerebrospinal fluid effusion/leak	3.3,[23] 4.9[11]	Revise wound, consider purse string stitch at the fascia, measure intracranial pressure with a lumbar puncture before pump implantation if hydrocephalus is suspected
Catheter malfunction	8.5,[23] 15.1[11]	Revise catheter
Pump malfunction	1.8,[23] 1[11]	Interrogate pump, replace pump if stalling
All-cause adverse events	37[23] (23 severe), 25[11]	Monitor outcomes with a quality registry. Use meticulous surgical technique.

- Consider partnering with a physical medicine and rehabilitation specialist that can offer a multimodal treatment environment for patients with dystonia/spasticity, including oral medications, botulinum toxin injections, and physical therapy recommendations.

SUMMARY

An intrathecal baclofen infusion is an accepted treatment for spasticity. Evidence also exists for the treatment of secondary generalized dystonia with intrathecal baclofen infusion. Benefits include decreased tone, improved positioning, and decreased decubitus ulcers. Despite these benefits, there are significant complications that can occur with this therapy, including drug withdrawal, catheter infection, drug overdose, failure, and pump failure. In some cases, practitioners encourage a trial dose of intrathecal baclofen by injection or catheter infusion before pump implantation. To improve patient selection and outcomes, many centers offering intrathecal baclofen therapy use a multidisciplinary team composed of physicians, surgeons, and physical therapists.

REFERENCES

1. Brashear A. Spasticity: diagnosis and management. Springer Publishing Company; 2015.
2. Ward KA, Allan Ward K. Botox A and spasticity treatment. Arch Phys Med Rehabil 1996;77(10):1095.
3. Awaad Y, Rizk T, Vrak E. Management of spasticity and cerebral palsy. In: Cerebral palsy - challenges for the future. 2014.
4. Davidoff RA. Antispasticity drugs: mechanisms of action. Ann Neurol 1985;17(2):107–16.
5. Hasnat MJ, Rice JE. Intrathecal baclofen for treating spasticity in children with cerebral palsy. Cochrane Database Syst Rev 2015;(11):CD004552.
6. Winter G, Beni-Adani L, Ben-Pazi H. Intrathecal baclofen therapy-practical approach: clinical benefits and complication management. J Child Neurol 2018;33(11):734–41.
7. Knutsson E, Lindblom U, Mårtensson A. Plasma and cerebrospinal fluid levels of baclofen (Lioresal) at optimal therapeutic responses in spastic paresis. J Neurol Sci 1974;23(3):473–84.
8. Ertzgaard P, Campo C, Calabrese A. Efficacy and safety of oral baclofen in the management of spasticity: a rationale for intrathecal baclofen. J Rehabil Med 2017;49(3):193–203.
9. Berweck S, Lütjen S, Voss W, et al. Use of intrathecal baclofen in children and adolescents: interdisciplinary consensus table 2013. Neuropediatrics 2014;45(5):294–308.
10. Albright AL, Barry MJ, Shafton DH, et al. Intrathecal baclofen for generalized dystonia. Dev Med Child Neurol 2001;43(10):652–7.

11. Motta F, Antonello CE. Analysis of complications in 430 consecutive pediatric patients treated with intrathecal baclofen therapy: 14-year experience. J Neurosurg Pediatr 2014;13(3):301–6.
12. Vidailhet M, Jutras M-F, Grabli D, et al. Deep brain stimulation for dystonia. J Neurol Neurosurg Psychiatry 2013;84(9):1029–42.
13. Leland Albright A, Turner M, Pattisapu JV. Best-practice surgical techniques for intrathecal baclofen therapy. J Neurosurg Pediatr 2006;104(4):233–9.
14. Lake WB. Intrathecal baclofen infusion: a treatment for spasticity and secondary generalized dystonia. Contemp Neurosurg 2018;40(14):6.
15. Albright AL, Cervi A, Singletary J. Intrathecal baclofen for spasticity in cerebral palsy. JAMA 1991; 265(11):1418–22.
16. Van Schaeybroeck P, Nuttin B, Lagae L, et al. Intrathecal baclofen for intractable cerebral spasticity: a prospective placebo-controlled, double-blind study. Neurosurgery 2000;46(3):603–9 [discussion: 609–12].
17. Albright AL, Leland Albright A. Continuous intrathecal baclofen infusion for spasticity of cerebral origin. JAMA 1993;270(20):2475.
18. Azouvi P, Mane M, Thiebaut JB, et al. Intrathecal baclofen administration for control of severe spinal spasticity: functional improvement and long-term follow-up. Arch Phys Med Rehabil 1996;77(1):35–9.
19. Lambrecq V, Muller F, Joseph P-A, et al. Intrathecal baclofen in hereditary spastic paraparesis: benefits and limitations. Ann Readapt Med Phys 2007; 50(7):577–81 [in French].
20. Meythaler JM, Steers WD, Tuel SM, et al. Continuous intrathecal baclofen in spinal cord spasticity. A prospective study. Am J Phys Med Rehabil 1992;71(6): 321–7.
21. Turner M, Nguyen HS, Cohen-Gadol AA. Intraventricular baclofen as an alternative to intrathecal baclofen for intractable spasticity or dystonia: outcomes and technical considerations. J Neurosurg Pediatr 2012;10(4):315–9.
22. Moeini-Naghani I, Hashemi-Zonouz T, Jabbari B. Botulinum toxin treatment of spasticity in adults and children. Semin Neurol 2016;36(1):64–72.
23. Taira T, Ueta T, Katayama Y, et al. Rate of complications among the recipients of intrathecal baclofen pump in Japan: a multicenter study. Neuromodulation 2013;16(3):266–72 [discussion: 272].

Occipital Nerve Stimulation

Konstantin V. Slavin, MD[a,*], Emil D. Isagulyan, MD, PhD[b], Christy Gomez, APN[a], Dali Yin, MD, PhD[a]

KEYWORDS

• Peripheral nerve stimulation • Occipital nerve stimulation • Classical occipital neuralgia • Occipital neuroma • Headache • Migraine

KEY POINTS

- Although the first publications on clinical use of peripheral nerve stimulation for treatment of chronic pain came out in mid-1960s, it took another 10 years before this approach was used to stimulate the occipital nerves.
- Since then, occipital nerve stimulation has been successfully used in countless patients for a variety of indications, including classical occipital neuralgia, both idiopathic and posttraumatic, pain owing to occipital neuroma, so-called cervicogenic headaches, migraines, cluster headaches, and fibromyalgia.
- Based on results of a large multicenter randomized controlled study, occipital nerve stimulation was granted CE mark for the treatment of migraines, and a set of guidelines published by the Congress of Neurologic Surgeons came up with Level III recommendation supporting use of occipital nerve stimulation as a treatment option for patients with medically refractory occipital neuralgia.

Although the first publications on clinical use of peripheral nerve stimulation for treatment of chronic pain came out in mid-1960s,[1–3] it took another 10 years before this approach was used to stimulate the occipital nerves.[4–6] It seems that the main reason for clinicians' reluctance to stimulate the occipital nerve was a combination of the relatively small size of the targeted nerve and high mobility of the stimulated region. In those early days, the nerve had to be surgically dissected to place a stimulation electrode directly over (or under) it, and therefore the approach was reserved for larger nerves in the extremities with the occipital nerve stimulation (ONS) reported in only a handful of cases. Such surgery required surgical skills and certain commitment of the implanting team making it available in only few highly specialized centers. The situation changed dramatically—both in terms of the number of specialists feeling comfortable with ONS procedure and in the number of patients willing to undergo ONS intervention—with introduction of percutaneous ONS technique by Weiner and Reed in 1999.[7] Soon after that, multiple other publications described minor modifications in the Weiner technique with the use of cylindrical percutaneous electrode leads,[8–11] and then the open surgical approach with flat paddle-type electrodes was reintroduced and popularized.[12–14]

Since then, ONS has been successfully used in countless patients for a variety of indications, including classical occipital neuralgia (ON), both idiopathic and posttraumatic, pain owing to occipital neuroma, so-called cervicogenic headaches,

Disclosure: Dr. Slavin has received honoraria and research support from Abbott, ATI, Bioness, Biotronik, Boston Scientific, Medtronic, Neuramodix, Neuros, Nevro, Nuvectra, Pfizer, ROM3, SPR Therapeutics, Stimwave, Theraquil. The rest of the authors have no relevant disclosures.
[a] Department of Neurosurgery, University of Illinois at Chicago, 912 South Wood Street, M/C 799, Chicago, IL 60612, USA; [b] Burdenko Neurosurgical Institute, Moscow, Russian Federation, 4th Tverskaya-Yamskaya Str, dom 16, Moscow 125047, Russia
* Corresponding author.
E-mail address: kslavin@uic.edu

Neurosurg Clin N Am 30 (2019) 211–217
https://doi.org/10.1016/j.nec.2018.12.004

migraines, cluster headaches, and fibromyalgia.[3] At some point, based on results of a large multicenter randomized controlled study,[15–17] ONS was granted CE mark (Conformite Europeene) for the treatment of migraines,[18] and a set of guidelines published by the Congress of Neurologic Surgeons came up with Level III recommendation supporting the use of ONS as a treatment option for patients with medically refractory ON.[19]

INDICATIONS

The original indication for ONS was ON, a chronic pain syndrome that is characterized by sharp pain in the distribution of the occipital nerve(s). The pain tends to be a combination of underlying constant or almost constant dull pain and discomfort and intermittent shooting pain that is sometimes described as burning or jolting. As opposed to classical trigeminal neuralgia, which presents with short-lived and triggerable pain attacks, the pain in ON usually comes without obvious reasons and lasts for minutes or hours. In some cases, the pain may be aggravated by a head movement or some position of the neck, or with a specific type of activity. Sensory impairment in the occipital nerve distribution is rare in cases of ON, but may be present as a result of previous surgical or ablative interventions aimed at the occipital nerve(s), upper cervical nerve roots, and ganglia.

ONS for ON has been investigated in multiple centers worldwide and found to be both safe and effective.[7,13,14,20–22] The target for ONS in ON patients is the nerve or nerves that seem to be responsible for the pain generation and therefore the electrodes are usually placed over the course of the greater, lesser, and the third occipital nerves on 1 or both sides, depending on the pain pattern. A similar approach is used for patients with pain owing to occipital neuroma and those with postoperative ON.

Another set of indications includes various headache disorders—the so-called cervicogenic headaches that refer to a pain that originates in the occipital region and then spreads to the back of the head or the entire head and originates from upper cervical radiculopathy, cervical instability, or cervical spondylosis[10,23–27]; the migraine headaches (a common condition that is sometimes refractory to medical treatments)[13,15–17,28–36]; and the cluster headaches (relatively uncommon condition from the category of trigeminal autonomic cephalalgias).[37–41] In each of these conditions, the ONS electrodes are usually placed on both sides and there are multiple reports where ONS was used for these conditions in conjunction with unilateral or bilateral supraorbital nerve stimulation.

Finally, there is increasing experience with the use of ONS for diffuse body pain owing to fibromyalgia.[42–46] This indication came out from original experience with treatment of occipital pain in patients with fibromyalgia, where whole body pain improved in response to ONS. Since then, this indication was investigated in several clinical series and the results were very encouraging.

PATIENT SELECTION

Just like in every other functional neurosurgical intervention—and even more so in neuromodulation—the success of surgery in ONS is primarily determined by proper patient selection. The process of choosing appropriate surgical candidates for ONS starts with a determination of the severity and chronicity of their pain as well as the level of associated disability. Surgery is normally not indicated for those whose pain is not severe (usually, at least 6 or 7 out of 10 on a numeric rating scale), not chronic (the minimal duration is 3–6 months), and not disabling (the pain that is simply a nuisance does not justify the associated surgical risks and treatment-related costs).

The usual criteria for medical refractoriness have been defined in the literature in the past. They include (1) history of a trial of treatment with at least 4 drugs of known effectiveness in neuropathic pain; (2) each of these drugs has been tried for at least 3 months or until adverse effects prevent adequate dosage or continued treatment; (3) despite this treatment, the intensity of pain has not been reduced by more than 30%, or remained at a level of at least 5 on a 0 to 10 scale; and/or (4) it continued to contribute significantly to poor quality of life.[47] For ONS patient selection, we do not insist on a mandatory failure of 4 drugs, but the experience shows that by the time of neurosurgical referral, the patients have already tried, and failed, multiple medications, physical and behavioral treatments, and so on.

The location of the pain is of significant importance when ONS is used for neuropathic pain as in ON, and postoperative and posttraumatic occipital pain. There is no consensus on whether occipital pain dominance or the occipital onset of pain in migraine presentation makes patients better candidates for ONS, whereas for cluster headache management with ONS the pain does not reach occiput at all, and in patients with fibromyalgia the occipital pain is only a minor part diffuse pain distribution.

It is generally agreed that pain relief with local anesthetic blocks of the occipital nerve(s) does not predict success of ONS, but we still use these blocks for confirmation of the involvement of the occipital nerves in pain generation, particularly when there is a concern that sensory impairment from previous trauma or surgery may be a result of an altered innervation pattern.

The next step in patient selection is a formal psychological evaluation. We routinely use it to screen out those patients who are unlikely to benefit from neuromodulation owing to somatization disorder, malingering, untreated (or undertreated) depression, personality disorders, drug-seeking behavior, as well as cognitive impairment. These red flags have not been formally investigated for most ONS indications, but most of them are more of common sense predictors of failure.

Finally, there is an issue of medical fitness for surgery—because our general practice is to implant ONS devices under general anesthesia, it is important to make sure that the patients are safe to undergo general anesthesia and are medically cleared for surgical intervention.

The ultimate test for ONS appropriateness is the trial of stimulation. The purpose of the trial is to determine ONS effectiveness and presence of any stimulation-related side effects, including unpleasant stimulation and focal discomfort that becomes intolerable for some patients. Normally, patients are able to determine the success of ONS within a few days of electrode insertion; therefore, we perform 5- to 7-day-long stimulation trials. There is an exception, however—ONS for cluster headache tends to exhibit clinical effect after several weeks of stimulation, and because side effects of ONS are generally rare, there is a question whether the trial is even needed for this particular indication.

The opponents of trialing argue that the neuromodulation community has accepted proceeding directly with permanent implantation in other peripheral nerve stimulation procedures, such as vagal nerve stimulation for both epilepsy and depression, hypoglossal nerve stimulation for sleep apnea, and phrenic nerve stimulation for diaphragmal palsy, and therefore it is time to abandon the trial in ONS as well.

Technical Description of Occipital Nerve Stimulation

There is no universally accepted approach to the ONS technique. A brief survey of implanting physicians revealed significant difference in opinions as to the choice of electrodes (percutaneous vs paddles), number of contacts needed for optimal stimulation (4, 8, 12, or 16), direction for electrode placement (horizontal, vertical, or oblique), entry point and anchoring location (midline vs retromastoid), the need in dedicated anchors and anchor types (cylindrical, locking, with addition or glue, or simple suturing to the fascia), and generator location (infraclavicular, gluteal, abdominal, midaxillary, etc). We describe the technique that we routinely use in our practice and discuss the reasons for our choice on each of these issues. This technique has been used in dozens of patients in our practice and multiple other institutions. In essence, it follows the original description of Weiner and Reed[7] and has already been detailed in previous publications.[20,48]

Our experience indicates better clinical results with the use of cylindrical electrodes. Despite a higher incidence of electrode migrations, we observed better coverage and patient satisfaction with percutaneous electrodes than with paddle electrodes. To minimize the probability of muscle spasms in response to stimulation,[49] we place ONS electrodes above the fascia, and to decrease incidence of electrode erosion,[34,50] we position them at a depth of at least 8 mm from the skin surface. Furthermore, we advocate using curved insertion needles, preferably with blunt stylets, to follow the natural curvature of the occipital region. Another option is to use bendable needles with plastic stylets,[51] but the rigid metal stylets are essential for easy tunneling of the electrodes using a so-called needle-over-the-stylet technique.

Ever since 8-contact in-line electrodes became available, we have been using them routinely, with one 8-contact electrode for each stimulated side. Twelve-contact electrodes may be used for bilateral coverage, and longer 16-contact electrodes may eventually become acceptable for ONS applications; currently, the use of 16-contact electrodes is hindered by the need for special splitters because there are no 16-contact headers in the current implantable pulse generators (IPGs).

Although there are many different directions for electrode placement in ONS, the preferred direction is horizontal (**Fig. 1**). It allows one to cover all 3 occipital nerves on 1 side of the patient's head, the greater, the lesser, and the third occipital nerves,[52] because they travel parallel to each other in vertical direction and end up in the direct vicinity of 1 or 2 contacts, thereby facilitating coverage with lower stimulation parameters. Placing an electrode in other than a horizontal direction may be needed owing to the presence of surgical scars; in such situations, an individual decision has to be made regarding the safe and effective electrode location. The entire process of electrode insertion is done under fluoroscopic control; an alternative to fluoroscopy may be ultrasound guidance that, among other advantages, may help in ensuring a sufficient depth of electrode position.[53,54]

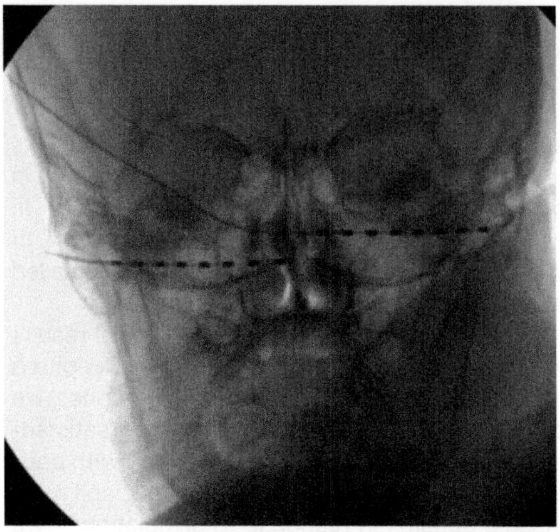

Fig. 1. Intraoperative radiographic image of bilateral 8-contact occipital nerve stimulation electrodes inserted for a week-long stimulation trial. Both electrodes are tunneled toward the parietooccipital region.

The choice of anchoring location and direction for electrode insertion is dictated by pragmatic considerations. The technical details of bilateral insertion of ONS electrodes have been described in detail in the past[48,55]—the anchoring takes place in the retromastoid region (**Fig. 2**). The contralateral electrode is inserted through the punctate midline incision toward the contralateral mastoid process and then the electrode tail is tunneled back toward the retromastoid incision. The ipsilateral electrode is inserted from the retromastoid incision toward the midline. As the result, the two 8-contact electrode leads are placed along the same horizontal line extending over the span of 10 to 15 cm between the mastoid processes, just below the occipital protuberance. The midline anchoring technique was abandoned owing to a higher incidence of electrode migrations and hardware fractures, most likely owing to high mobility of the posterior neck aspect, in favor of retromastoid placement, because the retromastoid area is remarkably stable and safe.

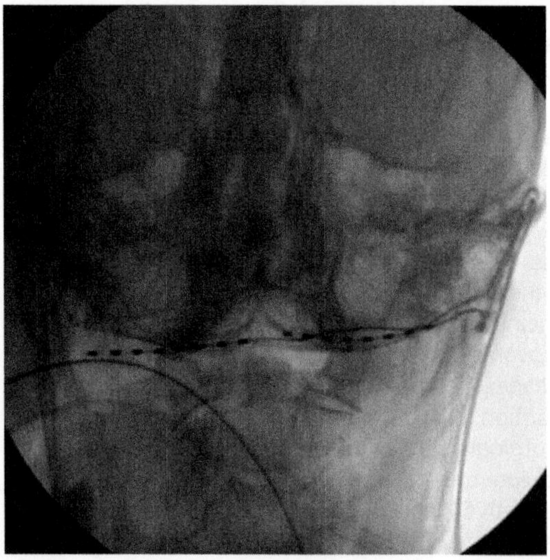

Fig. 2. Intraoperative radiographic image of bilateral 8-contact occipital nerve stimulation electrodes inserted during permanent implantation surgery. Both electrodes are anchored in the retroauricular region.

Because the electrodes have to be secured in place to minimize the probability of migration, various options have been proposed over the years—all the way from direct suturing the electrode leads to the underlying fascia to the use of specially designed locking and injectable anchors that immobilize the electrodes by holding them within soft tissues.[56,57] Our practice has evolved from suturing the large and robust anchors to the fascia to suturing the loops of electrodes to the fascia itself to our current technique where smaller cylindrical anchors are buried under the fascia. This step is done to decrease irritation of the overlying skin and minimize the risk of hardware erosion.

The final step of ONS implantation is insertion of the IPG. The recommended IPG location is the ipsilateral infraclavicular region, the same area that is used for routine placement of vagal nerve stimulation and deep brain stimulation generators, as well as countless cardiac pacemakers and defibrillators. The alternative locations for ONS IPG include the gluteal and abdominal areas, but these locations require more than 1 pass with the tunneling tool and/or are associated with a significant change in the pathway length in response to the patient movement.[58]

OUTCOMES AND COMPLICATIONS OF OCCIPITAL NERVE STIMULATION

The most attractive features of ONS are its low invasiveness, adjustability of the settings, reversibility of action, and testability. The outcomes tend to vary by indication, but there are no large and long-term series of ONS for ON, postoperative neuropathic occipital pain, or cluster headaches. Several large-scale trials of ONS for chronic migraines have been completed, and the results were encouraging overall, but not significant enough to justify regulatory approval in the United States. Nevertheless, a recent critical analysis of published studies of ONS for ON yielded 9 qualifying publications and resulted in a Level III recommendation that supports ONS as a treatment option for this particular indication.[19] In a large retrospective series, 76 patients with ON were treated ONS, and in vast majority of patients ONS resulted in a long-term improvement of the pain.[7,13,14,20–22,59–61]

The side effects and complications of ONS have also been analyzed previously—in patients with ON and the complication rate varied between 0% and 40% and included lead migrations, lead breakages, infections, wound dehiscence, hardware connection problems, and skin reactions.[50] An in-depth analysis of a large group of patients with chronic migraines who participated in a multicenter, prospective, randomized study of ONS showed that, of 157 patients who underwent permanent implantation (20 of 177 trialed patients did not proceed with implantation of permanent device), 111 (71%) experienced 1 or more adverse events.[34] The most common of the serious events were persistent pain or numbness at the IPG or lead site (17.8% of patients), lead migrations (16.6%), undesirable or unintended changes in stimulation (10.8%), battery failure or passivation (7.0%), and infection (6.4%). There were also lead fractures, skin erosions, wound site complications, device malfunctions, allergic reactions, expected postoperative pain, and normal battery depletions. The 64 adverse events in 51 patients (32.5%) resulted in additional surgery that included replacement or revision of device components or system explantation.[34] An expected finding of this analysis was the predominant occurrence of complications in patients who were implanted by surgeons with insufficient experience in ONS, and those surgeons with previous experience with fewer than 5 implants had a significantly higher incidence of patients with migrations, persistent pain at implant site, and infections. The analysis also showed that the incidence of surgery-related adverse events decreased with increasing surgical experience.[34]

FUTURE DIRECTIONS FOR OCCIPITAL NERVE STIMULATION

The future for ONS is likely to bring new indications, new devices, new stimulation paradigms, and, most certainly, further reduction of invasiveness[9,62]—with the eventual disappearance of ONS altogether, being replaced by completely noninvasive approaches. As the experience increases, one may expect that ONS will eventually gain regulatory approval for a number of indications, most likely for ON, migraines and cluster headaches. This process may require additional studies, at least for approval from the US Food and Drug Administration.

One of the major obstacles to greater acceptance of ONS is the lack of dedicated devices; the electrodes, anchors, and generators that are currently used for it are designed and marketed for spinal cord stimulation. Technological developments resulting in smaller, softer, more flexible, stretchable, less prone to migration, and kink-resistant electrodes, with better anchoring options. Simpler and miniaturized generators or receivers are expected to revolutionize ONS. An example of such innovation was a miniaturized rechargeable stimulation device, introduced in early 2000s and used in ONS for primary headaches and hemicranias continua.[63,64]

Similarly, the recent introduction of wireless miniaturized neurostimulation systems may be particularly beneficial for craniofacial applications, including ONS, because it eliminates the need for tunneling across the mobile areas and implanting the internal power source for pulse generation.[65] The preliminary results are indeed very encouraging and there is an expectation that this type of device will be approved for ONS use in the near future.

In the meantime, efforts are aimed at maximizing the beneficial effects of ONS by refining patient selection and keeping complications to a minimum. As the past research has conclusively showed, surgical experience correlates with safer ONS procedures,[34] and therefore it makes sense to develop proper surgical training, perhaps with the help of simulation approaches.[66] At the same time, one must consider the creation of dedicated centers of ONS excellence that would serve as means of access to novel technologies and facilitate research and education to further promote clinical acceptance and regulatory approval.[67]

REFERENCES

1. Shelden CH. Depolarization in the treatment of trigeminal neuralgia. Evaluation of compression and electrical methods; clinical concept of neurophysiological mechanism. In: Knighton RS, Dumke PR, editors. Pain. Boston: Little, Brown; 1966. p. 373–86.
2. Wall PD, Sweet WH. Temporary abolition of pain in man. Science 1967;155:108–9.
3. Slavin KV. History of peripheral nerve stimulation. Prog Neurol Surg 2011;24:1–5.
4. Picaza JA, Cannon BW, Hunter SE, et al. Pain suppression by peripheral nerve stimulation. II. Observations with implanted devices. Surg Neurol 1975;4:115–26.
5. Long DM, Erickson D, Campbell J, et al. Electrical stimulation of the spinal cord and peripheral nerves for pain control. A 10-year experience. Appl Neurophysiol 1981;44:207–17.
6. Waisbrod H, Panhans C, Hansen D, et al. Direct nerve stimulation for painful peripheral neuropathies. J Bone Joint Surg Br 1985;67:470–2.

7. Weiner RL, Reed KL. Peripheral neurostimulation for control of intractable occipital neuralgia. Neuromodulation 1999;2:217–21.
8. Slavin KV, Burchiel KJ. Use of long-term nerve stimulation with implanted electrodes in the treatment of intractable craniofacial pain. J Neurosurg 2000;92:576.
9. Weiner RL. The future of peripheral nerve stimulation. Neurol Res 2000;22:299–304.
10. Weiner RL, Aló KM, Reed KL, et al. Subcutaneous neurostimulation for intractable C-2–mediated headaches. J Neurosurg 2001;94:398A.
11. Hammer M, Doleys DM. Perineuromal stimulation in the treatment of occipital neuralgia: a case study. Neuromodulation 2001;4:47–51.
12. Jones RL. Occipital nerve stimulation using a Medtronic Resume II ® electrode array. Pain Physician 2003;6:507–8.
13. Oh MY, Ortega J, Bellotte JB, et al. Peripheral nerve stimulation for the treatment of occipital neuralgia and transformed migraine using a C1-2-3 subcutaneous paddle style electrode: a technical report. Neuromodulation 2004;7:103–12.
14. Kapural L, Mekhail N, Hayek SM, et al. Occipital nerve electrical stimulation via the midline approach and subcutaneous surgical leads for treatment of severe occipital neuralgia: a pilot study. Anesth Analg 2005;101:171–4.
15. Saper JR, Dodick DW, Silberstein SD, et al, ONSTIM Investigators. Occipital nerve stimulation for the treatment of intractable chronic migraine: ONSTIM feasibility study. Cephalalgia 2011;31:271–85.
16. Lipton RB, Goadsby PJ, Cady RK, et al. PRISM study: occipital nerve stimulation for treatment-refractory migraine. Cephalalgia 2009;29(Suppl 1):30.
17. Silberstein SD, Dodick DW, Saper J, et al. Safety and efficacy of peripheral nerve stimulation of the occipital nerves for the management of chronic migraine: results from a randomized, multicenter, double-blinded, controlled study. Cephalalgia 2012;32:1165–79.
18. Birk DM, Yin D, Slavin KV. Regulation of peripheral nerve stimulation technology. Prog Neurol Surg 2015;29:225–37.
19. Sweet JA, Mitchell LS, Narouze S, et al. Occipital nerve stimulation for the treatment of patients with medically refractory occipital neuralgia: Congress of Neurological Surgeons systematic review and evidence-based guideline. Neurosurgery 2015;77:332–41.
20. Slavin KV, Nersesyan H, Wess C. Peripheral neurostimulation for treatment of intractable occipital neuralgia. Neurosurgery 2006;58:112–9.
21. Johnstone CS, Sundaraj R. Occipital nerve stimulation for the treatment of occipital neuralgia—eight case studies. Neuromodulation 2006;9:41–7.
22. Magown P, Garcia R, Beauprie I, et al. Occipital nerve stimulation for intractable occipital neuralgia: an open surgical technique. Clin Neurosurg 2009;56:119–24.
23. Weiner RL. Occipital neurostimulation (ONS) for treatment of intractable headache disorders. Pain Med 2006;7:S137–9.
24. Schwedt TJ, Dodick DW, Hentz J, et al. Occipital nerve stimulation for chronic headache—Long-term safety and efficacy. Cephalalgia 2007;27:153–7.
25. Rodrigo-Royo MD, Azcona JM, Quero J, et al. Peripheral neurostimulation in the management of cervicogenic headaches: four case reports. Neuromodulation 2005;4:241–8.
26. Burns B. 'Dual' occipital and supraorbital nerve stimulation for primary headache. Cephalalgia 2010;30:257–9.
27. Royster EI, Crumbley K. Initial experience with implanted peripheral nerve stimulation for the treatment of refractory cephalgia. Ochsner J 2011;11:147–50.
28. Rogers LL, Swidan S. Stimulation of the occipital nerve for the treatment of migraine: current state and future prospects. Acta Neurochir Suppl 2007;97(Pt 1):121–8.
29. Popeney CA, Aló KM. Peripheral neurostimulation for the treatment of chronic, disabling transformed migraine. Headache 2003;43:369–75.
30. Hagen JE, Bennett DS. Occipital nerve stimulation for treatment of migraine. Pract Pain Manag 2007;7(6):43–5, 56.
31. Reed KL, Black SB, Banta CJ II, et al. Combined occipital and supraorbital neurostimulation for the treatment of chronic migraine headaches: initial experience. Cephalalgia 2010;30:260–71.
32. Matharu MS, Bartsch WN, Frackowiak RSJ, et al. Central neuromodulation in chronic migraine patients with suboccipital stimulators: a PET study. Brain 2004;127:220–30.
33. Serra R, Marchioretto R. Occipital nerve stimulation for chronic migraine: a randomized trial. Pain Physician 2012;15:245–53.
34. Sharan A, Huh B, Narouze S, et al. Analysis of adverse events in the management of chronic migraine by peripheral nerve stimulation. Neuromodulation 2015;18:305–12.
35. Dodick DW, Silberstein SD, Reed KL, et al. Safety and efficacy of peripheral nerve stimulation of the occipital nerves for the management of chronic migraine: long-term results from a randomized, multicenter, double-blinded, controlled study. Cephalalgia 2015;35:344–58.
36. Schwedt TJ, Green AL, Dodick DW. Occipital nerve stimulation for migraine: update from recent multicenter trials. Prog Neurol Surg 2015;29:117–26.

37. Schwedt TJ, Dodick DW, Trentman TL, et al. Occipital nerve stimulation for chronic cluster headache and hemicrania continua: pain relief and persistence of autonomic features. Cephalalgia 2006;26:1025–7.
38. Burns B, Watkins L, Goadsby PJ. Treatment of medically intractable cluster headache by occipital nerve stimulation: long-term follow-up of eight patients. Lancet 2007;369:1099–106.
39. Magis D, Allena M, Bolla M, et al. Occipital nerve stimulation for drug-resistant chronic cluster headache: a prospective pilot study. Lancet Neurol 2007;6:314–21.
40. Leone M, Franzini A, Cecchini AP, et al. Stimulation of occipital nerve for drug-resistant chronic cluster headache. Lancet Neurol 2007;6:289–91.
41. Burns B, Watkins L, Goadsby PJ. Treatment of intractable chronic cluster headache by occipital nerve stimulation in 14 patients. Neurology 2009; 72:341–5.
42. Thimineur M, De Ridder D. C2 area neurostimulation: a surgical treatment for fibromyalgia. Pain Med 2007;8:639–46.
43. Slavin KV. Peripheral neurostimulation in fibromyalgia: a new frontier?! Pain Med 2007;8:621–2.
44. Plazier M, Vanneste S, Dekelver I, et al. Peripheral nerve stimulation for fibromyalgia. Prog Neurol Surg 2011;24:133–46.
45. Plazier M, Dekelver I, Vanneste S, et al. Occipital nerve stimulation in fibromyalgia: a double-blind placebo-controlled pilot study with a six-month follow-up. Neuromodulation 2014;17:256–64.
46. Plazier M, Ost J, Stassijns G, et al. C2 nerve field stimulation for the treatment of fibromyalgia: a prospective, double-blind, randomized, controlled cross-over study. Brain Stimul 2015;8:751–7.
47. Smith BH, Torrance N, Ferguson JA, et al. Towards a definition of refractory neuropathic pain for epidemiological research. An international Delphi survey of experts. BMC Neurol 2012;12:29.
48. Trentman TL, Slavin KV, Freeman JA, et al. Occipital nerve stimulator placement via a retromastoid to infraclavicular approach: a technical report. Stereotact Funct Neurosurg 2010;88:121–5.
49. Jasper JF, Hayek SM. Implanted occipital nerve stimulators. Pain Physician 2008;11:187–200.
50. Falowski S, Wang D, Sabesan A, et al. Occipital nerve stimulator systems: review of complications and surgical techniques. Neuromodulation 2010; 13:121–5.
51. Massie L, Ali R, Slavin KV, et al. Concurrent placement of bilateral suboccipital and supraorbital nerve stimulators using On-Q* tunneler: technical note. Oper Neurosurg (Hagerstown) 2018. https://doi.org/10.1093/ons/opy036.
52. Tubbs RS, Mortazavi MM, Loukas M, et al. Anatomical study of the third occipital nerve and its potential role in occipital headache/neck pain following midline dissections of the craniocervical junction. J Neurosurg Spine 2011;15:71–5.
53. Skaribas I, Aló K. Ultrasound imaging and occipital nerve stimulation. Neuromodulation 2010;13:126–30.
54. Eldrige JS, Obray JB, Pingree MJ, et al. Occipital neuromodulation: ultrasound guidance for peripheral nerve stimulator implantation. Pain Pract 2010; 10:580–5.
55. Slavin KV, Colpan ME, Munawar N, et al. Trigeminal and occipital peripheral nerve stimulation for craniofacial pain: a single-institution experience and review of the literature. Neurosurg Focus 2006;21(6):E5.
56. Gofeld M. Anchoring of suboccipital lead: case report and technical note. Pain Pract 2004;4:307–9.
57. Franzini A, Messina G, Leone M, et al. Occipital nerve stimulation (ONS). Surgical technique and prevention of late electrode migration. Acta Neurochir (Wien) 2009;151:861–5.
58. Trentman TL, Mueller JT, Shah DM, et al. Occipital nerve stimulator lead pathway length changes with volunteer movement: an in vitro study. Pain Pract 2010;10:42–8.
59. Palmisani S, Al-Kaisy A, Arcioni R, et al. A six year retrospective review of occipital nerve stimulation practice - controversies and challenges of an emerging technique for treating refractory headache syndromes. J Headache Pain 2013;14:67–76.
60. Abhinav K, Park ND, Prakash SK, et al. Novel use of narrow paddle electrodes for occipital nerve stimulation—technical note. Neuromodulation 2013;16:607–9.
61. Melvin EA Jr, Jordan FR, Weiner RL, et al. Using peripheral stimulation to reduce the pain of C2-mediated occipital headaches: a preliminary report. Pain Physician 2007;10:453–60.
62. Slavin KV. Peripheral nerve stimulation for neuropathic pain. Neurotherapeutics 2008;5:100–6.
63. Burns B, Watkins L, Goadsby PJ. Treatment of hemicrania continua by occipital nerve stimulation with a Bion device: long-term follow-up of a crossover study. Lancet Neurol 2008;7:1001–12.
64. Trentman TL, Rosenfeld DM, Vargas BB, et al. Greater occipital nerve stimulation via the Bion microstimulator: implantation technique and stimulation parameters. Clinical trial: NCT00205894. Pain Physician 2009;12:621–8.
65. Perryman LT, Speck B, Weiner RL. A novel wireless minimally invasive neuromodulation device for the treatment of chronic intractable occipital neuralgia: case illustrations. J Neurol Stroke 2017;6:00213.
66. Slavin KV, Yin D. The use of simulation in the training for spinal cord stimulation for treatment of chronic pain. In: Alaraj A, editor. Comprehensive healthcare simulation: neurosurgery. New York: Springer Intl; 2018. p. 131–7.
67. Levy RM. Centers of excellence for neuromodulation: a critical proposal. Neuromodulation 2014;17: 1–9.

Vagus Nerve Stimulation for the Treatment of Epilepsy

Hernán F.J. González, MS[a,b,*], Aaron Yengo-Kahn, MD[c], Dario J. Englot, MD, PhD[a,b,d,e]

KEYWORDS

• Epilepsy • Seizures • Epilepsy surgery • Neuromodulation • Vagus nerve stimulator

KEY POINTS

- Vagus nerve stimulation (VNS) treatment is an efficacious surgical intervention for patients aged 4 years and older with pharmacoresistant epilepsy who cannot receive or failed resective surgery.
- After more than 2 years of VNS, approximately 8% of patients achieve seizure freedom, and approximately 50% have at least 50% reduced seizure frequency.
- Serious adverse events with VNS, such as device infection, are rare.

INTRODUCTION

Approximately 50 million people worldwide suffer from epilepsy, and approximately 30% to 40% of these persons have seizures that are refractory to treatment with antiepileptic medication.[1–3] Surgical resection or ablation can result in seizure freedom in well-chosen patients; however, not all persons with epilepsy are candidates for epilepsy surgery.[3] Furthermore, despite careful selection, some patients may continue to experience seizures postoperatively.[4–6] In patients whose seizures are inadequately controlled, neuromodulation-based interventions should be considered.[7] Vagus nerve stimulation (VNS) is one of the most common neuromodulation-based approaches. The VNS system is a battery-powered device that resembles a cardiac pacemaker (**Fig. 1**). The VNS consists of an implanted pulse generator implanted below the clavicle and lead that is wrapped around the left vagus nerve in the carotid sheath. Although complete seizure freedom with VNS therapy is rare, it may be beneficial in reducing seizure frequency and improving quality of life (QOL).[7]

Several important and early studies of VNS on brain activity were conducted by Bailey and Bremmer in 1938 and by Dell and Olson in 1951.[8–10] These studies proposed that stimulation of the vagus nerve affected cortical activity by way of nucleus tractus solitarii projections to other brainstem nuclei, such as the locus coeruleus and raphe magnus, which project diffusely to the cortex.[8] It has been proposed that VNS exhibits antiepileptic therapy by decreasing interictal events and by desynchronizing cortical activity.[11–13]

Disclosure Statement: This work was supported by the NIH-NINDS R00NS097618 and NIH-NINDS F31NS106735.
[a] Department of Biomedical Engineering, Vanderbilt University Medical Center, 1500 21st Avenue South, 4340 Village at Vanderbilt, Nashville, TN 37232-8618, USA; [b] Vanderbilt University Institute of Imaging Science, Vanderbilt University Medical Center, 1500 21st Avenue South, 4340 Village at Vanderbilt, Nashville, TN 37232-8618, USA; [c] Department of Neurological Surgery, Vanderbilt University Medical Center, 1121 21st Avenue South, Medical Center North, T4224, Nashville, TN 37232, USA; [d] Department of Neurological Surgery, Vanderbilt University Medical Center, 1500 21st Avenue South, 4340 Village at Vanderbilt, Nashville, TN 37232-8618, USA; [e] Department of Radiology and Radiological Sciences, Vanderbilt University Medical Center, 1500 21st Avenue South, 4340 Village at Vanderbilt, Nashville, TN 37232-8618, USA
* Corresponding author. 1500 21st Avenue South, 4340 Village at Vanderbilt, Nashville, TN 37232-8618.
E-mail address: hernan.gonzalez@vanderbilt.edu

Neurosurg Clin N Am 30 (2019) 219–230
https://doi.org/10.1016/j.nec.2018.12.005

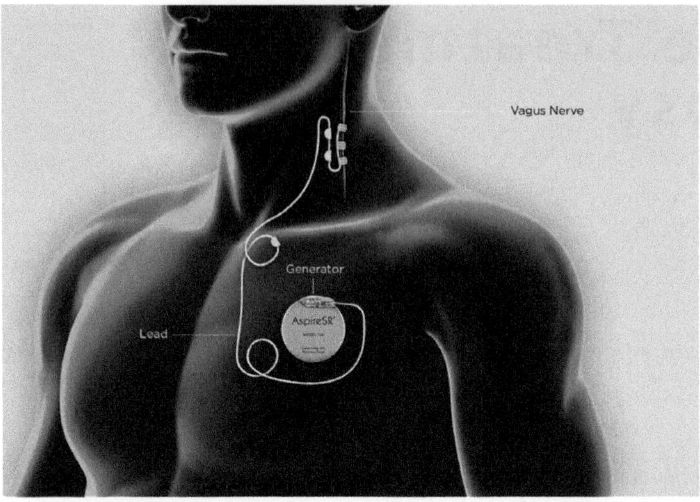

Fig. 1. AspireSR VNS system consists of implanted pulse generator surgically implanted beneath clavicle and lead wrapped around left vagus nerve. (*Courtesy of* LivaNova, Inc, Houston, TX.)

Zabara additionally showed that anticonvulsant effects of VNS lasted at least 4 times the duration of stimulation.[12,14,15] Zabara and Reese developed the first generation of the vagus nerve stimulator through their newly incorporated company Cyberonics in 1987 (now LivaNova). In 1988, Bell implanted the first VNS, the neurocybernetic prosthesis, at Wake Forest University.[8,16] In July 1997, the United States Food and Drug Administration (FDA) approved VNS as adjunctive therapy for adults and adolescents (older than 12 years old) with partial-onset seizures that are refractory to antiepileptic medications. More recently, the FDA has expanded VNS approval as an adjunctive treatment in patients 4 years and older with partial-onset seizures refractory to medications.[17] Since its original approval more than 20 years ago, more than 100,000 patients have been implanted with VNS.[18]

SHORT-TERM OUTCOMES OF VAGUS NERVE STIMULATION FROM RANDOMIZED CONTROLLED TRIALS

Efficacy of VNS for the treatment of epilepsy has been examined in 4 blinded, randomized controlled trials (class I data), which are summarized in **Table 1**.[19–23] In a 1994 study led by Ben-Menachem and colleagues,[19] 114 patients with partial epilepsy were randomized at multiple centers. These patients received either high-frequency (therapeutic) or low-frequency (sham) stimulation paradigms. At a 3-month follow-up, this study reported that high-frequency stimulation reduced seizure frequency by 25% and low-frequency stimulation reduced seizure frequency by 6%. A responder to VNS therapy is commonly defined as seizure frequency reduction by at least 50%, a definition used from this point forward.[24] In this study, 31% of patients receiving high-frequency stimulation achieved responder status.[19]

In a subsequent multicenter randomized controlled trial, Handforth and colleagues[20] randomized 196 patients with partial epilepsy to receive either high-frequency stimulation or sham stimulation. Patients with high-frequency stimulation achieved 28% reduced seizure frequency whereas those with sham stimulation had a 15% decrease. Overall, 23% of those receiving therapeutic stimulation (high-frequency) achieved responder status at the 3-month postoperative follow-up.[20] Amar and colleagues[21] provided further evidence of VNS efficacy with the publication of a randomized controlled trial of VNS implantation in 17 persons, resulting in 57% of patients achieving responder status.

In the first randomized controlled trial for children with intractable epilepsy, Klinkenberg and colleagues[23] randomized patients with partial (N = 35) or generalized epilepsy (N = 6) to high-output stimulation (maximum 1.75 mA) or low-output stimulation (0.25 mA) for 20 weeks, followed by an add-on period of 19 weeks of high-output stimulation for all patients. At the end of the randomized controlled blinded period, 16% of patients receiving high stimulation and 21% of patients receiving low stimulation achieved responder status. After the add-on phase, 26% of patients experienced at least 50% reduced seizure frequency.[23] In summary, blinded randomized controlled trials for both children and adults with intractable epilepsy have demonstrated that

Table 1
Class I, class II, and class III evidence of vagus nerve stimulation efficacy in epilepsy treatment

Class I Evidence: Blinded, Randomized Controlled Trials							
Study	**N**	**Seizure Type**	**Comparison**	**Follow-up**	**Number of Centers**	**Mean Seizure Reduction, %**	**Patients With Greater Than 50% Reduction, %[a]**
Ben-Menachem et al,[19] 1994	114	Partial	High vs low stim.	3 mo	Multi	25 (high) vs 6 (low)	31
Handforth et al,[20] 1998	196	Partial	High vs low stim.	3 mo	Multi	28 (high) vs 15 (low)	23
Amar et al,[21] 1998	17	Partial	High vs low stim.	3 mo	Single	71 (high) vs 6 (low)	57
Klinkenberg et al,[23] 2012	41	Mixed	High vs low stim.	3 mo	Single	16 (high) vs 21 (low)	26[b]
Class II Evidence: Nonblinded, Randomized Controlled Trials							
Study	**N**	**Seizure Type**	**Comparison**	**Follow-up**	**Number of Centers**	**Median Seizure Reduction, %**	**Patients with Greater Than 50% Reduction, %**
Scherrmann et al,[25] 2001	28	Mixed	2 Stim. paradigms	NR	Single	30 (overall)	45
DeGiorgio et al,[26] 2005	61	Partial	3 Stim. paradigms	3 mo	Multi	26 (overall)	29
Class III Evidence: Prospective Observational Studies (>10 Patients)							
Study	**N**	**Seizure Type**	**Notes**	**Follow-up**	**Number of Centers**	**Mean or Median Seizure Reduction, %**	**Patients with Greater Than 50% Reduction, %**
Ben-Manachem et al,[56] 1999	64	Mixed		3–64 mo	Single	NR	45
Parker et al,[57] 1999	15	Mixed	Children with encephalopathy	1 y	Single	17	27
Labar et al,[58] 1999	24	Gen		3 mo	Single	46	46
DeGiorgio et al,[44] 2000	195	Mixed		12 mo	Multi	45	35
Chavel et al,[59] 2003	29	Partial		1–2 y	Single	53	54 (at 1 y)
Vonck et al,[60] 1999; Vonck et al,[61] 2004	118	Mixed		>6 mo	Multi	55	50
Majoie et al,[62] 2001; Majoie et al,[63] 2005	19	Mixed	Children with encephalopathy	2 y	Single	20.6	21
Huf et al,[64] 2005	40	NR	Low IQ adults	2 y	Single	26	28

(continued on next page)

Table 1
(continued)

Class III Evidence: Prospective Observational Studies (>10 Patients)							
Study	**N**	**Seizure Type**	**Notes**	**Follow-up**	**Number of Centers**	**Mean or Median Seizure Reduction, %**	**Patients with Greater Than 50% Reduction, %**
Kang et al,[65] 2006	16	Mixed	children	>1 y	Multi	50	50
Ardesch et al,[66] 2007	19	Partial		>2 y	Single	25 (at 2 y)	33 (at 2 y)
Ryvlin et al,[67] 2014	112	Partial	VNS + BMP vs BMP	2 y	Multi	23 (at 1 y)	32 (at 1 y)
Fisher et al,[42] 2016	20	Mixed	AutoStim trial	1 y	Multi	47.3	50
Boon et al,[43] 2015	31	Mixed	AutoStim trial	1 y	Multi	NR	29.6

Abbreviations: BMP, best medical practice; Gen, generalized; Multi, multiple; NR, not reported; Stim, Stimulation.
[a] Refers to "high" stimulation group only.
[b] Refers to add-on period results with all participants switched to high-stimulation.
Adapted from Englot DJ, Chang EF, Auguste KI. Vagus nerve stimulation for epilepsy: a meta-analysis of efficacy and predictors of response. J Neurosurg 2011;115(6):1250; with permission.

23% to 57% of patients typically achieve 50% seizure reduction with VNS implantation in short-term follow-up.[19–21,23]

Additionally, these conclusions are supported by 2 nonblinded randomized controlled trials (class II data [**Table 1**]) comparing VNS stimulation parameters. The first, a single-center study, was conducted by Scherrmann and colleagues[25] and included 28 patients, and the second, a multicenter study, was performed by DeGiorgio and colleagues[26] and included 61 patients. Scherrmann and colleagues[25] reported median seizure reduction of 30% and that 45% of patients achieved responder status. DeGiorgio and colleagues[26] reported a median seizure reduction of 26% and that 29% of patients achieved responder status.

LONG-TERM SEIZURE OUTCOMES FOR VAGUS NERVE STIMULATION FROM RETROSPECTIVE AND PROSPECTIVE COHORT STUDIES

Long-term studies, including 13 prospective observational studies (class III data [see **Table 1**]), have shown progressive increases in response to VNS with increased duration of implant.[22,24,27] These studies included between 16 patients and 95 patients and follow-up periods of 3 months to 64 months. As seen in **Table 1**, results from these studies report a median seizure reduction rate between 17% and 55% and responder rates between 21% and 54%. To further evaluate VNS response rate over time, 1 group conducted a review of VNS therapy patient outcome registry data and literature review, including 5554 patients and 2869 patients respectively.[27] From registry data, 49% of patients were responders to therapy and 5.1% of patients were seizure-free at zero to 4 months postimplantation. Subsequently, at 24 months to 48 months, 63% of patients were responders with 8.2% achieving seizure freedom. The authors' literary review yielded similar results (**Fig. 2**), with 40% of patients responders at zero to 4 months (2.6% seizure-free), and 60.1% of patients responded to therapy at last follow-up (8.0% seizure-free).[27] These studies, however, are not controlled in nature and, therefore, may be susceptible to selection bias and can overestimate long-term favorable outcomes, because patients not receiving response may be less likely to continue therapy.

QUALITY-OF-LIFE OUTCOMES IN VAGUS NERVE STIMULATION

The most important predictor for QOL in patients with epilepsy is freedom from seizures.[28] As discussed previously, VNS only leads to seizure

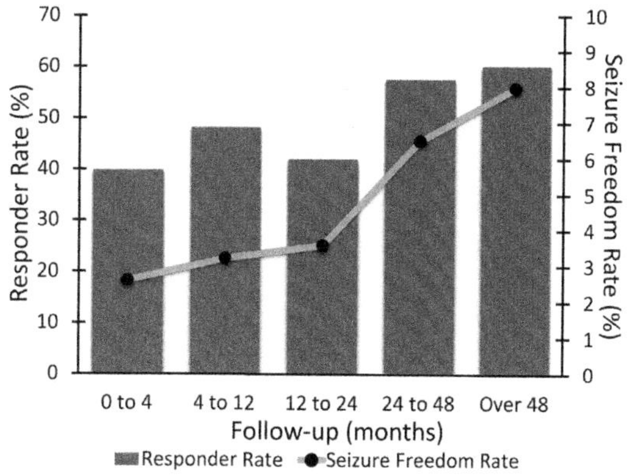

Fig. 2. VNS seizure freedom rate and responder rate from systematic literature review. These data, from 2869 patients across 78 studies, show increases in both responder rate and seizure freedom rate over time. At last follow-up, 60% of patients achieved responder status to VNS and 8% of patients were seizure-free. N = 650 patients, 405 patients, 1503 patients, 876 patients, and 326 patients at each follow-up period, respectively. (*From* Englot DJ, Rolston JD, Wright CW, et al. Rates and predictors of seizure freedom with vagus nerve stimulation for intractable epilepsy. Neurosurgery 2015;79(3):348; with permission.)

freedom in approximately 8% of patients.[27] Therefore, understanding other QOL outcomes in epilepsy patients with VNS has helped providers to better advise patients about this treatment. One study specifically evaluated QOL metrics in 5000 patients using the VNS therapy patient outcome registry.[29] In general, this group reported that use of VNS for medically refractory epilepsy was associated with many QOL improvements. These findings were based, however, on data subjectively recorded by treating physicians and, therefore, are susceptible to bias. Specifically, this study reported that patients experienced improvements in alertness (58%–63%), postictal state (55%–62%), cluster seizures (48%–62%), mood change (43%–49%), verbal communications (38%–45%), school/professional achievements (29%–39%), and memory (29%–38%).[29] Additional benefits include reduced sudden unexpected death in epilepsy rates over time with VNS therapy.[30] Improvements in QOL metrics have been seen in both responders and nonresponders and in adults and children.[29,31] Unlike seizure frequency, QOL metrics were not found to improve over time (as seen in **Fig. 3**),[29] which may imply that benefit from VNS is not due solely to effects on seizure frequency or may reflect study bias.

FACTORS ASSOCIATED WITH OUTCOME

As with resective surgery, optimal patient selection plays a central role in predicting outcomes of VNS

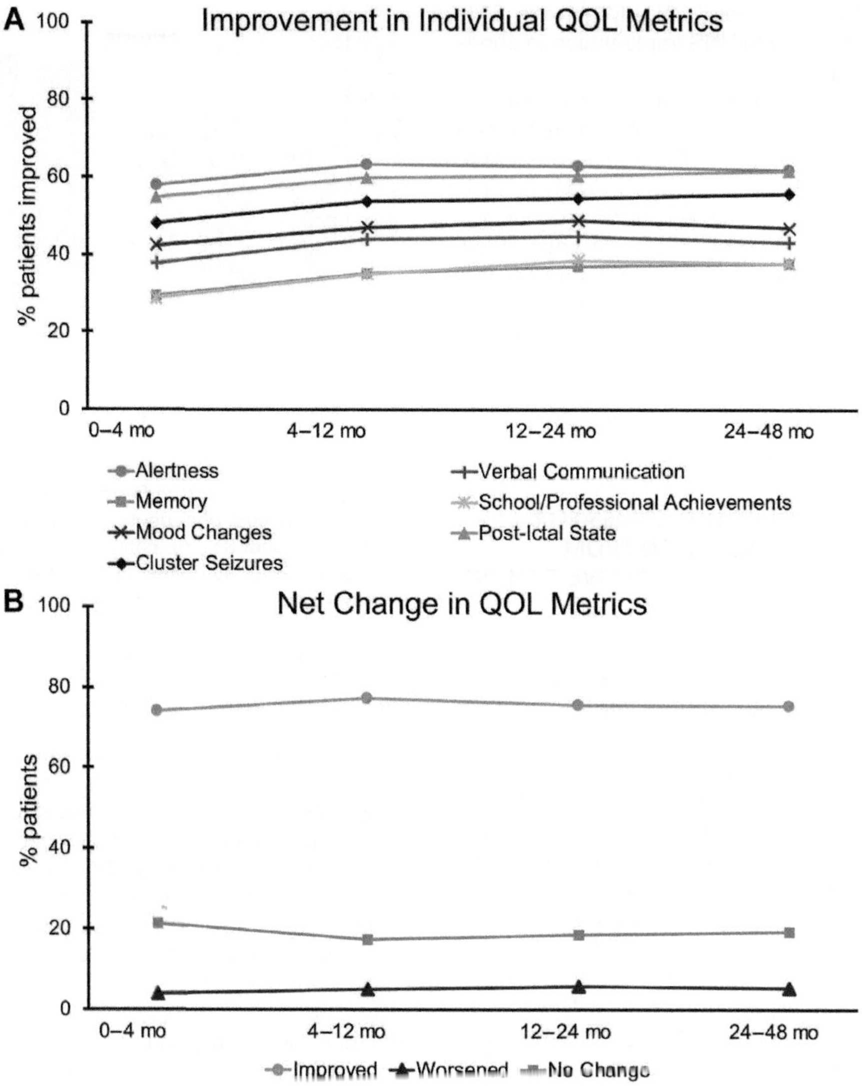

Fig. 3. QOL metrics for patients with VNS. (*A*) When examined individually, multiple metrics of QOL show improvement in patients with VNS as rated subjectively by the treating physician. (*B*) Overall, across all 7 subject QOL metrics, there was no trend toward improvement over time with increased time of treatment. For (*A*) and (*B*), no significant trends over time were observed (F <11, *P*>.05 per metric, Bonferroni corrected). The "F value" statistics test the overall significance of the regression model. N = 4666 (0–4 months), 3277 (4–12 months), 3182 (12–24 months), and 1194 (24–48 months) patients. (*From* Englot DJ, Hassnain KH, Rolston JD, et al. Quality-of-life metrics with vagus nerve stimulation for epilepsy from provider survey data. Epilepsy Behav 2017;66:6; with permission.)

implantation, so understanding factors associated with outcome is imperative.[7,27,32] Currently, VNS is approved as adjunctive therapy in patients 4 years of age and older with partial-onset seizures refractory to medication.[17] Despite the narrow indications for use, VNS has been implemented for treatment of many types of patients with medically refractory epilepsy. A 2015 study of predictors of seizure freedom found that at 4 months to 48 months 8.2% of implanted patients became seizure-free.[27] Seizure freedom was predicted by age of epilepsy onset greater than 12 years of age (odds ratio [OR] 1.89%; 95% CI, 1.01–1.82) and by having a generalized seizure type (OR 1.38; 95% CI, 1.06–1.81). Overall patient response (greater than 50% seizure frequency reduction) was predicted by having nonlesional epilepsy (OR 1.38; 95% CI, 1.06–1.81) and approximately 60% all of patients were responders at last follow-up.[27]

Studies of patient groups not included in the original FDA approval (greater than 12 years of age with medically intractable partial epilepsy) have shown that VNS may be beneficial in a wide range of patients with medically refractory epilepsy. An example population that merits consideration are patients with posttraumatic epilepsy (PTE). PTE is a common consequence of traumatic brain injury and accounts for approximately 20% of symptomatic epilepsy cases.[33,34] These patients are often resistant to treatment with antiepileptic medications and may be unlikely to have a localizable lesion.[35] In a retrospective study, summarized in **Fig. 4**, patients with PTE who received VNS achieved greater seizure frequency reduction than patients with nontraumatic epilepsy both at 3-month follow-up (50% vs 46% fewer seizures) and 24-month follow-up (73% vs 57% fewer seizures).[36] Furthermore, patients with PTE had an overall responder rate of 78% at 24 months versus 61% in the nontraumatic epilepsy group.[36] Additionally, children (<18 years of age) and patients with less than 10 years of seizures have shown better response to VNS than adults or those with duration greater than 10 years respectively.[22] Another group that has shown favorable outcome with VNS is patients with Lennox-Gastaut syndrome, whose seizure types are typically considered primary generalized.[24,30] These findings indicate that further study of different patient characteristics may yield insight regarding which patients may have greater probability of experiencing a positive response to VNS therapy.

ICTAL TACHYCARDIA

Modern VNS systems have multiple programming options allowing customization of therapy delivery for individual patients. One common initial programming of VNS stimulation parameters consists

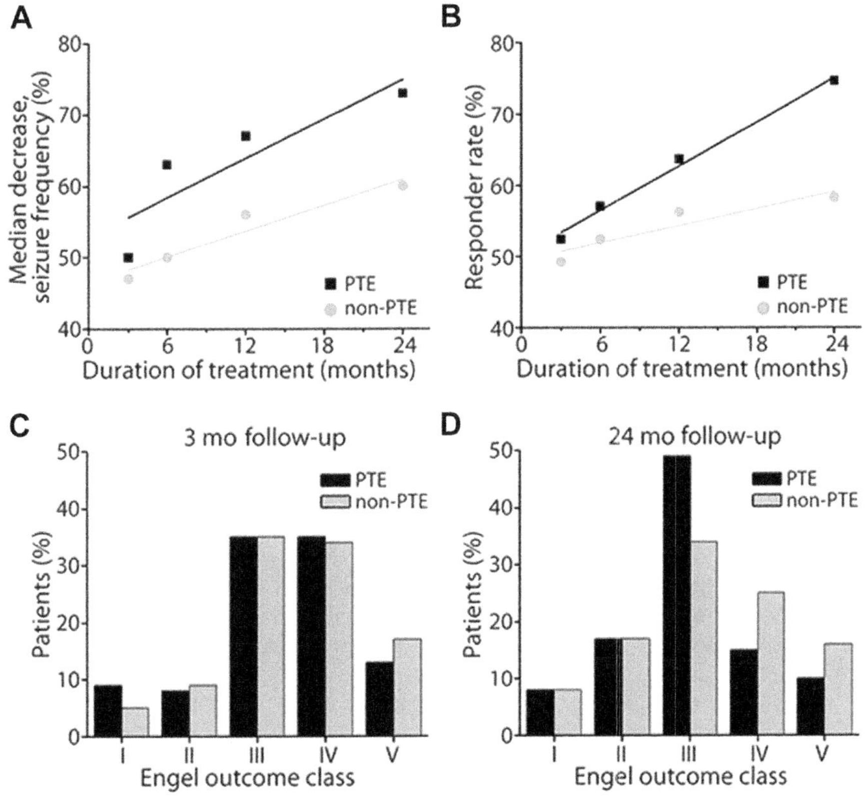

Fig. 4. Seizure outcomes after VNS treatment in patients with PTE versus patients with non–posttraumatic epilepsy. The median percent seizure frequency decrease (*A*) and the responder rates (*B*) are seen with VNS therapy at 3 months, 6 months, 12 months, and 24 months. Over time, the data show a trend toward improved seizure outcomes in PTE versus non-PTE patients. When examining Engel outcomes classes, little difference is found when comparing PTE with non-PTE patients at 3 months after VNS implantation (*C*). Twenty-four months after VNS (*D*), patients with PTE exhibit Engel class III more frequently and Engel class IV–V less frequently, when compared with non-PTE patients. The numbers of patients are 254, 158, 154, and 71 for those with PTE and 1449, 975, 878, and 364 for those with non-PTE at 3 months, 6 months, 12 months, and 24 months, respectively. (*From* Englot DJ, Rolston JD, Wang DD, et al. Efficacy of vagus nerve stimulation in posttraumatic versus nontraumatic epilepsy. J Neurosurg 2012;117(5):972; with permission.)

of open-loop stimulation cycles of 30 seconds of stimulation every 5 minutes.[37] Additionally, VNS allows user-initiated stimulation at or before the time of seizure onset with the VNS manual magnet mode.[37] With this manual stimulation initiated by patients or caregivers, some patients may experience benefits, such as aborted seizures or decreased postictal state.[30,38] Manual triggering of stimulation, however, may not always be feasible for a variety of reasons, such as lack of premonitory symptoms or seizures in sleep. An automated trigger for stimulation would address some barriers to manual stimulation at time of seizure. Heart rate is an easily measured extracranial biomarker for seizure detection that has been recently implemented into a VNS model.

Ictal tachycardia is defined as increase in heart rate above baseline that is associated with ictal events.[39,40] In a review of 34 articles, Eggleston and colleagues[40] reported that approximately 82% of patients with epilepsy experience ictal tachycardia. Furthermore, when examined by seizure type, 64% of generalized seizures and 71% of partial-onset seizures were associated with significant heart rate changes.[40] Previous research suggests that propagation of epileptic activity to the right insular cortex may be one mechanism for autonomic nervous system perturbations resulting in ictal heart rate fluctuations.[41] Using this knowledge of ictal tachycardia, the Model 106 VNS Therapy System (LivaNova) includes an automatic stimulation mode (AutoStim) that stimulates the vagus nerve on detecting tachycardia.[37,42,43]

The efficacy of the AutoStim mode has been studied in 2 multisite trials: 1 in the United States (E–37) and 1 in Europe (E–36).[42,43] Both of these studies defined ictal tachycardia as a heart rate of greater than 100 beats per minute during a seizure, with at least a 55% increase or 35 beats per minute increase from baseline heart rate.[42,43] The E–37 protocol was a prospective, unblinded United States multisite study of this feature in 20 patients with medically refractory partial-onset seizures and history of ictal tachycardia. At 12 months, Fisher and colleagues[42] report that QOL and seizure severity scores may improve with a responder rate of 50%. They noted that, during an inpatient observation period, approximately 43% of all seizures occurred with at least a 20% increase in heart rate compared with baseline heart rate and that complex partial seizures were most likely associated with higher heart rate increases.[42] During the E–36 trial, responder rate at 12 months was reported as 29.6%.[43] Extra stimulations triggered by ictal tachycardia did not significantly affect battery life, with measured duty cycles increasing from 11% to 16% with AutoStim activated in the E–37 trial.[42] There are 2 mechanisms to avoid false-positive results in the Model 106. First, to avoid false-positive results due to exercise, AutoStim is triggered by an increase from a baseline heart rate that is continually updated from a moving average. Therefore, although false-positive stimulations are possible at the beginning of an exercise session, these should subside once the baseline heart rate is updated to reflect increased heart rate of exercise. Second, a tachycardia detection threshold can be can be customized for each patient as increase from baseline heart rate of 20% to 70%.[37] Additionally, false-positive stimulations would not incur any additional risk of adverse events compared with the regularly scheduled stimulations patients receive with standard open-loop VNS. In summary, ictal tachycardia triggered VNS is at least as effective as standard open-loop VNS and may help abort or reduce severity of seizures in some patients.

ADVERSE EFFECTS AND COMPLICATIONS

Adverse events associated with VNS fall into 2 categories: (1) those associated with surgical implantation and (2) those associated with electrical stimulation.[14] The most common adverse effects of VNS, as summarized by 4 studies, are shown in **Table 2**.[19,20,23,44] In a recent large retrospective study of 247 primary VNS implants, Ben-Menachem and colleagues[45] examined adverse effects specific to the surgical implantation. This group reported a surgical complication rate of 8.6%, with the most common complications postoperative hematoma in 1.9%, infection in 2.6%, and vocal cord palsy in 1.4% of cases.[45] Across the studies in **Table 2** and others, hoarseness is the most prevalent adverse effect reported from stimulation.[22] Additionally, asystole or severe bradycardia has been described in few cases of VNS intraoperatively and postoperatively (0.06 events per 1000 patient years from July 1997 to March 2011).[24,46] Finally, some recent studies have suggested that there may be an association between VNS and sleep apnea; however, the latest American Academy of Neurology guidelines on VNS state that the clinical importance of this effect is still unclear.[30,47]

NONINVASIVE VAGUS NERVE STIMULATION

Implantable VNS is a safe and efficacious treatment of medically refractory epilepsy. Newer noninvasive VNS (nVNS) systems, however, posit to offer the advantage of avoiding most common

Table 2
Incidence of adverse effects of vagus nerve stimulation for epilepsy

	Ben-Menachem et al,[19] 1994	Handforth et al,[20] 1998	DeGiorgio et al,[44] 2000	Klinkenberg et al,[23] 2012
No. patients	114	196	195	41
Follow-up	3 mo	3 mo	1 y	3 mo
Hoarseness	37	62	55	19.5
Cough	7	21	15	7.3
Paresthesia	6	25	15	4.8
Pain	6	17	15	7.3
Dyspnea	6	16	13	NR
Headache	2	20	16	2.4
Infection	NR	4	6	4.8

Abbreviation: NR, not reported

Adapted from Englot DJ, Chang EF, Auguste KI. Vagus nerve stimulation for epilepsy: a meta-analysis of efficacy and predictors of response. J Neurosurg 2011;115(6):1253; with permission.

VNS-associated adverse events.[48] The primary advantage of the noninvasive-based treatment is avoiding surgery and therefore avoiding implantation-associated adverse events, such as infection and vocal cord paresis.[49] Additionally, nVNS claims to limit stimulation-related adverse events by allowing greater customization of stimulation paradigm.[48] NEMOS (cerbomed, Erlangen, Germany) is an external transcutaneous VNS available in Germany, Austria, Switzerland, and Italy.[49] NEMOS stimulates the auricular branch of the vagus nerve using an intra-auricular electrode. Patients can control their VNS stimulation during treatment sessions, which occur 3 times to 4 times a day, and may each last 1 hour to 4 hours, or they may stimulate before a seizure. In a proof-of-concept trial involving 10 patients with medically refractory epilepsy using 1-hour treatments 3 times a day, 5 patients reported some seizure frequency reductions, but none achieved 50% reduced seizure frequency.[50] A second nVNS device is the gammaCore device (electroCore, Basking Ridge, New Jersey), which has been studied for patients with chronic headache and migraine but not in patients with epilepsy.[51–53] The gammaCore device is a handheld portable stimulator with 2 stainless steel round discs that are placed on the skin to deliver electrical stimulation to the vagus nerve. In summary, the advantages of nVNSs are they avoid any adverse events associated with surgery for implantable VNSs and with less frequent stimulation may reduce the amount of stimulation-associated adverse events.[49] True efficacy of these nVNS devices, however, has yet to be proved for medically refractory epilepsy; therefore, implantable VNS currently remain the superior choice for seizure control.

FUTURE DIRECTIONS FOR VAGUS NERVE STIMULATION

Future directions for usage of VNS therapies are extensive. For the first 20 years of its use, VNS was FDA approved only for patients 12 years and older with medically refractory partial epilepsy. Recent changes, however, have expanded this approval to patients as young as 4 years old with medically refractory partial epilepsy.[17] As discussed previously, multiple studies have shown efficacy in patients outside of these categories, such as patients with generalized types of epilepsy or nonlocalizable PTE, and future approval for these patients may increase the number of people who benefit from VNS.[24,27,36] Additionally, future VNS systems with closed-loop seizure detection and responsive stimulation may provide additional benefit.[38] These VNS systems may resemble the responsive neurostimulation system (RNS) (Neuropace, Mountain View, California). Like the RNS, a closed-loop VNS not only may offer the benefits of seizure-onset–induced stimulation but also may also record and provide objective data on seizure frequency to help clinicians accurately assess response to treatment.[54]

SUMMARY

Patients with epilepsy are defined as medically refractory when they have failed to achieve seizure control with 2 or more antiepileptic medications.[3] These patients should be referred to a comprehensive epilepsy center for surgical evaluation.[7] Surgery remains underutilized, however, and on average, patients who are referred have already suffered from 20 years of poorly controlled seizures.[3,55] For patients with certain types of epilepsy, resective epilepsy surgery may result in seizure freedom.[3] Unfortunately, not all patients are candidates for resective surgery. Despite lower rates of seizure freedom, patients who are not candidates for resective surgery should still be offered surgical treatment with neuromodulation techniques, such as VNS therapy. With 2 years to 4 years of VNS therapy, approximately 8% of patients reach seizure freedom, and approximately 50% to 60% have at least 50% reduction in seizure frequency.[27] VNS has been used for more than 20 years in clinical practice and serves a vital role for patients with epilepsy who are poor surgical candidates, such as those with generalized or nonlocalizable epilepsy and individuals who have failed resection.[27]

REFERENCES

1. Behr C, Goltzene MA, Kosmalski G, et al. Epidemiology of epilepsy. Rev Neurol (Paris) 2016;172(1):27–36.
2. Engel J. What can we do for people with drug-resistant epilepsy? The 2016 Wartenberg Lecture. Neurology 2016;87(23):2483–9.
3. Wiebe S, Jette N. Pharmacoresistance and the role of surgery in difficult to treat epilepsy. Nat Rev Neurol 2012;8(12):669–77.
4. Englot DJ, Raygor KP, Molinaro AM, et al. Factors associated with failed focal neocortical epilepsy surgery. Neurosurgery 2014;75(6):648–56.
5. Englot DJ, Han SJ, Rolston JD, et al. Epilepsy surgery failure in children: a quantitative and qualitative analysis. J Neurosurg Pediatr 2014;14(4):386–95.
6. Englot DJ, Lee AT, Tsai C, et al. Seizure types and frequency in patients who "fail" temporal lobectomy for intractable epilepsy. Neurosurgery 2013;73(5):838–44.
7. Englot DJ. A modern epilepsy surgery treatment algorithm: Incorporating traditional and emerging technologies. Epilepsy Behav 2018;80:68–74.
8. Lulic D, Ahmadian A, Baaj AA, et al. Vagus nerve stimulation. Neurosurg Focus 2009;27(3):E5.
9. Bailey P, Bremer F. A sensory cortical representation of the vagus nerve: with a note on the effects of low blood pressure on the cortical electrogram. J Neurophysiol 1938;1(5):405–12.
10. Dell P, Olson R. Projections thalamiques, corticales et cérébelleuses des afférences viscérales vagales. Comptes rendus des séances de la Société de biologie et de ses filiales 1951;145(13–1):1084–8.
11. Zanchetti A, Wang SC, Moruzzi G. The effect of vagal afferent stimulation on the EEG pattern of the cat. Electroencephalogr Clin Neurophysiol 1952; 4(3):357–61.
12. Zabara J. Peripheral control of hypersynchronous discharge in epilepsy. Electroencephalogr Clin Neurophysiol 1985;61(3):S162.
13. Blum B, Magnes J, Bental E, et al. Electroencephalographic studies in cats with experimentally produced hippocampal epilepsy. Clin Neurophysiol 1961;13(3):340–53.
14. George MS, Aston-Jones G. Noninvasive techniques for probing neurocircuitry and treating illness: vagus nerve stimulation (VNS), transcranial magnetic stimulation (TMS) and transcranial direct current stimulation (tDCS). Neuropsychopharmacology 2010;35(1):301–16.
15. Zabara J. Inhibition of experimental seizures in canines by repetitive vagal stimulation. Epilepsia 1992;33(6):1005–12.
16. Terry RS, Tarver WB, Zabara J. The implantable neurocybernetic prosthesis system. Pacing Clin Electrophysiol 1991;14(1):86–93.
17. Medscape. FDA okays VNS therapy for epilepsy in children as young as 4 years 2017. Available at: https://www.medscape.com/viewarticle/882346.
18. Browne G. Cyberonics announces 100,000th patient implant of VNS therapy® 2012.
19. Ben-Menachem E, Manon-Espaillat R, Ristanovic R, et al. Vagus nerve stimulation for treatment of partial seizures: 1. A controlled study of effect on seizures. Epilepsia 1994;35(3):616–26.
20. Handforth A, DeGiorgio CM, Schachter SC, et al. Vagus nerve stimulation therapy for partial-onset seizures: a randomized active-control trial. Neurology 1998;51(1):48–55.
21. Amar AP, Heck CN, Levy ML, et al. An institutional experience with cervical vagus nerve trunk stimulation for medically refractory epilepsy: rationale, technique, and outcome. Neurosurgery 1998;43(6):1265–80.
22. Englot DJ, Chang EF, Auguste KI. Vagus nerve stimulation for epilepsy: a meta-analysis of efficacy and predictors of response. J Neurosurg 2011;115(6): 1248–55.
23. Klinkenberg S, Aalbers MW, Vles JS, et al. Vagus nerve stimulation in children with intractable epilepsy: a randomized controlled trial. Dev Med Child Neurol 2012;54(9):855–61.
24. Englot DJ, Chang EF, Auguste KI. Efficacy of vagus nerve stimulation for epilepsy by patient age, epilepsy duration, and seizure type. Neurosurg Clin N Am 2011;22(4):443–8.
25. Scherrmann J, Hoppe C, Kral T, et al. Vagus nerve stimulation: clinical experience in a large patient series. J Clin Neurophysiol 2001;18(5):408–14.
26. DeGiorgio C, Heck C, Bunch S, et al. Vagus nerve stimulation for epilepsy: randomized comparison of three stimulation paradigms. Neurology 2005;65(2):317–9.
27. Englot DJ, Rolston JD, Wright CW, et al. Rates and predictors of seizure freedom with vagus nerve stimulation for intractable epilepsy. Neurosurgery 2015; 79(3):345–53.
28. Taylor RS, Sander JW, Taylor RJ, et al. Predictors of health-related quality of life and costs in adults with

epilepsy: a systematic review. Epilepsia 2011; 52(12):2168–80.
29. Englot DJ, Hassnain KH, Rolston JD, et al. Quality-of-life metrics with vagus nerve stimulation for epilepsy from provider survey data. Epilepsy Behav 2017;66:4–9.
30. Morris GL, Gloss D, Buchhalter J, et al. Evidence-based guideline update: vagus nerve stimulation for the treatment of epilepsy Report of the Guideline Development Subcommittee of the American Academy of Neurology. Neurology 2013;81(16):1453–9.
31. Orosz I, McCormick D, Zamponi N, et al. Vagus nerve stimulation for drug-resistant epilepsy: a European long-term study up to 24 months in 347 children. Epilepsia 2014;55(10):1576–84.
32. Englot DJ, Chang EF. Rates and predictors of seizure freedom in resective epilepsy surgery: an update. Neurosurg Rev 2014;37(3):389–405.
33. Agrawal A, Timothy J, Pandit L, et al. Post-traumatic epilepsy: an overview. Clin Neurol Neurosurg 2006; 108(5):433–9.
34. Annegers JF, Coan SP. The risks of epilepsy after traumatic brain injury. Seizure 2000;9(7):453–7.
35. Garga N, Lowenstein DH. Posttraumatic epilepsy: a major problem in desperate need of major advances. Epilepsy Curr 2006;6(1):1–5.
36. Englot DJ, Rolston JD, Wang DD, et al. Efficacy of vagus nerve stimulation in posttraumatic versus nontraumatic epilepsy. J Neurosurg 2012;117(5): 970–7.
37. LivaNova-Inc. VNS therapy physician's manual 2017. Houstan (TX).
38. Fisher RS, Eggleston KS, Wright CW. Vagus nerve stimulation magnet activation for seizures: a critical review. Acta Neurol Scand 2015;131(1):1–8.
39. Stefanidou M, Carlson C, Friedman D. The relationship between seizure onset zone and ictal tachycardia: an intracranial EEG study. Clin Neurophysiol 2015;126(12):2255–60.
40. Eggleston KS, Olin BD, Fisher RS. Ictal tachycardia: the head-heart connection. Seizure 2014;23(7): 496–505.
41. Oppenheimer SM, Gelb A, Girvin JP, et al. Cardiovascular effects of human insular cortex stimulation. Neurology 1992;42(9):1727–32.
42. Fisher RS, Afra P, Macken M, et al. Automatic vagus nerve stimulation triggered by ictal tachycardia: clinical outcomes and device performance–the U.S. E-37 trial. Neuromodulation 2016;19(2):188–95.
43. Boon P, Vonck K, van Rijckevorsel K, et al. A prospective, multicenter study of cardiac-based seizure detection to activate vagus nerve stimulation. Seizure 2015;32:52–61.
44. DeGiorgio CM, Schachter SC, Handforth A, et al. Prospective long-term study of vagus nerve stimulation for the treatment of refractory seizures. Epilepsia 2000;41(9):1195–200.
45. Revesz D, Rydenhag B, Ben-Menachem E. Complications and safety of vagus nerve stimulation: 25 years of experience at a single center. J Neurosurg Pediatr 2016;18(1):97–104.
46. Iriarte J, Urrestarazu E, Alegre M, et al. Late-onset periodic asystolia during vagus nerve stimulation. Epilepsia 2009;50(4):928–32.
47. Marzec M, Edwards J, Sagher O, et al. Effects of vagus nerve stimulation on sleep-related breathing in epilepsy patients. Epilepsia 2003;44(7): 930–5.
48. Schulze-Bonhage A. Brain stimulation as a neuromodulatory epilepsy therapy. Seizure 2017;44: 169–75.
49. Ben-Menachem E, Revesz D, Simon BJ, et al. Surgically implanted and non-invasive vagus nerve stimulation: a review of efficacy, safety and tolerability. Eur J Neurol 2015;22(9):1260–8.
50. Stefan H, Kreiselmeyer G, Kerling F, et al. Transcutaneous vagus nerve stimulation (t-VNS) in pharmacoresistant epilepsies: a proof of concept trial. Epilepsia 2012;53(7):e115–8.
51. Barbanti P, Grazzi L, Egeo G, et al. Non-invasive vagus nerve stimulation for acute treatment of high-frequency and chronic migraine: an open-label study. J Headache Pain 2015;16:61.
52. Goadsby PJ, Grosberg BM, Mauskop A, et al. Effect of noninvasive vagus nerve stimulation on acute migraine: an open-label pilot study. Cephalalgia 2014;34(12):986–93.
53. Nesbitt AD, Marin JCA, Tompkins E, et al. Initial use of a novel noninvasive vagus nerve stimulator for cluster headache treatment. Neurology 2015; 84(12):1249–53.
54. Hoppe C, Poepel A, Elger CE. Epilepsy: accuracy of patient seizure counts. Arch Neurol 2007;64(11): 1595–9.
55. Englot DJ. The persistent under-utilization of epilepsy surgery. Epilepsy Res 2015;118:68.
56. Ben-Menachem E, Hellstrom K, Waldton C, et al. Evaluation of refractory epilepsy treated with vagus nerve stimulation for up to 5 years. Neurology 1999;52(6):1265–7.
57. Parker AP, Polkey CE, Binnie CD, et al. Vagal nerve stimulation in epileptic encephalopathies. Pediatrics 1999;103(4):778–82.
58. Labar D, Murphy J, Tecoma E. Vagus nerve stimulation for medication-resistant generalized epilepsy. E04 VNS Study Group. Neurology 1999;52(7): 1510–2.
59. Chavel SM, Westerveld M, Spencer S. Long-term outcome of vagus nerve stimulation for refractory partial epilepsy. Epilepsy Behav 2003;4(3): 302–9.
60. Vonck K, Boon P, D'Have M, et al. Long-term results of vagus nerve stimulation in refractory epilepsy. Seizure 1999;8(6):328–34.

61. Vonck K, Thadani V, Gilbert K, et al. Vagus nerve stimulation for refractory epilepsy: a transatlantic experience. J Clin Neurophysiol 2004;21(4):283–9.
62. Majoie HJ, Berfelo MW, Aldenkamp AP, et al. Vagus nerve stimulation in children with therapy-resistant epilepsy diagnosed as Lennox-Gastaut syndrome: clinical results, neuropsychological effects, and cost-effectiveness. J Clin Neurophysiol 2001;18(5): 419–28.
63. Majoie HJ, Berfelo MW, Aldenkamp AP, et al. Vagus nerve stimulation in patients with catastrophic childhood epilepsy, a 2-year follow-up study. Seizure 2005;14(1):10–8.
64. Huf RL, Mamelak A, Kneedy-Cayem K. Vagus nerve stimulation therapy: 2-year prospective open-label study of 40 subjects with refractory epilepsy and low IQ who are living in long-term care facilities. Epilepsy Behav 2005;6(3):417–23.
65. Kang HC, Hwang YS, Kim DS, et al. Vagus nerve stimulation in pediatric intractable epilepsy: a Korean bicentric study. Acta Neurochir Suppl 2006;99:93–6.
66. Ardesch JJ, Buschman HP, Wagener-Schimmel LJ, et al. Vagus nerve stimulation for medically refractory epilepsy: a long-term follow-up study. Seizure 2007;16(7):579–85.
67. Ryvlin P, Gilliam FG, Nguyen DK, et al. The long-term effect of vagus nerve stimulation on quality of life in patients with pharmacoresistant focal epilepsy: the PuLsE (open prospective randomized long-term effectiveness) trial. Epilepsia 2014; 55(6):893–900.

Responsive Neurostimulation for the Treatment of Epilepsy

Caio M. Matias, MD, PhD[a,b,*], Ashwini Sharan, MD[a],
Chengyuan Wu, MD, MSBME[a]

KEYWORDS

• Responsive stimulation • Closed-loop neurostimulation • Neuromodulation • Cortical stimulation
• Partial seizures • Focal seizures • Focal stimulation

KEY POINTS

- The RNS System is a programmable and responsive device that consists of depth or subdural strip leads, a pulse generator and an external programmer.
- The RNS System has an algorithm capable of detecting specific patterns of epileptogenic activity and triggering focal stimulation to interrupt the seizure.
- Responsive neurostimulation (RNS) is indicated for individuals greater than or equal to 18 years old, who have partial-onset seizures with no more than 2 epileptogenic foci, and who have 3 or more disabling seizures per month.
- The RNS System is an effective and safe treatment tool that works as an adjunctive therapy.
- In addition to seizure frequency reduction, RNS may have other applications, such as drug response evaluation and long-term electrocorticography recording.

INTRODUCTION

Approximately 1% of the world population is affected by epilepsy.[1] Antiepileptic drug (AED) treatment is considered the gold standard, but one-third of these patients do not achieve seizure freedom or they experience intolerable side effects from medical treatment.[2] For these patients with drug-resistant epilepsy (DRE), epilepsy surgery can be a therapeutic option and may lead to seizure freedom. Unfortunately, for a significant portion of DRE patients, the zone of ictal onset cannot be identified or lies within eloquent areas, precluding resective procedures. For this subset of patients, neuromodulation has emerged as an alternative treatment modality and includes vagal nerve stimulation, open-loop stimulation (eg, anterior thalamic deep brain stimulation), and closed-loop stimulation, such as the RNS System (NeuroPace, Mountain View, California). This review summarizes the available data in the literature regarding RNS for the treatment of DRE.

Disclosure Statement: Dr C.M. Matias has no conflicts of interest. Dr A.D. Sharan has the following disclosures: Cerebral Therapeutics (owner), Neurotargeting (owner), Mudjala (owner), Tigerlabs (owner), Neuspera (consultant), Boston Biomedical Association (consultant), Medtronic (fellowship support), Abbot (fellowship support), DARPA (grant), NIH (grant), Groff Foundation (grant), CNS (president), and NANS (past president). Dr C. Wu has the following disclosures: Medtronic Inc. (advisory board), Micro Systems Engineering Inc. (advisory board), NeuroPace Inc. (consultant), and Nevro Corp. (consultant).

[a] Department of Neurological Surgery, Thomas Jefferson University Hospitals, Philadelphia, PA, USA; [b] Department of Surgery and Anatomy, Ribeirão Preto Medical School, University of São Paulo, Ribeirão Preto, São Paulo, Brazil
* Corresponding author. Department of Neurological Surgery, Thomas Jefferson University Hospitals, 909 Walnut Street, Third Floor, Philadelphia, PA 19107.
E-mail address: caio.matias@jefferson.edu

Neurosurg Clin N Am 30 (2019) 231–242
https://doi.org/10.1016/j.nec.2018.12.006

THE RNS SYSTEM

The RNS System (**Fig. 1**A) comprises both implantable components—including a responsive neurostimulator (pulse generator) and depth and subdural strip leads—and external products, including a programmer, a patient remote monitor and magnet, and a database and Web-based database application:[3,4]

- The leads are platinum-iridium, with 4 contacts, and are available as depth leads (see **Fig. 1**B), designed for stereotactic implantation, and as strip leads (see **Fig. 1**C), designed for subdural implantation. **Fig. 1**D and E demonstrates an implantation combining 1 depth lead and 1 subdural strip lead.
- The pulse generator contains the electronics, battery, telemetry coil, and connection ports to the leads. The case of the pulse generator is curved to mimic the skull convexity. The pulse generator has several functions, including
  - Recording of electrographic activity. Electrocorticography (ECoG) storage can be set to specific start times or can be triggered by different mechanisms. For example, a magnet can be swiped by the patient over the neurostimulator when clinical symptoms occur, initiating ECoG capture. Other common mechanisms include the long episode, which initiates ECoG capture when a detected episode exceeds the

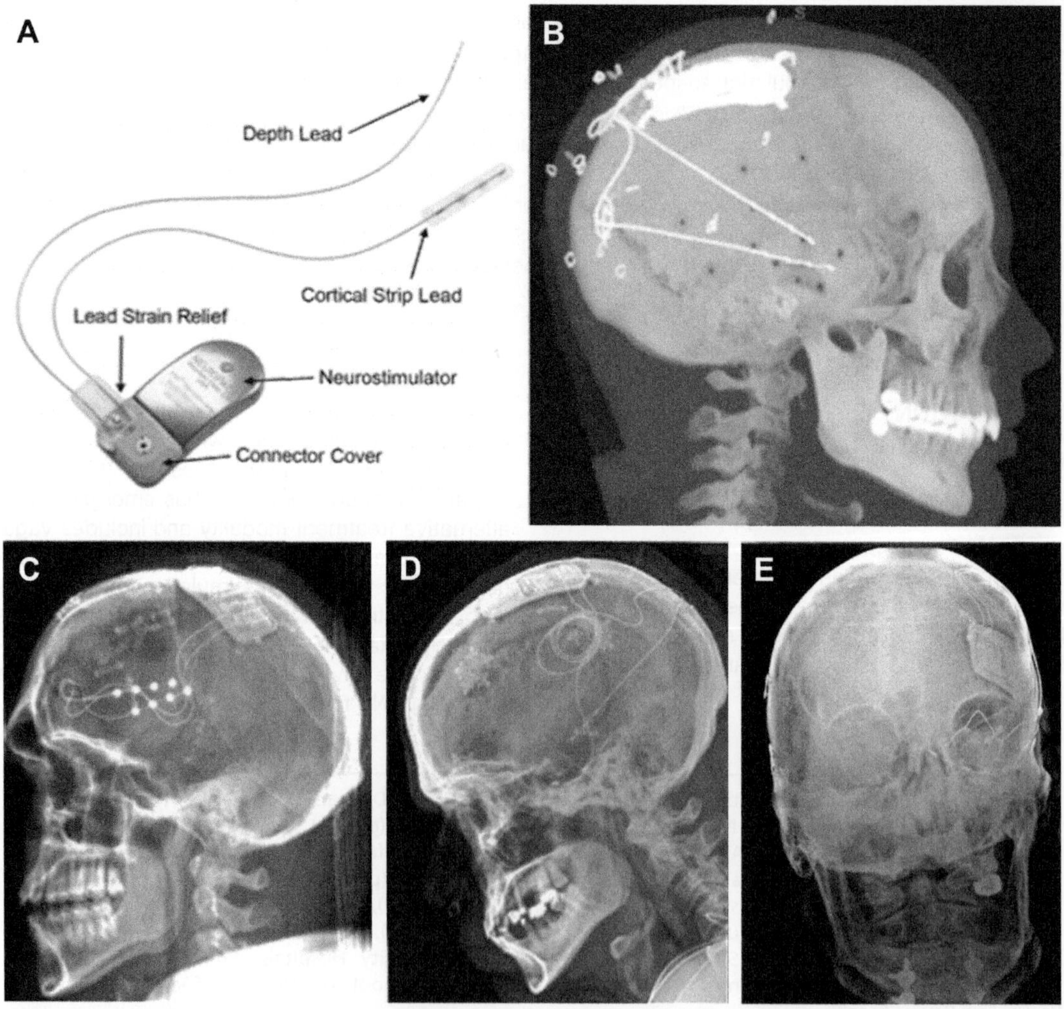

Fig. 1. (*A*) RNS System. (*B*) CT reconstruction showing a RNS System with depth leads implanted in the right insula and right hippocampus. (*C*) Radiograph (lateral view) of a RNS System with subdural strip leads implanted over the lateral surface the left frontal lobe. Radiographs: (*D*) lateral view and (*E*) anterior-posterior view of a RNS System with one subdural strip lead implanted under the left temporal lobe and one depth lead implanted in the left hippocampus. (*Courtesy of* [*A*] NeuroPace Inc., Mountain View, CA.)

episode length previously set, and the saturation mechanism, which triggers recording when ECoG amplitude exceeds a predefined threshold.[5] The RNS System has a limited memory capacity; however, several events can be recorded and analyzed by the clinician during follow-up visits:

- Detection of epileptogenic activity. The RNS System has an algorithm capable of detecting specific patterns of electrographic activity as defined by the clinician. Three seizure detection tools are available: line length, area, and bandpass (**Fig. 2**).
  - The line-length tool works by measuring the total length of the signal in a window of time and comparing it to line-length measurements of the recent past. Therefore, if there is a signal frequency or amplitude increase compared with the recent past, a detection is made.
  - The area tool works by measuring the area under the curve between the ECoG signal and the baseline. Similar to the line-length tool, the area tool works by measuring the area between the ECoG signal and baseline and compares it to the area measurements of the recent past.
  - The bandpass tool acts as a bandpass filter. The upper and lower frequencies of the filter and the minimum amplitude for detection are set by the clinician. Once the frequency and amplitude threshold requirements have been met for the selected window of time, a detection occurs.
- Therapeutic stimulation. Stimulation consists of biphasic square waves. Parameters, such as polarity, amplitude (0.5–12 mA), pulse width (40–1000 microseconds [μsec]), and frequency (1–333 Hz), can be adjusted and applied as monopolar or bipolar stimulation to any of the electrode contacts. Stimulation is triggered after the algorithm detects epileptogenic activity (**Fig. 3**).

• The programmer is a computer with a dedicated software and has a telemetry wand that communicates with the pulse generator. The software allows the clinician to analyze ECoG data, define electrographic patterns as interictal activity or ictal activity, and define stimulation thresholds. Data obtained from the device can be stored in the Patient Data Management System (PDMS), which can be accessed by authorized clinicians via a secure Web site.[5]

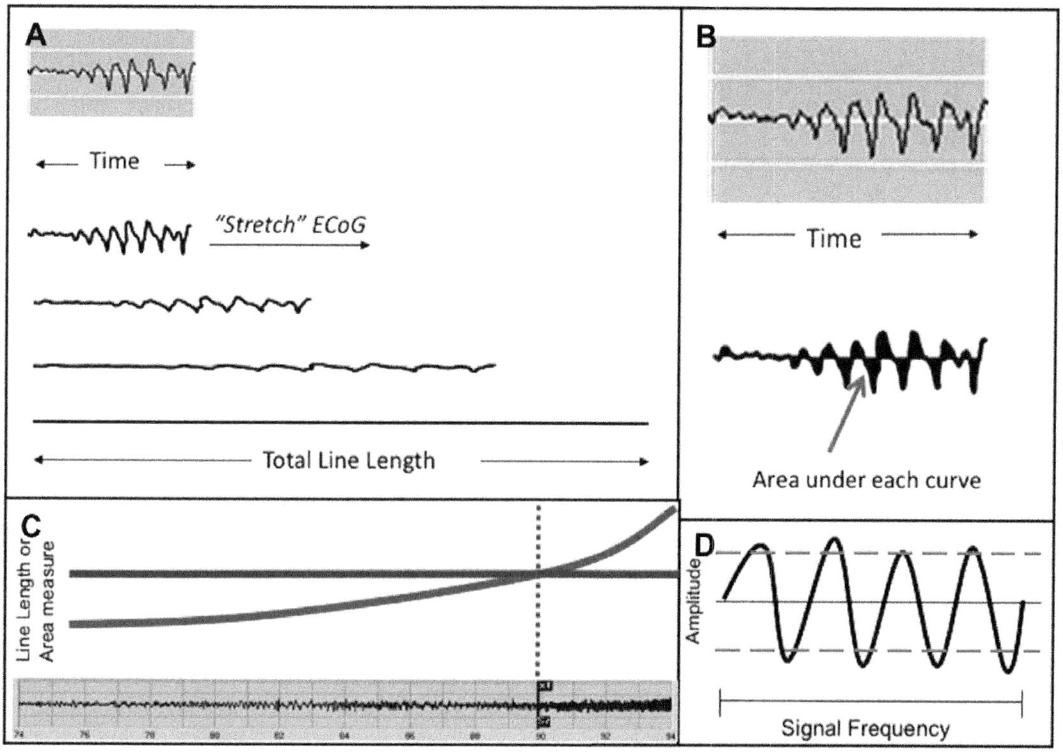

Fig. 2. Seizure detection tools. (*A*) Line-length tool. (*B*) Area tool. (*C*) Line-length and area tools comparing the current measurements to measurements of the recent past or the long-term trend. (*D*) Bandpass tool.

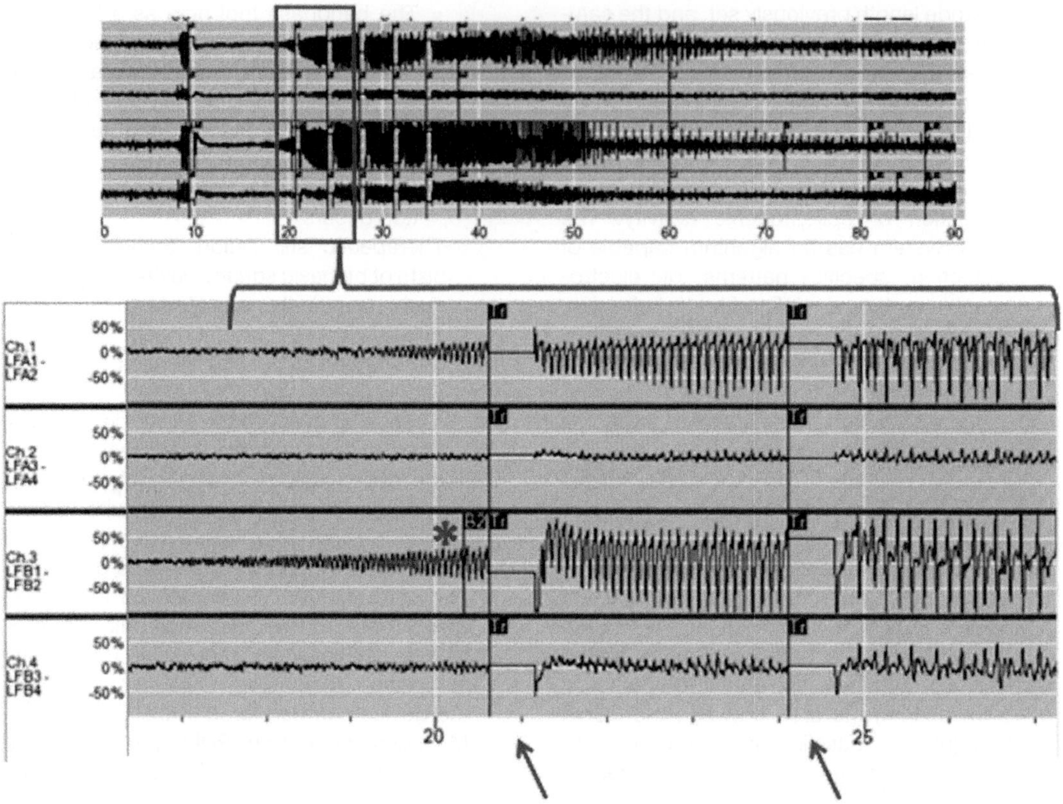

Fig. 3. ECoG example of detection of seizure onset (*asterisks*), triggering 2 sets of therapeutic stimulation (*arrows*).

SELECTION OF CANDIDATES FOR RESPONSIVE NEUROSTIMULATION

The RNS System is approved by the Food and Drug Administration (FDA)[5,6] for individuals with age equal or greater than 18 years old, as an adjunctive therapy in reducing the frequency of seizures. These patients must

- Be refractory to 2 or more AEDs
- Have frequent (average of 3 or more seizures per month, over the 3 most recent months) and disabling seizures, classified as motor partial seizures, complex partial seizures, and/or secondary generalized seizures
- Have undergone diagnostic testing that localized no more than 2 epileptogenic foci

Diagnostic work-up includes interictal surface electroencephalography (EEG), video-EEG monitoring, brain MRI, detailed neuropsychological evaluation, and, when necessary, ictal single-photon emission CT (SPECT), subtraction ictal SPECT coregistered with MRI studies, interictal PET (positron emission tomography), Wada tests, and invasive EEG (with depth and/or subdural electrodes).[3]

IMPLANTATION TECHNIQUE

The procedure is typically performed under general endotracheal anesthesia; however, for some cooperative patients, sedation with local anesthesia or field blocks of the scalp can be used.[3] The skin incisions are determined by the localization of the epileptogenic focus/foci and the entry point for the lead/leads, except for patients with previous incisions, which can be utilized or occasionally have to be adapted.

Depth Lead Implantation

The implantation of depth leads is performed with the aid of frame-based systems (eg, Leksell frame)[3] or frameless systems (eg, Nexframe [Medtronic Inc, Minneapolis, Minnesota]),[7] including robotic-assisted systems.[8,9] Using stereotactic planning software, the target is defined based on previous work-up, which defines the ictal onset zone and, consequently, the area to be stimulated to stop the seizure or to prevent its initiation. Planning is conducted following general stereotactic principles, such as a trajectory avoiding sulci, blood vessels, and ventricles, to prevent hemorrhage and brain shift. A burr hole is made using a high-speed drill and a plastic or peek secure device is fixed to the skull.[3,8] Alternatively, small-caliber holes, from previous stereo-EEG monitoring can be used with the advantage of keeping the bone opening aligned with the desired electrode trajectory.[10] For this technique, the lead can be secured using titanium miniplates. The depth lead is then implanted with the aid of a slotted canulla[8] or after the introduction of an insertion tool.[3] The stylet of the lead is removed and the implanted lead is then secured. The final position of the lead can be verified using fluoroscopy[3] or intraoperative CT.[11]

Subdural Lead Placement

The subdural strip is implanted through a burr hole or by using previous craniotomy sites. The dura is opened in a linear fashion and the lead strip is inserted through the dura and positioned over the desired cortical area. Finally, the lead is secured to the skull.[3,4]

Pulse Generator Implantation

To implant the pulse generator, a partial-thickness or ful- thickness craniectomy is shaped using a high-speed drill, to match the ferrule format (**Fig. 4**). For patients with a previous craniotomy/craniectomy, the bone defect can be adapted to accommodate the generator.[3,4] The ferule is bolted to the skull using miniscrews. Finally, the implanted leads are connected to the pulse generator and then secured in the implanted ferrule.

OUTCOMES

Seizure Control

The RNS System Pivotal trial was a randomized, double-blind, multicenter, sham-stimulation controlled study, from which results have been extensively reported.[12–19] The initial results published in 2011 by Morrell and colleagues[12] included 191 patients who underwent actual or sham programming of the neurostimulator during a blinded period of 4 weeks and reported the difference in the reduction of mean seizure frequency. Patients were relatively young (mean 34.9 years old, range 18–66 years old), with a long duration of epilepsy (mean 20.5 years old, range 2–57 years old). At baseline, patients were using 0 to 8 different AEDs, with seizures ranging from 0.1 events/d to 12.1 events/d. There were 2 seizure foci in 55% of the patients, whereas the rest had a single epileptogenic focus. Approximately one-third of the patients had had prior therapeutic surgery. One month after implantation, seizure frequency was reduced for both stimulation (34.2%) and sham groups (25.2%) without a statistically significant difference (P = .279). This finding is in line with seizure reduction previously described to follow surgical procedures,[20,21] which may simply result from anesthesia or the surgical procedure itself.[12] Over time, the difference between groups increased (37.8% with stimulation vs 17.3% in the sham group) demonstrating significant efficacy of RNS (P = .012). Additional analyses showed a higher responder rate (percentage of subjects with $\geq$50% reduction in seizures) for the stimulation group. Patients receiving actual stimulation had 27% fewer days with seizures whereas the sham group experienced 16% fewer days (P = .048).

After the blinded phase, all patients received stimulation during an open label evaluation period. Outcomes results were subsequently published by Heck and colleagues[13] and by Bergey and colleagues[15] During this period, stimulation was applied at a frequency of 200 Hz, pulse width of 160 μsec, and burst duration of 100 milliseconds (ms), whereas amplitude was titrated upward to less than 4.0 mA in 53.8% of the patients, 4.0 mA to 7.9 mA in 34.8% of the patients, 8.0 mA to 11.9 mA in 8.7% of the patients, and 12.0 mA in 2.7% of the patients.[13] These studies

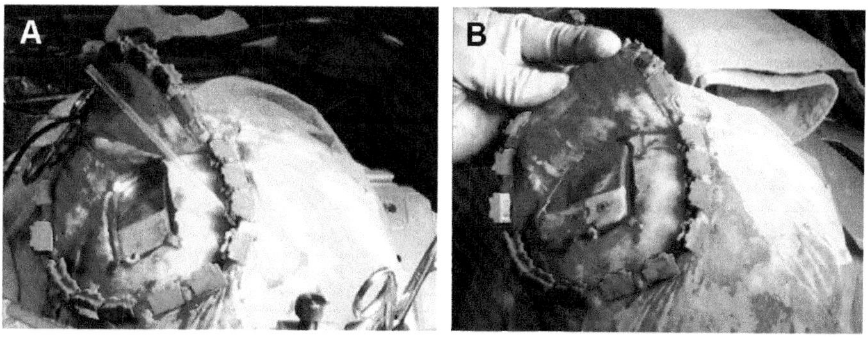

Fig. 4. Pulse generator implantation. (*A*) Ferrule bolted at the craniectomy site. (*B*) Pulse generator connected to the leads and secured to the implanted ferrule.

demonstrated that both percentage of seizure reduction and responder rate continued to improve over time. After 1 year, there was 44% seizure reduction, whereas after 6 years, patients reported a median reduction of 66% in seizure frequency. Likewise, responders rate increased from 44% at the 1-year follow-up visit to 59% after 6 years of follow-up (**Table 1**). Bergey and colleagues[15] also demonstrated that 36.7% of the patients had at least 1 seizure-free period of 3 months or longer during his treatment, whereas 23% of the patients reported 6 months or longer, and 12.9% reported 1 year or longer period of seizure-freedom since the beginning of the treatment. None of them had been seizure-free the entire follow-up (**Table 2**).

Quality of Life

Quality-of-life outcomes of the same cohort of patients from the pivotal trial were thoroughly analyzed by Meador and colleagues.[16] The Quality of Life in Epilepsy Inventory–89 (QOLIE-89) scoring manual[22] was used to evaluate changes in quality of life based on the overall score as well as on 4 derived subscales consisting of epilepsy-targeted, cognitive, mental health, and physical health. At baseline, overall scores from patients receiving RNS were lower than epilepsy patients in general (mean [SD]: 45.1 [9.6] versus 67.9 [15.6]).[23] Improvement in quality of life occurred at different time points. At the end of the blinded period, both stimulation and sham groups had significant improvement in the QOLIE-89 scores. The stimulation group had an average increment of 2.0 (9.4) (P = .040), whereas the sham group score was increased by 2.2 points (9.4) in average (P = .032). Thereafter, quality of life continued to improve during the open label period, remaining higher than baseline. At 2 years, quality-of-life scores had an increment of 4.0 points (10.4) on average (P<.001). In addition, 44% of the patients receiving RNS reported meaningful improvements in quality of life, whereas 44% reported no change, and 16% reported declines. Significant improvement also occurred for each subscale at 1 year and at 2 years of follow-up. **Table 2** summarizes the stimulation parameters and overall outcomes at 2 years of follow-up.

Mood and Cognition

Although quality of life was the primary endpoint in a study by Meador and colleagues,[16] mood was also evaluated but as a secondary endpoint. Mood changes were measured using the Beck Depression Inventory–II (BDI-II)[24] and the Profile of Mood States (POMS)[25] scores. During the baseline period, 16% of the patients had moderately severe symptoms of depression and 10% acknowledged suicidality, corroborating that patients with DRE are at risk for mood disturbances. There were no adverse mood changes at the end of the blinded period nor over the following 2 years of the trial. There was actually a modest improvement in the BDI-II (−1.9 points; P<.008) and POMS (−5.8; P = .04) total scores, which indicates that there is not an increased risk of mood issues after RNS.

The same cohort of patients was thoroughly analyzed by Loring and colleagues,[17] with regard to cognitive function. Language and verbal memory were assessed using the Boston Naming Test (BNT)[26] and the Rey Auditory Verbal Learning Test (RAVLT),[27,28] respectively. There was no significant cognitive decline for any neuropsychological measure over 2 years. There was a significant improvement in naming across all patients (P<.0001); 23.5% of the patients had better scores and 6.7% had worse scores compared with baseline. Auditory verbal learning test (AVLT) also had a favorable outcome, with 6.9% of the patients

Table 1
Change in seizure frequency and responder rate of responsive neurostimulation implantation over time

			Seizure Reduction, %		50% Responder Rate, %	
Author, year	**n**	**Follow-up**	**Stim**	**Sham**	**Stim**	**Sham**
Morrel,[12] 2011	191	4 mo	−37.9	−17.3	27.0	16.0
		1 y	44.0		44.0	
Heck et al,[13] 2014	191	2 y	53.0		55.0	
		3 y	60.0		58.0	
Bergey et al,[15] 2015	256	6 y	66.0		59.0	

Abbreviations: 50% Responder Rate, percentage of subjects with a 50% reduction in seizures; Sham, group of patients receiving sham stimulation during blinded period; Stim, group of patients receiving actual stimulation during blinded period.

Table 2
Seizure freedom periods during 6-years' follow-up

Author, Year	
Bergey et al,[15] 2015 (n)	256
Period of seizure freedom	**%**
At least 1 period of 3 mo or longer	36.7
At least 1 period of 6 mo or longer	23.0
At least 1 period of 12 mo or longer	12.9
Seizure freedom during the entire follow up	0.0

demonstrating improvement and 1.4% demonstrating decline in the scores. In addition, Loring and colleagues[17] evaluated cognition outcomes as function of seizure-onset area. Patients with neocortical seizure onsets exhibited improvement after 2 years of RNS (*P*<.0001), whereas patients with mesial temporal lobe (MTL) seizure onset did not (*P* = .679). Conversely, there was a significant improvement in verbal learning for patients with MTL seizure onsets (*P* = .005) but there was not for patients with neocortical onsets (*P* = .403).

Mesial Temporal Lobe Onset

To evaluate the efficacy of RNS specifically for MTL epilepsy, 111 patients were analyzed separately by Geller and colleagues[18] On average, these patients were young (mean 37.3 years old), with a long history of epilepsy (mean 19.8 years old), taking 1 to 6 different AEDs, with an average monthly seizure frequency of 15.1 events. Bilateral onset was present in 72% of the patients and 55% of them had unilateral or bilateral MTS. Most commonly the patients underwent implantation of 2 depth leads along the longitudinal axis of the hippocampus. At 6 years, there was a median decrease of 70% seizure frequency with a responder rate of 66% (**Tables 3** and **4**), based on the most recent 3 months of available seizure diary data (last observation carried forward method). Over the follow-up period, 45% of the patients reported seizure-free intervals of 3 months or longer, 29% reported seizure-free intervals of 6 months or longer, and 15% reported seizure-free interval of 1 year or longer. Moreover, no seizures were reported by 20.8% of the patients in the last 3 months of follow-up; 62 patients had high-resolution postoperative imaging, which allowed verification of lead location. Only 50% (n = 31) of the leads were inside the hippocampus, and seizure reduction was not dependent on the location of depth leads. Additional analyses showed that there was no difference in seizure control in patients with MTS, bilateral onsets, prior resection, prior intracranial monitoring, or prior vagus nerve stimulation.

Neocortical Onset

The outcomes of RNS for patients with neocortical seizure onset were published in 2017 by Jobst and colleagues.[19] These patients were also young (mean 30.4 years old), with a long history of epilepsy (mean 19.5 years), taking 1 to 6 different AEDs, with an average monthly seizure frequency of 88.0 events. Seizure onset was located in the frontal lobe (31%), temporal lobe (25%), parietal lobe (13%), occipital lobe (3%), or multiple lobes (27%). There was a visible lesion on MRI in 55% of the patients. Two seizure foci were present in 26% of the patients, whereas only 1 focus was identified in the remaining patients. At 6 years of follow-up, there was an overall median seizure reduction of 58% and 55% responder rate (see **Table 3**), based on the last observation carried forward method. In average, there was a median 70% reduction in seizure frequency for patients with frontal onsets as well as for patients with parietal seizure onsets, 58% for those with temporal neocortical onsets, and 51% for those with multilobar onsets. Over the follow-up period, 37% of the patients reported seizure-free intervals of 3 months or longer, 26% reported intervals of 6 months or longer, and 14% reported seizure-free interval of 1 year or longer. There was a higher reduction rate for patients with lesions on MRI compared with those with normal MRI findings (*P* = .02), although both groups benefitted from the treatment (77% reduction and 45% reduction, respectively).

SAFETY AND COMPLICATIONS

Clinical trials have demonstrated that the procedure to place the RNS System is safe procedure.[12,13,15] Major complications reported were hemorrhage, infections, increased seizure frequency, hardware-related complications, and death.

Hemorrhage and Infection

Intracranial hemorrhage occurred in 12 of the 256 patients (4.7%) on the long-term treatment study,[15] mostly within the first days after implantation (4 patients) or due to seizure-related head trauma (5 patients), yielding no neurologic sequelae. The remaining 3 patients experienced

Table 3
Summary of 2-years follow-up outcomes

Stimulation Parameters		Frequency		Pulse Width	Burst Duration	Amplitude[a]			Author, Year
						<4.0 mA	8.0–11.9 mA	12.0 mA	
		200 Hz		160 μs	100 ms	53.80%	8.70%	2.70%	
Change in seizure frequency		**Seizure reduction, %**		**50% responder rate, %**					Heck et al,[13] 2014
		53.0		55.0					
		Baseline Average	**SD**	**Two years postimplantation Average**	**SD**	**Change from baseline Average**	**SD**	***P* value**	
Quality of life	QOLIE-89 overall	45.3	9.9	49.3	10.3	4.0	10.4	<.001	Meador et al,[16] 2015
Mood	BDI-II	10.6	8.4	8.7	8.9	−1.9	8.8	.008	
Mood	POMS	27.8	33.0	22.0	36.5	−5.8	35.1	.040	
		Improvement, %		**With no change, %**		**With decline, %**		***P* value**	
Cognition	BNT	6.7		69.8		23.5		<.001	Loring et al,[17] 2015
	AVLT learning	1.4		91.7		6.9		.03	
	AVLT delayed recall	0.7		92.5		6.8		.07	

Abbreviation: 50% responder rate, percentage of subjects with a 50% reduction in seizures.
[a] Amplitude, percentage of patients on each amplitude range.

Table 4
Comparison of seizure outcomes between patients with mesial temporal lobe and neocortical onsets

	Mesial Temporal Lobe			Neocortical	
Author, Year	Geller et al,[18] 2017			Jobst et al,[19] 2017	
n	111			126	
	Mean	SD		Mean	SD
Age (y)	37.3	11.3		30.4	10.1
Duration (y)	19.8	12.7		19.5	10.2
AED (n)	2.7	1.1		3.1	1.1
Seizure frequency (n/month)	15.1	25		88	246.7
Overall seizure reduction, %	70			58	
50% responder rate, %	66			55	
				Seizure onset, %	Seizure reduction, %
Bilateral MTS onset	72		Frontal	31	70
Unilateral MTS onset	28		Temporal	25	58
Left	68		Parietal	13	70
Right	32		Occipital	3	—
			Multilobar	27	51
Seizure-free interval					
≥3 mo	45			37%	
≥6 mo	29			26%	
≥12 mo	15%			14%	

Abbreviations: MTS, mesial temporal sclerosis; 50% responder rate, percentage of subjects with a 50% reduction in seizures.

intracranial hemorrhages that were not related to seizures and that occurred between 2.5 years and 3.0 years after implantation. Unfortunately, these 3 patients suffered permanent sequelae of mild right-hand paresis, exacerbation of a preexisting memory deficit, and persistent headache. Although RNS System implantations include additional surgical steps (subdural lead implantation and craniectomy), the perioperative hemorrhage rate (9 patients, 3.5%) was similar to the hemorrhage rate in stereotactic implantations (3.9%).[29,30]

With regard to infections, 28 patients (11%) had a total of 31 events[31]; 14 of the 31 infections (45%) occurred within the first postoperative month and the remaining infections ranged from 35 days to 3.5 years after implantation. All patients were treated with antibiotics and 61% also underwent débridement; 6 patients (21.5%) continued to receive therapy with no explantations or replacements. Another 6 patients (21.5%) had only the neurostimulator replaced. Thirteen patients (46.5%) had the entire system removed and 2 of these patients were subsequently reimplanted with the neurostimulator and leads. Finally, 3 patients (10.7%) had only the neurostimulator explanted and none of them presented meningitis or needed a subsequent surgery to remove the remaining leads during follow-up (range 59–1336 days). Although a vast majority of infections were superficial skin infections (27 of 28 patients),[31] there is risk of deeper and more complicated infections, such as osteomyelitis and epidural infections.[32] Wei and colleagues[32] report 3 cases from a single center of implant site infection that developed osteomyelitis and epidural infections. All patients had undergone multiple surgeries, such as resections, subdural grids implantation, and RNS battery replacements. For all 3 patients, the RNS had to be removed.

Death

Devinsky and colleagues[33] reported the causes of death in 14 of 707 patients treated with RNS (256 patients from clinical trials and 451 patients after FDA approval). The causes of death included suicide (n = 2), status epilepticus (n = 1), lymphoma (n = 1), colon cancer (n = 1), respiratory failure (n = 1), aspiration pneumonia (n = 1), and related to sudden unexpected death in epilepsy (SUDEP) (n = 7). There were 2 possible, 1 probable, and 4 definite SUDEP events. The RNS System was enabled in 5 of these 7 patients, whereas 2 patients had the system disabled. One patient had the system disabled to collect additional detection information and the other patient had the system disabled to evaluate the effect of RNS on seizure frequency. There was increased epileptiform activity in the hours prior to death in 3 of the 5 probable/definite SUDEP patients. One of them had both had both clinical and electrographic evidence of seizures before death. Although the other 2 patients had increased detections supportive of electrographic seizures, confirmation was precluded due to lack of witnessed clinical seizures or stored ECoG data. This population exhibited a SUDEP rate of 2.0 per 1000 patient-stimulation years. As a point of comparison, patients referred for epilepsy surgery and patients with recurrent seizures after epilepsy surgery have a SUDEP rate 6.3 for 1000 patient years. Although these groups include different and heterogeneous populations, seizure reduction seen with RNS may reduce the risk of SUDEP.

Other Complications

Forty-four patients (7.2%) required admission for intravenous antiseizure medication or admission to an epilepsy unit monitoring due to changes in seizure frequency. There was an increase in tonic-clonic seizures in 15 patients (5.9%) and an increase in complex partial seizures in 20 patients (7.8%). During follow-up, 8 patients (3.1%) had nonconvulsive status epilepticus and 7 patients (2.7%) presented with convulsive status epilepticus.

Other complications included hardware related complications, such as device lead damage (n = 9, 3.5%), device lead revision (n = 8, 3.1%), and premature battery depletion (n = 11, 4.3%).[15]

FUTURE PERSPECTIVES

In addition to seizure frequency reduction, RNS may have other applications. One important feature of the RNS System is that epileptiform activity and electrographic seizures can be recorded and stored. As such, 1 possible application is to evaluate changes in brain activity in response to a specific substance[34] as well as to different or additional AEDs.[35,36]

Another possible application is to provide additional long-term ECoG to complement video-EEG monitoring.[14,37] King-Stephens and colleagues[14] reported independent electrographic seizures in 84% of the patients with bilateral MTL implanted with RNS Systems, whereas 16% had only unilateral electrographic seizures after an average of 4.6 years of recording. The average time to record bilateral electrographic seizures was 41.6 days.

Furthermore, surgical strategies can emerge from the RNS ECoG data. DiLorenzo and colleagues[38] reported 5 patients who initially were not candidates for resective surgery due eloquent cortex involvement or bilateral temporal onset. Although RNS was ineffective in these cases, information obtained from the chronic intracranial recordings allowed for a better understanding of the seizure onset zone. These patients, who had previously been considered not candidates for surgery, then underwent resective surgery, with 4 of them achieving seizure freedom. Finally, future explorations with RNS recordings may enhance the understanding of epilepsy physiopathology.[33]

SUMMARY

The RNS System is an effective and safe adjunctive therapy in reducing the frequency of seizures in a specific subset of patients. New applications, such as evaluation of epileptiform activity in response to new medications and additional long-term ECoG recording to complement video-EEG monitoring, may increase the benefits and indications of RNS in the future.

REFERENCES

1. Engel J, Pedley TA, Aicardi J. Epilepsy: a comprehensive textbook. New York: Lippincott Williams & Wilkins; 2008.
2. Kwan P, Arzimanoglou A, Berg AT, et al. Definition of drug resistant epilepsy: consensus proposal by the ad hoc task force of the ILAE commission on therapeutic strategies. Epilepsia 2010;51(6):1069–77.
3. Fountas KN, Smith JR, Murro AM, et al. Implantation of a closed-loop stimulation in the management of medically refractory focal epilepsy: a technical note. Stereotact Funct Neurosurg 2005;83(4):153–8.
4. Anderson WS, Kossoff EH, Bergey GK, et al. Implantation of a responsive neurostimulator device in patients with refractory epilepsy. Neurosurg Focus 2008;25(3):E12.
5. Neuropace website. Available at: http://www.neuropace.com/manuals/RNS_System_Physician_Manual.pdf. Accessed August 8, 2018.
6. Food & Drug Administration website. Available at: https://www.accessdata.fda.gov/scripts/cdrh/cfdocs/cfpma/pma.cfm?id=P100026. Accessed August 8, 2018.
7. Gupta K, Raskin JS, Raslan AM. Intraoperative computed tomography and nexframe-guided placement of bilateral hippocampal-based responsive

neurostimulation: technical note. World Neurosurg 2017;101:161–9.
8. Rohatgi P, Jafrani RJ, Brandmeir NJ, et al. Robotic-guided bihippocampal and biparahippocampal depth placement for responsive neurostimulation in bitemporal lobe epilepsy. World Neurosurg 2018; 111:181–9.
9. Mcgovern RA, Bingaman WE, Gonzalez-martinez J. Robot-assisted responsive neurostimulator system placement in medically intractable epilepsy: instrumentation and technique. Oper Neurosurg (Hagerstown) 2018. https://doi.org/10.1093/ons/opy112.
10. Miller K, Halpern CH. Stereotactic bony trajectory preservation for responsive neurostimulator lead placement following depth EEG recording. Cureus 2016;8(3):3–8.
11. Kerolus MG, Kochanski RB, Rossi M, et al. Implantation of responsive neurostimulation for epilepsy using intraoperative computed tomography: technical nuances and accuracy assessment. World Neurosurg 2017;103:145–52.
12. Morrell MJ. Responsive cortical stimulation for the treatment of medically intractable partial epilepsy. Neurology 2011;77(13):1295–304.
13. Heck CN, King-Stephens D, Massey AD, et al. Two-year seizure reduction in adults with medically intractable partial onset epilepsy treated with responsive neurostimulation: final results of the RNS system pivotal trial. Epilepsia 2014;55(3): 432–41.
14. King-Stephens D, Mirro E, Weber PB, et al. Lateralization of mesial temporal lobe epilepsy with chronic ambulatory electrocorticography. Epilepsia 2015; 56(6):959–67.
15. Bergey GK, Morrell MJ, Mizrahi EM, et al. Long-term treatment with responsive brain stimulation in adults with refractory partial seizures. Neurology 2015; 84(8):810–7.
16. Meador KJ, Kapur R, Loring DW, et al. Quality of life and mood in patients with medically intractable epilepsy treated with targeted responsive neurostimulation. Epilepsy Behav 2015;45: 242–7.
17. Loring DW, Kapur R, Meador KJ, et al. Differential neuropsychological outcomes following targeted responsive neurostimulation for partial-onset epilepsy. Epilepsia 2015;56(11):1836–44.
18. Geller EB, Skarpaas TL, Gross RE, et al. Brain-responsive neurostimulation in patients with medically intractable mesial temporal lobe epilepsy. Epilepsia 2017;58(6):994–1004.
19. Jobst BC, Kapur R, Barkley GL, et al. Brain-responsive neurostimulation in patients with medically intractable seizures arising from eloquent and other neocortical areas. Epilepsia 2017;58(6):1005–14.
20. Katariwala NM, Bakay RAE, Pennell PB, et al. Remission of intractable partial epilepsy following implantation of intracranial electrodes. Neurology 2001. https://doi.org/10.1212/WNL.57.8.1505.
21. Lesser RP. Remission of intractable partial epilepsy following implantation of intracranial electrodes. Neurology 2002;58(8):1317. Available at: http://n.neurology.org/content/58/8/1317.2.abstract.
22. Vickrey BG, Perrine KR, Hays RD, et al. Quality of life in epilepsy QOLIE-89 (Version 1.0): scoring manual and patient inventory. Santa Monica (CA): Rand; 1993.
23. Devinsky O, Vickrey BG, Cramer J, et al. Development of the quality of life in epilepsy inventory. Epilepsia 1995. https://doi.org/10.1111/j.1528-1157.1995.tb00467.x.
24. Beck AT, Steer RA, Brown GK. BDI-II, beck depression inventory: manual; 1996.
25. McNair DM, Lorr M, Droppleman LF. Edits manual for the profile of mood states. San Diego (CA): Edits/Educational and Industrial Testing Service; 1992.
26. Kaplan E, Goodglass H, Weintraub S, et al. Boston naming test. Philadelphia: Lea & Febiger; 1983.
27. Rey A. L'examen psychologique dans les cas d'encéphalopathie traumatique. (Les problems.). [The psychological examination in cases of traumatic encepholopathy. Problems.]. Arch Psychol (Geneve) 1941;28:215–85.
28. Schmidt M. Rey auditory verbal learning test: RAVLT: a Handbook. Los Angeles (CA): Western Psychological Services; 1996.
29. Hamani C, Richter E, Schwalb JM, et al. Bilateral subthalamic nucleus stimulation for Parkinson's disease: a systematic review of the clinical literature. Neurosurgery 2005;56(6):1313–4.
30. Kleiner-Fisman G, Herzog J, Fisman DN, et al. Subthalamic nucleus deep brain stimulation: summary and meta-analysis of outcomes. Mov Disord 2006; 21(Suppl 14):S290–304.
31. Weber PB, Kapur R, Gwinn RP, et al. Infection and erosion rates in trials of a cranially implanted neurostimulator do not increase with subsequent neurostimulator placements. Stereotact Funct Neurosurg 2017;95(5):325–9.
32. Wei Z, Gordon CR, Bergey GK, et al. Implant site infection and bone flap osteomyelitis associated with the neuropace responsive neurostimulation system. World Neurosurg 2016;88: 687.e1–6.
33. Devinsky O, Friedman D, Duckrow RB, et al. Sudden unexpected death in epilepsy in patients treated with brain-responsive neurostimulation. Epilepsia 2018;59(3):555–61.
34. Mackow MJ, Krishnan B, Bingaman WE, et al. Increased caffeine intake leads to worsening of electrocorticographic epileptiform discharges as recorded with a responsive neurostimulation device.

Clin Neurophysiol 2016. https://doi.org/10.1016/j.clinph.2016.03.012.
35. Warner NM, Gwinn RP, Doherty MJ. Individualizing therapies with responsive epilepsy neurostimulation — A mirtazapine case study of hippocampal excitability. Epilepsy Behav Case Rep 2016;6:70–2.
36. Skarpaas TL, Tcheng TK, Morrell MJ. Clinical and electrocorticographic response to antiepileptic drugs in patients treated with responsive stimulation. Epilepsy Behav 2018;83:192–200.
37. Spencer D, Gwinn R, Salinsky M, et al. Laterality and temporal distribution of seizures in patients with bitemporal independent seizures during a trial of responsive neurostimulation. Epilepsy Res 2011;93(2–3):221–5.
38. DiLorenzo DJ, Mangubat EZ, Rossi MA, et al. Chronic unlimited recording electrocorticography–guided resective epilepsy surgery: technology-enabled enhanced fidelity in seizure focus localization with improved surgical efficacy. J Neurosurg 2014;120(6):1402–14.

Deep Brain Stimulation for Depression

An Emerging Indication

Megan M. Filkowski, PhD, Sameer A. Sheth, MD, PhD*

KEYWORDS

• Deep brain stimulation • Neuromodulation • Mood disorders • Depression

KEY POINTS

- Depression is a heterogenous disorder involving a constellation of symptoms, including depressed mood; anhedonia; changes in appetite and sleep; feelings of helplessness, hopelessness, and worthlessness; thoughts of suicide; and psychomotor changes.
- In cases of treatment-resistant depression, neurosurgical interventions such as lesion procedures or deep brain stimulation offer possible therapeutic options.
- Neuroimaging studies support the involvement of multiple interconnected regions that modulate different neural networks associated with various depressive symptoms; involved structures are both cortical and subcortical and include the subgenual cingulate, orbitofrontal cortex, medial prefrontal cortex, medial temporal lobe, ventral striatum containing the nucleus accumbens, and regions of the thalamus and brainstem.

INTRODUCTION

Depression is a heterogenous disorder involving a constellation of symptoms including depressed mood; anhedonia; changes in appetite and sleep; feelings of helplessness, hopelessness, and worthlessness; thoughts of suicide; and psychomotor changes. With a lifetime prevalence of 15% to 20% in the United States,[1] depression is the leading cause of years lost to disability worldwide[2] and is 1 of the top 3 contributors to global burden of disease.[3] Although most depressive episodes are successfully treated with psychopharmacologic interventions and/or psychotherapy, a significant fraction of patients (approximately 30%) remain symptomatic.[4] Moreover, for patients who do benefit from standard treatments, relapse is common and increases with each episode: there is a 60% relapse rate after the first episode, 70% after the second episode, and 90% after the third.[5,6] Electroconvulsive therapy, the most effective acute treatment,[7] is also progressively less effective in these patients.[8] Moreover, a greater number of previous psychopharmacologic treatments seem to be associated with increased resistance to medications prescribed in future episodes.[4] All these factors contribute to a roughly 30% prevalence of so-called treatment-resistant depression (TRD).[9] In these cases, neurosurgical interventions such as lesional procedures or deep brain stimulation (DBS) offer possible therapeutic options.

Rather than a disorder involving a single brain region or single neurotransmitter system, depression is certainly an example of a systems-level disorder.[10,11] Neuroimaging studies support the involvement of multiple interconnected regions that modulate different neural networks associated with various depressive symptoms. Involved structures are both cortical and subcortical and

Disclosure: The authors have nothing to disclose.
Department of Neurosurgery, Baylor College of Medicine, One Baylor Plaza, Houston, TX 77030, USA
* Corresponding author.
E-mail address: sheth@post.harvard.edu

Neurosurg Clin N Am 30 (2019) 243–256
https://doi.org/10.1016/j.nec.2018.12.007

include the subgenual cingulate (SgC), orbitofrontal cortex, medial prefrontal cortex (mPFC), medial temporal lobe, ventral striatum (VS) containing the nucleus accumbens (NaC), and regions of thalamus and brainstem.[10,12] Noninvasive neuromodulatory treatments such as transcranial magnetic stimulation or transcranial direct current stimulation have also shown promise, but these treatments are limited by poor targeting precision, especially to deeper subcortical structures, and stimulation cannot be delivered continuously. Herein, we review neurosurgical interventions for TRD, focusing on the recent advancements and future directions of DBS.

Historical Development of Neurosurgery for Treatment-Resistant Depression

Neurosurgical ablative procedures have been used for decades to treat a variety of psychiatric disorders. Indeed, the first neurosurgical stereotactic procedures were developed for psychiatric/behavioral indications. The medial thalamotomy, performed by Spiegel and Wycis in the late 1940s, was used to treat "emotional reactivity."[13] Additional stereotactic procedures were developed during the latter half of the 20th century for various psychiatric disorders as well as pain and movement disorders. Ablative procedures in use today, namely, the anterior capsulotomy, dorsal anterior cingulotomy, subcaudate tractotomy, and limbic leucotomy, aim to disrupt white matter tracts between prefrontal cortical regions and subcortical regions of the basal ganglia and thalamus. These procedures can be performed using radiofrequency techniques, stereotactic radiosurgery, laser interstitial thermal therapy, or high-intensity focused ultrasound, and have been successfully used to treat TRD, obsessive–compulsive disorder (OCD), and other psychiatric disorders.

Success and use of ablative treatments opened the door for further neurosurgical/stereotactic intervention in psychiatric disorders and allowed for better understanding of the circuitry involved in depression. Efficacy of ablative treatments for depression is suggested to be due to the targeting of connections in the corticostriatothalamocortical network,[14] which includes the orbitofrontal cortex, cingulate cortex, mPFC, mediodorsal thalamus, and basal ganglia.[15] Although sham-controlled randomized trials have not been performed with these methods, results from open-label series have shown a roughly 40% to 50% response rate for TRD.[3,16–18] These response rates are notable given the level of treatment resistance in these patients.

DBS evolved out of the experience of treating movement disorders (such as Parkinson's disease, essential tremor) with lesion procedures. The success of DBS for movement disorders led to its application for psychiatric disorders in the late 1990s.[19] Several DBS targets have been tested for the treatment of TRD including the ventral capsule (VC)/VS, NaC, SgC, superolateral branch of the medial forebrain bundle (slMFB), and lateral habenula (LHb; **Table 1**).

VENTRAL CAPSULE AND VENTRAL STRIATUM TARGET

The antidepressant effect of neurosurgical procedures in the VC/VS region has been recognized for both capsulotomy, as described elsewhere int his article, as well as for DBS. VC/VS DBS was initially developed for OCD in the late 1990s given the positive capsulotomy experience.[20] A subsequent multiinstitutional study refined the implantation site to its current location near the junction of the anterior limb of the internal capsule, anterior commissure, and posterior VS.[21] As with capsulotomy, patients receiving VC/VS stimulation also reported alleviation of depressive symptoms, often occurring before a decrease in OCD symptoms.[21,22] OCD and depression are theorized to involve overlapping networks, and imaging studies suggest that VC/VS DBS engages a widespread frontolimbic network, engaging multiple regions involved in depressive symptomology, including other regions that have also been targeted for DBS (NaC and SgC).[23–25] These initial reports of reduced depressive symptoms in OCD patients paved the way for the application of VC/VS DBS for TRD.[25]

The first open-label trial of VC/VS DBS for TRD reported by Malone and colleagues[26] in 2009 reported promising results. The chosen VC/VS target was 1 to 2 mm anterior to the posterior border of the anterior commissure and 3 to 4 mm inferior to the anterior commissure–posterior commissure line, based on prior DBS for OCD work. Using the Hamilton Depression Rating Scale (HDRS) as the primary outcome measure, response rates (a $\geq$50% decrease in HDRS) were reported as 46.7%, 40%, and 53.3% at 3 months, 6 months, and last follow-up, respectively (**Fig. 1**). Remission rates (HDRS of <10) were also significant, with 20% of patients achieving remission at 3 and 6 months and 40% in remission at last follow-up.[26] The impressive response rate in such refractory patients prompted initiation of an industry-sponsored randomized clinical trial (RCT).[27]

Table 1
Demographic and outcomes from various DBS targets

Study, Year	Target	N	Age (mean ± SD)	Outcome Measure	Response (%)/Remission (%)				
					1 mo	3 mo	6 mo	12 mo	Last Follow-Up
Mayberg et al,[39] 2005	SgC	6	46 ± 8	HDRS-17	33/N/A	83/N/A	66/N/A	N/A	N/A
Lozano et al,[41] 2008	SgC	20	47.4 ± 10.4	HDRS-17	35/10	N/A	60/35	55/35	N/A
Lozano et al,[42] 2012	SgC	21	47.3 ± 6.1	HDRS-17	57/N/A	N/A	48/N/A	29/N/A	N/A
Holtzheimer et al,[29] 2012	SgC	17	42.0 ± 8.9	HDRS-17	N/A	N/A	41/18	36/36	92/58
Puigdemont et al,[43] 2012	SgC	8	47.4 ± 11.3	HDRS-17	37.5/0	N/A	87.5/37.5	62.5/50	N/A
Merkl et al,[77] 2013	SgC	6	50.7 ± 9.2	HDRS-24	N/A	N/A	33/33	N/A	33/33
Ramasubbu et al,[73] 2013	SgC	4	50.3 ± 4.2	HDRS-17	17/0	0/0	33/0	N/A	N/A
Holtzheimer et al,[45] 2017	SgC	60[a]	50.3 ± 9.7	MADRS	N/A	12/2	22/10	30/18	48/25
Riva-Posse et al,[49] 2018	SgC	11	48.7 ± 10.1	HDRS17	9/9	27/0	55/18	45/36	N/A
Malone et al,[26] 2009	VC/VS	15	46.3 ± 10.8	HDRS-24	20/7	27/20	20/20	20/7	20/40
Dougherty et al,[27] 2015	VC/VS	15	47.7 ± 12.0	MADRS	N/A	20/N/A[b]	N/A	20/13	23.3/20
Bergfeld et al,[28] 2016	VC/VS	25	53.2 ± 8.4	HDRS-17	N/A	N/A	N/A	40/20	N/A
Schlaepfer et al,[57] 2013; Bewernick et al,[58] 2017	slMFB	7/8	42.6 ± 9.8	MADRS	71/N/A	85/N/A	100/N/A	75/50	85/57[c]
Fenoy et al,[59] 2016	slMFB	4	43.6 ± 8.9	MADRS	N/A	N/A	50/40	N/A	N/A

Abbreviations: DBS, deep brain stimulation; HDRS, hamilton depression rating scale (17 item or 24 item); MADRS, montgomery-asberg depression rating scale; N/A, not applicable; SD, standard deviation; SgC, subgenual cingulate; slMFB, supralateral branch of the medial forebrain bundle; VC/VS, ventral capsule/ventral striatum.

[a] Number of patients receiving active stimulation.
[b] Measurement at 4 months.
[c] Measurement at 33 weeks.

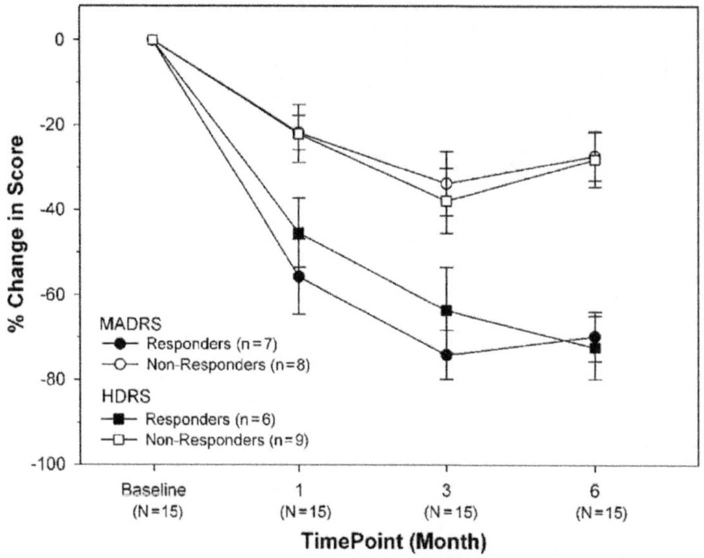

Fig. 1. Change in the Montgomery-Asberg Depression Rating Scale (MADDRS) and Hamilton Depression Rating Scale (HDRS) over 6 months in responders versus non-responders. (*From* Malone DA Jr, Dougherty DD, Rezai AR, et al. Deep brain stimulation of the ventral capsule/ventral striatum for treatment-resistant depression. Biol Psychiatry 2009;65(4):270; with permission.)

The RECLAIM trial, sponsored by Medtronic, was a multiinstituional US RCT.[27] In this double-blind, sham-controlled, randomized trial, patients received sham versus active stimulation for 16 weeks followed by an open-label period for up to 2 years. Stimulation parameters were initially optimized for settings that induced acute effects during testing, and the primary end point was a 50% decrease in the Montgomery-Asberg Depression Rating Scale (MADRS). In contrast with expectations from the previous open-label study, no significant difference in response rates were found between patients receiving active (20%) versus sham (14%) stimulation. The study was designed and powered to enroll a total of 200 patients, however, an interim analysis was performed by the sponsor after a total of 30 patients had enrolled. Although this interim analysis was not sufficiently powered to detect a difference between groups at only 30 participants, the findings resulted in the sponsor halting the study early. During the open-label portion of the trial, 20% to 27% of patients achieved response at some point during the 2-year follow-up phase. A subsequent analysis of this study has suggested that the lack of difference between the active and sham stimulation could be a result of several aspects of study design. First, stimulation parameters during the blinded phase were restricted to a specified range and changed only in a prescribed fashion. Therefore, patients receiving active stimulation may not necessarily have received optimized therapy. This fact, however, does not explain the lower response rate during the open-label phase. Second, the implantation site of the electrodes was based off of anatomic locations. Recent tractography research suggests that the optimal target location may need to be adjusted for each patient given interindividual variations in anatomy. It is, therefore, feasible that the electrodes were not optimally placed to engage the fiber pathways and network regions necessary to induce antidepressant effects.[27]

A nearly contemporaneous RCT from the Netherlands reported different results. The 25 patients in this trial were enrolled using a different trial structure. They initially received an average of 12 months of open-label VC/VS stimulation. During this time, stimulation parameters were optimized until patients exhibited a stable response for 4 weeks or reached the end of the phase. After this time, patients entered a double-blind randomized cross-over phase of either discontinuation of therapy or continued active stimulation. The open-label phase resulted in 40% full response, 20% partial response, and 20% remission rates. Notably, during the blinded cross-over phase, discontinuation of therapy resulted in recurrence of symptoms, whereas continued stimulation did not, demonstrating that DBS therapy was responsible for the observed antidepressant effect. This trial provided Level 1 evidence for the efficacy of VC/VS DBS for TRD.[28]

The reasons why this trial succeeded and RECLAIM "failed" could be due to several factors. First, slight differences in surgical targeting may have resulted in stimulation and activation of the necessary fiber pathways not engaged in the RECLAIM trial. Second, in RECLAIM, the investigators were unable to fully explore varying combinations of stimulation parameters because of the strict trial regulations. In contrast, Bergfeld and colleagues[28] initially treated all patients with open-label active stimulation, allowing investigators more leeway to test various parameters according to their best clinical judgment. Furthermore, the extended optimization phase presumably allowed acute implantation or placebo effects to wear off. Up-front randomization to active versus sham stimulation, as in RECLAIM, would have been subject to both of these early effects.[29]

VC/VS DBS remains investigational, but recent evidence has shown promise in the form of Level 1 evidence from a single-institution trial. We have learned that issues related to surgical targeting and stimulation parameter exploration are essential to positive outcomes. Details of trial design, including the use of an initial open-label phase, may also play a significant role.[28] Stimulation-related adverse effects of DBS in this region include incidences of hypomania (up to 50% over the course of treatment),[30] even in patients without bipolar disorder or prior drug-induced manic/hypomanic symptoms.[30] This adverse event usually responds to programming adjustments, but patients must be monitored carefully given the possibility of hypomania-induced deleterious behaviors.

TARGETING THE SUBGENUAL CINGULATE CORTEX

The SgC, also called Brodmann area 25, is another widely studied target for DBS for TRD. Stimulation of this region, particularly the SgC white matter, is thought to affect a widespread network of regions implicated in depression pathology.[31] The SgC is a highly interconnected region that acts as a hub between cortical and subcortical regions with reciprocal pathways to the mPFC, mesial temporal regions, cingulate cortex, insula, brainstem, and hypothalamus.[14] Initial work using PET demonstrated increased SgC blood flow in depressed patients and decreased flow with antidepressant treatment.[32–34] Furthermore, the decrease in SgC hypermetabolism was sustained in fully remitted patients prescribed maintenance treatment with selective serotonin reuptake inhibitors.[35] Studies incorporating mood induction paradigms with healthy controls also suggest that transient normal sadness increases metabolism in SgC, mimicking results observed in depressed patients, which suggests that the SgC is associated with sadness in particular.[36–38] This region was, therefore, suggested as a possible DBS target with the goal of downregulating activity to ameliorate depressive symptoms.

In an initial open-label trial performed in Toronto,[39] 6 patients with TRD received bilateral SgC DBS. At the 6-month end point, 4 of the 6 patients (67%) exhibited antidepressant response (≥50% reduction in HDRS score), and 3 of the 6 were in remission (HRDS of <7).[39] Long-term results (2–6 years) were also encouraging, with roughly a 62.5% response at 1 year, 46.2% at 2 years, 75% at 3 years, and 64.3% at the last follow-up.[40] In a follow-up study adding another 14 patients to the original cohort of 6 (N = 20), Lozano and colleagues[41] in 2008 (**Fig. 2**) reported response/remission rates of 35% and 10% at 1 month and 60% and 35% at 6 months, with a sustained benefit through l2 months. Additional open-label studies were conducted with positive results. In a multicenter trial, Lozano and colleagues[42] implanted DBS systems in 21 patients and reported response rates of 57% at 1 month, 48% at 6 months, 29% at 12 months, and 62% at last follow-up. Puigdemont and colleagues[43] conducted a separate open-label study in 8 patients and reported response/remission rates of 87.5% and 37.5% at 6 months and 62.5% and

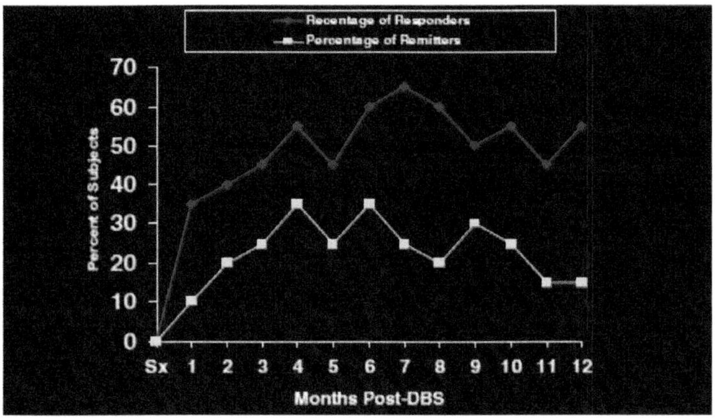

Fig. 2. Patients meeting response of remission criteria after deep brain stimulation (DBS). The proportion of patients responding or reaching submission increased over time to plateau from 6 to 12 months. (*From* Lozano AM, Mayberg HS, Giacobbe P, et al. Subcallosal cingulate gyrus deep brain stimulation for treatment-resistant depression. Biol Psychiatry 2008;64(6):463; with permission.)

50.0% at 1 year, respectively. Responses were variable across centers, but the overall encouraging results led to attempts at controlled trials.

In the first sham-controlled trial,[29] 17 unipolar and bipolar type II patients first received single-blind sham stimulation for 1 month followed by active stimulation for 6 months. After the primary end point (6 months), patients then entered a single-blind discontinuation phase. Results from the initial single-blind sham phase of the study showed a significant decrease in HDRS scores between the preoperative baseline and immediate postoperative period, but no significant difference from the postoperative period to the end of sham. These results suggest an implant effect, perhaps owing to microlesion effect or carryover effect from intraoperative stimulation, but only a modest placebo effect from sham stimulation. Active stimulation was associated with response/remission rates of 41% and 18%, respectively, at 6 months, 36% and 36% at 1 year, and 92% and 58% at 2 years. In the 3 patients who received single-blind discontinuation, depressive symptoms increased over a 2-week period. Upon reinitiation of stimulation, symptoms improved, albeit more gradually than the initial improvement. This pattern further suggests therapeutic efficacy of stimulation. Owing to the distress and increase in suicidal ideation associated with discontinuation, however, this phase was halted after the third patient. Importantly, there were no instances of mania or hypomania in either the group with major depressive disorder or the group with bipolar type II.[29] Puigdemont and colleagues[44] investigated the potential for relapse in a double-blind, crossover study of 5 remitted patients who received SgC DBS. At the end of the active stimulation phase, 4 of 5 patients remained in remission. When crossed to the sham phase, 2 patients remained in remission, 2 relapsed, and 1 exhibited worsening symptoms that did not meet the criteria for relapse, highlighting both efficacy and the need for chronic stimulation in SgC TRD. Based on the promising results from all these studies, a large multiinstitutional RTC was conducted.

The BROADEN trial was an industry-sponsored, multisite, double-blind, sham-controlled RTC funded by St. Jude Neuromodulation, now Abbott. After implantation, patients were randomly assigned to 6 months of active treatment or sham stimulation followed by 6 months of open-label stimulation.[45] The primary end point was a 50% decrease in MADRS scores at the end of the blinded phase. The study was powered with the expectation of a 40% true response rate, and up to an 18.5% sham response rate, with a total of 201 patients to be enrolled. A planned interim analysis was performed after the first 90 patients had completed the 6-month sham-controlled phase, at which point they observed a 20% response in the active group and a 17% response rate in the sham group. An ensuing futility analysis suggested that there was a 17% chance that continuing the study would result in a significant difference between groups. Although the futility analysis did not meet the preset threshold (<10% chance) to end the study, the sponsor chose to close enrollment.[45] The results of the BROADEN trial and the number of nonresponders in prior trials highlighted the need to more carefully investigate factors affecting the efficacy of SgC DBS therapy. A number of factors have been discussed, including patient selection, surgical targeting, trial design, stimulation parameter exploration, and several others, as discussed elsewhere in this article.[46]

A key factor influencing successful SgC DBS that has emerged over the past several years is surgical targeting. Hamani and colleagues[47] compared electrode placement between responders and nonresponders and reported no differences in the anatomic location of the electrodes between the 2 groups in terms of simple x–y–z coordinates. However, another hypothesis proposes that the targeting of specific white matter tracts on an individualized basis, rather than "one size fits all" canonical coordinates, may improve outcomes.

Retrospective data consistent with this theory came from Riva-Posse and colleagues,[48] who obtained preoperative diffusion tensor imaging data from 16 SgC DBS patients (**Fig. 3**). Whole brain probabilistic tractography showed white matter tract convergence in all patients who responded to DBS at both 6 months and 2 years. These patients shared bilateral white matter pathways including forceps minor and uncinate fasciculus, cingulum bundle, and frontostriatal fibers.[48] In addition, as in the study by Hamani and colleagues,[47] the x–y–z coordinates of active contacts did not distinguish responders and nonresponders.

Using this targeting heuristic, a subsequent study tested the use of prospective white matter tracking to guide targeting.[49] Preoperative deterministic tractography was used to identify the implantation site in 11 patients. Active contacts were determined by combining the deterministic tractography with postoperative probabilistic tractography in each individual patient. All patients received open-label stimulation. At the end of 6 months, 72.7% of patients responded and, of those, 5 of the 11 achieved remission. By the end of 12 months, 81.8% responded with 5

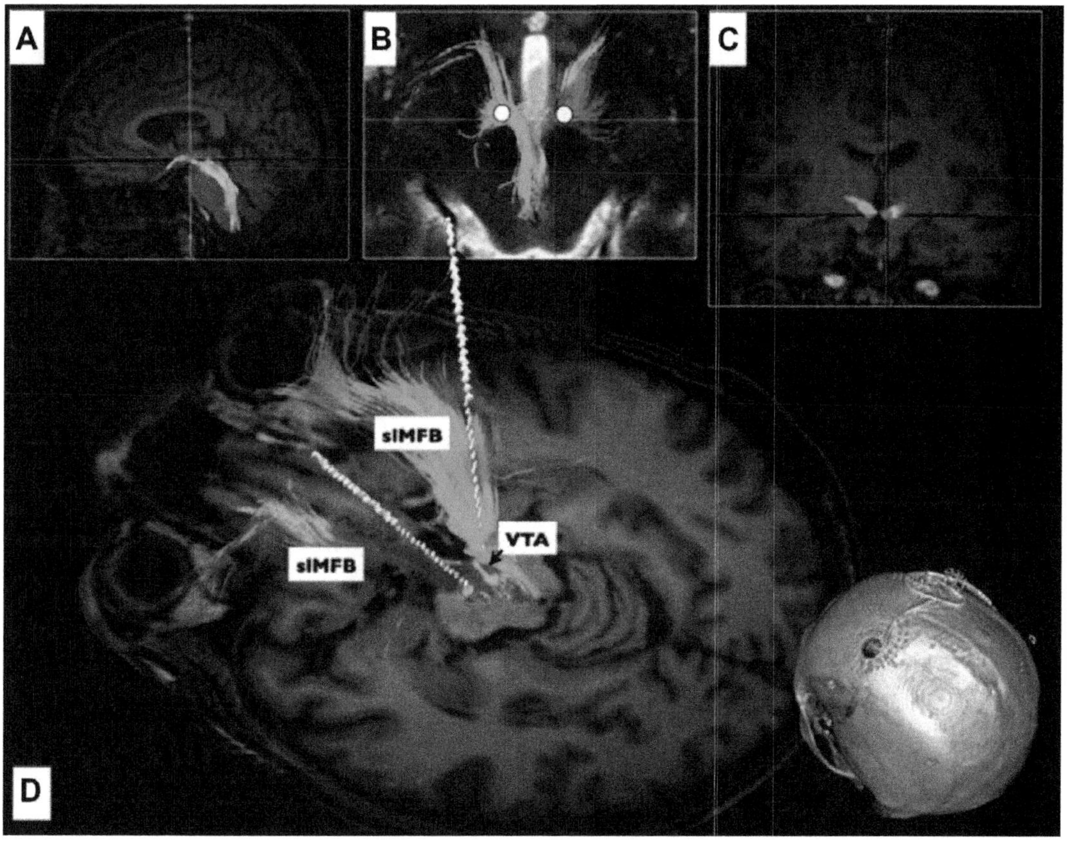

Fig. 3. Diffusion tensor imaging-based patient individual planning of bilateral superolateral medial forebrain bundle (slMFB) deep brain stimulation (DBS). (*A–C*) Projection of the S1MFB (*dark green, left side*) onto sagittal (*A*), axial (*B*), and coronal (*C*) sections. Note bilateral deep brain stimulation (DBS) electrode positions in B (*white circles*). (*D*) Three-dimensional rendering as seen from posterior and superior left includes final DBS electrode positions (*white rods*). VTA, ventral tegmental area. (*From* Schlaepfer TE, Bewernick BH, Kayser S, et al. Rapid effects of deep brain stimulation for treatment-resistant major depression. Biol Psychiatry 2013;73(12):1207; with permission.)

achieving remission (**Fig. 4**).[49] Findings from this study are encouraging and suggest that stimulation of specific white matter pathways is pivotal to positive outcomes in SgC DBS. In addition, using diffusion tensor imaging tractography can enable patient-specific targeting to ensure stimulation of those pathways.

TARGETING THE SUPEROLATERAL BRANCH OF THE MEDIAL FOREBRAIN BUNDLE

Reward network dysfunction in depression is widely reported.[50–53] This network includes the NaC, ventral tegmental area, amygdala, and several nuclei of the hypothalamus connected via the medial forebrain bundle.[54,55] Similar to the hypermetabolism reported in the SgC neuroimaging, studies report an association of depression with dysfunction in the reward network.[51,56] These circuit-based arguments led to the hypothesis that stimulation of the medial forebrain bundle would modulate a dysfunctional reward network and engage motivational behavior to alleviate anhedonia in patients with TRD. The slMFB, in particular, was chosen as a possible target for DBS owing to its proximity to the ventral tegmental area and structural and functional connectivity to other DBS targets.

The first open-label pilot study of slMFB DBS reported encouraging results.[57] Because the slMFB is not readily seen on conventional MRI, 7 patients with TRD were implanted using deterministic tractography to locate the slMFB. Use of tractography-guided implantation also reduces the likelihood of stimulating nearby oculomotor nerve fibers and causing dose-limiting side effects. The effects of stimulation were rapid, with 4 of 7 patients (57%) responding at 1 week and 5 of 7 patients (71%) responding at 6 weeks (**Fig. 5**). At last follow-up, all but 1 patient reached

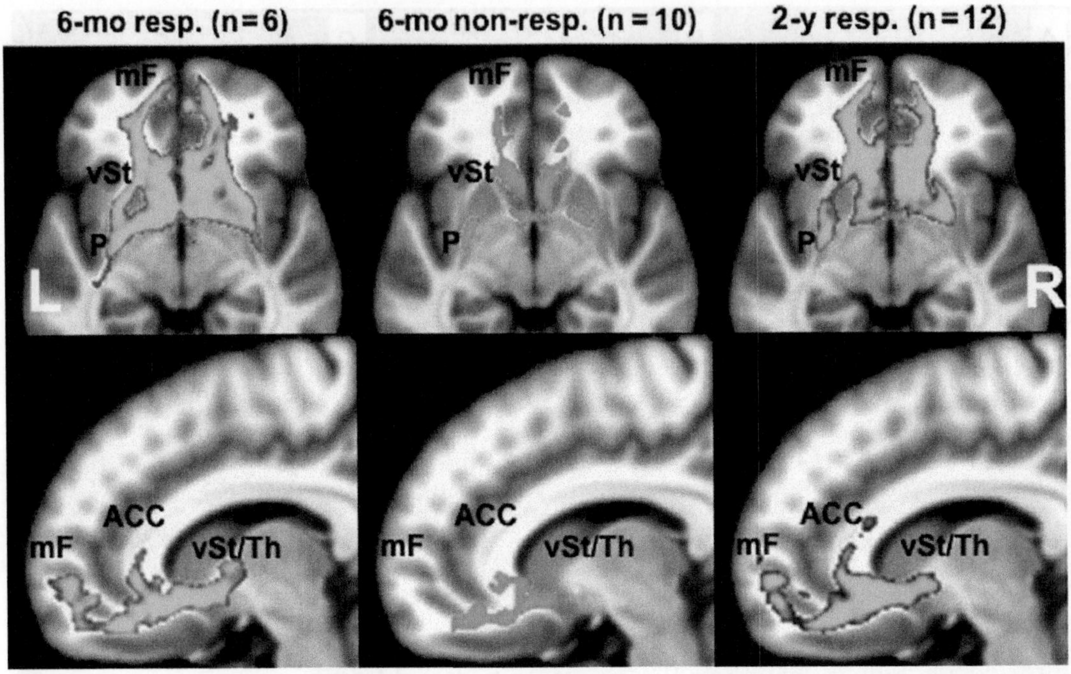

Fig. 4. Whole brain probabilistic tractography of shared fiber tract maps of subcallosal cingulate deep brain stimulation target. (*Left*) Six-month responders (resp.; n = 6). (*Middle*) Six-month nonresponders (non-resp.; n = 10). (*Right*) Two-year responders (n = 12). Responders (at 6 months and 2 years) noted in *blue*. Nonresponders (at 6 months) noted in *green*. Based on individual activation volume tract maps, all 6-month responders share bilateral pathways via forceps minor and uncinate fasciculus to medial frontal cortex (Brodmann area 10); via the cingulum bundle to subgenual, rostral, and dorsal anterior and midcingulate; and descending subcortical fibers to ventral striatum (NaC, ventral pallidum), putamen, hypothalamus, and anterior thalamus. Six-month nonresponders, although similar in some regions, lack connections to both medial frontal and subcortical regions seen in the responder group. All 2-year responders show a pattern that is nearly identical to the 6-month responder tract map. ACC, anterior cingulate cortex; L, left; mF, medial frontal; P, putamen; R, right; Th, thalamus; vSt, ventral striatum. (*From* Riva-Posse P, Choi KS, Holtzheimer PE, et al. Defining critical white matter pathways mediating successful subcallosal cingulate deep brain stimulation for treatment-resistant depression. Biol Psychiatry 2014;76(12):966; with permission.)

response criterion (86%), and 4 had achieved remission.[57] A long-term follow-up study of the same patients reported 6 of 8 patients (75%) as responders and 4 patients (50%) in remission, with stable effects for up to 4 years.[58]

Fenoy and colleagues[59] reported interim findings on 4 patients enrolled in a larger single-blind sham-controlled clinical trial assessing the safety and efficacy of slMFB DBS. After implantation, patients entered the sham-controlled phase for 1 month followed by active stimulation for 1 year. At the end of the sham-controlled phase, all patients exhibited a decrease in depressive symptoms, but the difference between baseline and the end of the sham phase was not significant. After 1 week of stimulation, patients exhibited a further and significant decrease in MADRS scores, with 3 of 4 patients classified as responders. One patient who completed 52 weeks by the time of the report had achieved an 85% decrease in depressive symptoms.[59] A subsequent study from the same group described results in 2 additional patients, with longer follow-up of the cohort.[60] With the inclusion of 2 more patients, the decrease in MADRS between preoperative baseline and the end of the sham period (28% decrease; $P = .02$) was significant. With active stimulation, MADRS scores further improved, with a mean response rate of 3 of 6 after 1 week of stimulation, and 4 of 5 (1 patient dropped out) after 52 weeks.

For patients with TRD, the slMFB seems to be a promising DBS target. The white matter tracts and prefrontal cortical targets to which they project are likely shared between this target and the ones previously discussed.[61] The proximity of other brainstem structures in the area, in particular the oculomotor fibers, can produce dose-limiting side effects. Future work with this target will need to incorporate sham and blinding strategies

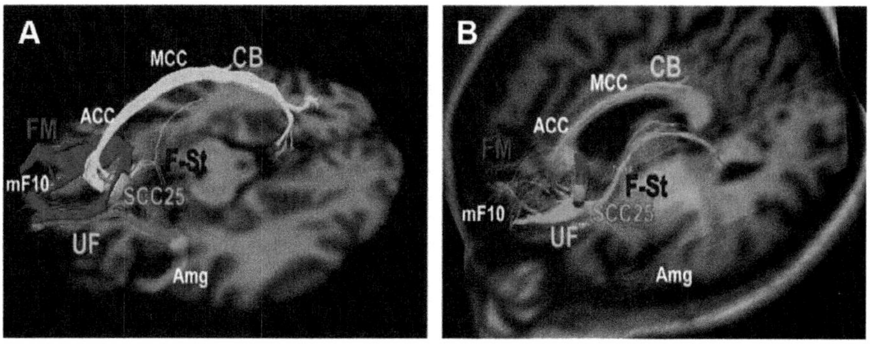

Fig. 5. Blueprint used for structural connectivity-based target selection. (*A*) The necessary 4 fiber bundles, namely forceps minor, uncinate fasciculus, cingulum bundle and fronto-striatal fibers, based on the common fibers impacted by DBS responders in Holtzheimer and colleagues[29] (2012). (*B*) An individualized deterministic tractography target selection in 1 participant: optimal target location within SCC region with modeled stimulation impacting necessary fiber bundles for effective SCC DBS. CB, Cingulum Bundle; DBS, deep brain stimulation; FM, forceps minor; F-St, fronto-striatal fibers; SCC, subcallosal cingulate; UF, uncinate fasciculus. (*From* Riva-Posse P, Choi K, Holtzheimer PE, et al. A connectomic approach for subcallosal cingulate deep brain stimulation surgery: prospective targeting in treatment-resistant depression. Mol Psychiatry 2018;23(4):843; with permission.)

to disentangle insertion, sham response, and other such effects from true response.

TARGETING THE LATERAL HABENULA

Catecholamines, specifically serotonin and norepinephrine, are hypothesized to play a significant role in the pathogenesis of depression.[62,63] The LHb is a small structure that modulates the dorsal raphe nucleus and locus coeruleus, regions from which serotonin fibers originate.[64,65] The dorsal raphe nucleus and locus ceruleus in turn project serotonin fibers to the mPFC, which also modulates activity of both regions.[66,67] One hypothesis proposes that increased activity within the LHb downregulates catelcholaminergic pathways between this network of structures resulting in depressive symptoms.[68] Both animal and human research has implicated the habenula in both reward network dysfunction and negative mood states. Recent irreversible learned helplessness animal models of depression[69] have provided fundamental understanding of the role of the LHb in regulating behaviors possibly related to mood.[70] In humans, depletion of the serotonin precursor tryptophan results in an increase in both LHb cerebral blood flow and depressive mood symptoms, further supporting the involvement of the region in human depression.[71] LHb inhibition with DBS has therefore been proposed as an antidepressant strategy.

In a case report describing the use of bilateral LHb DBS in a 65-year-old patient with TRD, stimulation of the LHb resulted in full remission after 4 months of treatment. The patient did relapse upon accidental discontinuation of stimulation, but symptoms resolved upon resumed stimulation, suggesting that benefit was not due to placebo effects.[72] The animal literature and the previously described case report spurred the initiation of the first open-label pilot trial that is currently underway to evaluate the safety and potential efficacy of bilateral DBS in LHb (NCT01798407).

LESSONS LEARNED FROM PREVIOUS TRIALS

The insignificant difference between sham and true response seen in the 2 large RCTs for the VC/VS and SgC targets contrasts with the observation of a significant number of patients who seem to have benefited from DBS therapy in the preceding open-label studies. Discussions involving several leaders in this field have identified a number of possibly contributing factors.[46] The first factor could be a true lack of efficacy of the treatment itself. However, data from several studies indicate that patients who have had unexpected battery failures[27,29] or were part of a blinded discontinuation after achieving response[28,44] experienced either a significant decline in mood or relapsed, which indicates that the device likely was providing an antidepressant effect.

The response rates could be due to a placebo effect. Roughly 14% to 17% of patients are placebo responders as reported by RECLAIM and BROADEN, which may indicate that some patients may simply derive benefit from the intensive care received from their treatment teams. A placebo effect would indeed obfuscate differences between active and sham stimulation, especially in trials with upfront randomization between the 2 groups. In addition to this effect, outcomes in the larger RCTs could be due to several issues including study design, patient selection, and targeting and stimulation optimization, as discussed elsewhere in this article.

Trial Design

Trial design strategy may play a significant role in the differences reported in response rates. First, some previous trials have relied on designs in which patients are randomized to sham or active stimulation with a primary end point of 3 to 6 months, which is relatively short compared with the 12- to 24-month end points in many open-label trials. In the most studied targets, the VC/VS and SgC, response can take several months to achieve. If the full effect of DBS requires more time, assessing outcomes at 3 or 6 months would not adequately capture true response rates. When up against a sham response rate of perhaps 15% to 20%, a short time window may not provide enough time for the curves to diverge. In the BROADEN study, for example, the initial interim analysis was performed with 90 participants who completed the 6-month blinded phase and found only a 20% response rate, but after 24 months with open-label stimulation, the response rate increased to 49%.

Second, increased time and flexibility for optimization of stimulation parameters may be needed before assessing primary end points. Both BROADEN and RECLAIM imposed strict limitations on parameter adjustments during the blinded phase of the study and reported increased response rates during the open-label portion when parameters could be manipulated fully. Ramasubbu and colleagues[73] also strictly controlled stimulation parameters, even when the current settings were ineffective. Importantly, at the end of that study, stimulation parameters were changed in a nonresponder and resulted in a 30% decrease in HDRS score in 1 month. The stimulation parameters typically used for TRD are derived from the movement disorder experience and therefore may not be optimal. Tight adherence to this narrow range of parameter space may not be ideal for TRD trials.

Another option following the design of the study from Bergfeld and colleagues[28] is the incorporation of an upfront extended open-label period during which stimulation parameters are individually optimized for each patient. In that trial, patients were then cross-over randomized to discontinuation or continued stimulation to assess the efficacy of stimulation. Other design options include device implantation on a staggered or waitlisted fashion or a stepped-wedge design during which patients receive treatment at different times allowing for between-participant analysis.

Patient Selection

Patient selection in psychiatric clinical trials, especially DBS trials, is notoriously difficult.[74] Depression is a heterogenous disorder characterized by a multitude of possible symptoms and combinations thereof. Patients with 1 constellation of symptoms may be better suited for 1 target over another. Knowing which symptoms are ameliorated by each target location could help to tailor treatment to patients with a specific set of symptoms. Further research is also needed to investigate possible biomarkers that may identify patients who may be more likely to respond to DBS. As an analogy, restricting DBS implants to Parkinson's disease patients who are levodopa responsive results in a much better overall response rate than including all patients.

Clinical trials generally incorporate strict inclusion and exclusion criteria to create a homogeneous sample, but as a result may exclude those who would have benefitted and, in real-world practice, comorbidities are the rule rather than the exception. TRD may mask underlying pathology, which may only surface when depressive symptoms regress. Recently, the National Institutes of Health has proposed a new transdiagnostic system design called the Research Domain Criteria to organize symptoms into functional domains. By focusing not only on behaviors and thought patterns, but also on neurobiology and genetics, the Research Domain Criteria approach aims to link functional domains with known neural circuitry that ideally can, in turn, be treated with more rationally designed treatments.[75] The implementation of Research Domain Criteria concepts into patient selection may help to better match patients with disorders such as depression with the most appropriate treatment.

Targeting

The 2 unsuccessful pivotal trials were conducted quickly and before sufficient research had been conducted to perfect targeting and dosing optimization procedures. The RECLAIM trial was initiated after only 1 multiinstitutional open-label trial. Shortly after initiation of the BROADEN study, the benefit of individualized white matter targeting began to be appreciated,[49] but the technique could not be incorporated into the trial. A similar tractographic analysis has not yet been published for the VC/VS target. Before the initiation of large trials, more investigation regarding the neural pathways involved in each target location and the symptoms associated with those pathways needs to be conducted.

FUTURE DIRECTIONS

From the trials discussed, it is clear that there are gaps in our knowledge that result in inconclusive results on the effectiveness of DBS for TRD. These gaps include a (1) lack of a comprehensive understanding of the brain networks involved in TRD both in general and specifically within an individual and (2) the present inability to adequately target and confirm engagement of these networks with current DBS technology. Ongoing efforts are bringing new technologies to bear on this yet investigational but promising therapy, including closed-loop approaches and individualized network targeting with intracranial recording.

Closed-Loop Approach

The closed-loop approach intends to investigate neural networks engaged by DBS using a system designed to both stimulate and record from the DBS lead.[76] A currently funded trail (NCT01984710) is using an experimental prototype DBS system that has this ability to both stimulate and chronically record local field potential data. These recordings can be wirelessly downloaded from the implanted device. This device may be a powerful research tool that can facilitate investigation of the neuronal changes associated with antidepressant response to chronic DBS. This study has the potential to provide insight into the fundamental neuronal processes that underlie depressive illness and antidepressant response.

Directional Current and Intracranial Recording Approach

Another recently initiated trial (NCT03437928) is using intracranial recordings to understand network physiology at the individual level, and a DBS system with directional steering that will allow specific targeting of the identified optimal subnetwork. Unlike previous studies, this study will implant at 2 target sites, the VC/VS and the SgC, which involve overlapping but distinct networks and hopefully will thus be able to address a wide range of depressive symptoms.[25] Furthermore, this study includes the implantation of intracranial depth electrodes to subchronically monitor neurophysiological changes in response to stimulation and to assist in tailoring stimulation parameters on a participant-by-participant basis. With these methods, the study hopes to gain insight into the networks underlying depression symptomatology, investigate the ability to predict the effects of DBS on network activity, and combine results to implement a network-guided approach for DBS for TRD.

SUMMARY

Given the prevalence and associated disability burden associated with TRD, new therapies are greatly needed. The initial enthusiasm for DBS was tempered by the 2 halted pivotal trials, but a recent resurgence in promise has been fueled by transdiagnostic approaches to patient evaluation, advances in imaging connectomics, and an increased appreciation of individualized network engagement. Future studies addressing key problems evident in the design and implementation of prior trials will help to disambiguate sham from true response and optimize stimulation parameters. With the recent resurgence in interest in this therapy and an infusion of National Institutes of Health funding through the BRAIN Initiative, the next several years should see significant advances in this therapy.

REFERENCES

1. Kessler RC, Berglund P, Demler O, et al. Lifetime prevalence and age-of-onset distributions of DSM-IV disorders in the National Comorbidity Survey Replication. Arch Gen Psychiatry 2005;62(6): 593–602.
2. World Health Organization. Depression and other common mental disorders: global health estimates. Geneva (Switzerland): World Health Organization; 2017.
3. World Health Organization. Global health estimates 2016: deaths by cause, age, sex, by country and by region, 2000-2016. Geneva (Switzerland): World Health Organization; 2016.
4. Rush AJ, Trivedi MH, Wisniewski SR, et al. Acute and longer-term outcomes in depressed outpatients requiring one or several treatment steps: a STAR* D report. Am J Psychiatry 2006;163(11):1905–17.
5. American Psychiatric Association. Diagnostic and statistical manual of mental disorders. 4th edition. Washington, DC: APA press; 2000.
6. Sackeim HA. The definition and meaning of treatment-resistant depression. J Clin Psychiatry 2001;62(Suppl 16):10–7.
7. Carney S, Cowen P, Geddes J, et al. Efficacy and safety of electroconvulsive therapy in depressive disorders: a systematic review and meta-analysis. Lancet 2003;361(9360):799–808.

8. Prudic J, Sackeim HA, Devanand DP. Medication resistance and clinical response to electroconvulsive therapy. Psychiatry Res 1990;31(3):287–96.
9. Nemeroff CB. Prevalence and management of treatment-resistant depression. J Clin Psychiatry 2007;68(8):17.
10. Mayberg HS. Limbic-cortical dysregulation: a proposed model of depression. J Neuropsychiatry Clin Neurosci 1997;9(3):471–81.
11. Nemeroff CB. Recent advances in the neurobiology of depression. Psychopharmacol Bull 2002; 36:6–23.
12. Mayberg HS. Modulating dysfunctional limbic-cortical circuits in depression: towards development of brain-based algorithms for diagnosis and optimised treatment. Br Med Bull 2003;65(1):193–207.
13. Spiegel EA, Wycis HT, Marks M, et al. Stereotaxic apparatus for operations on the human brain. Science 1947;106(2754):349–50.
14. Mayberg HS. Targeted electrode-based modulation of neural circuits for depression. J Clin Invest 2009; 119(4):717–25.
15. Rauch SL, Shin LM, Wright CI. Neuroimaging studies of amygdala function in anxiety disorders. Ann N Y Acad Sci 2003;985(1):389–410.
16. Sachdev P, Sachdev J. Sixty years of psychosurgery: its present status and its future. Aust N Z J Psychiatry 1997;31(4):457–64.
17. Christmas D, Eljamel MS, Butler S, et al. Long term outcome of thermal anterior capsulotomy for chronic, treatment refractory depression. J Neurol Neurosurg Psychiatry 2011;82(6):594–600.
18. Shields DC, Asaad W, Eskandar EN, et al. Prospective assessment of stereotactic ablative surgery for intractable major depression. Biol Psychiatry 2008; 64(6):449–54.
19. Gardner J. A history of deep brain stimulation: technological innovation and the role of clinical assessment tools. Soc Stud Sci 2013;43(5):707–28.
20. Nuttin B, Cosyns P, Demeulemeester H, et al. Electrical stimulation in anterior limbs of internal capsules in patients with obsessive-compulsive disorder. Lancet 1999;354(9189):1526.
21. Greenberg B, Gabriels L, Malone D Jr, et al. Deep brain stimulation of the ventral internal capsule/ventral striatum for obsessive-compulsive disorder: worldwide experience. Mol Psychiatry 2010; 15(1):64.
22. Goodman WK, Foote KD, Greenberg BD, et al. Deep brain stimulation for intractable obsessive compulsive disorder: pilot study using a blinded, staggered-onset design. Biol Psychiatry 2010; 67(6):535–42.
23. Figee M, Luigjes J, Smolders R, et al. Deep brain stimulation restores frontostriatal network activity in obsessive-compulsive disorder. Nat Neurosci 2013; 16(4):386.
24. Haber SN, Heilbronner SR. Translational research in OCD: circuitry and mechanisms. Neuropsychopharmacology 2013;38(1):252.
25. Nanda P, Banks GP, Pathak YJ, et al. Connectivity-based parcellation of the anterior limb of the internal capsule. Hum Brain Mapp 2017;38(12):6107–17.
26. Malone DA Jr, Dougherty DD, Rezai AR, et al. Deep brain stimulation of the ventral capsule/ventral striatum for treatment-resistant depression. Biol Psychiatry 2009;65(4):267–75.
27. Dougherty DD, Rezai AR, Carpenter LL, et al. A randomized sham-controlled trial of deep brain stimulation of the ventral capsule/ventral striatum for chronic treatment-resistant depression. Biol Psychiatry 2015;78(4):240–8.
28. Bergfeld IO, Mantione M, Hoogendoorn ML, et al. Deep brain stimulation of the ventral anterior limb of the internal capsule for treatment-resistant depression: a randomized clinical trial. JAMA Psychiatry 2016;73(5):456–64.
29. Holtzheimer PE, Kelley ME, Gross RE, et al. Subcallosal cingulate deep brain stimulation for treatment-resistant unipolar and bipolar depression. Arch Gen Psychiatry 2012;69(2):150–8.
30. Widge AS, Licon E, Zorowitz S, et al. Predictors of hypomania during ventral capsule/ventral striatum deep brain stimulation. J Neuropsychiatry Clin Neurosci 2016;28(1):38–44.
31. Tsolaki E, Espinoza R, Pouratian N. Using probabilistic tractography to target the subcallosal cingulate cortex in patients with treatment resistant depression. Psychiatry Res Neuroimaging 2017;261:72–4.
32. Mottaghy FM, Keller CE, Gangitano M, et al. Correlation of cerebral blood flow and treatment effects of repetitive transcranial magnetic stimulation in depressed patients. Psychiatry Res Neuroimaging 2002;115(1–2):1–14.
33. Nobler MS, Oquendo MA, Kegeles LS, et al. Decreased regional brain metabolism after ECT. Am J Psychiatry 2001;158(2):305–8.
34. Goodwin G, Austin M-P, Dougall N, et al. State changes in brain activity shown by the uptake of 99mTc-exametazime with single photon emission tomography in major depression before and after treatment. J Affect Disord 1993;29(4):243–53.
35. Liotti M, Mayberg HS, McGinnis S, et al. Unmasking disease-specific cerebral blood flow abnormalities: mood challenge in patients with remitted unipolar depression. Am J Psychiatry 2002;159(11):1830–40.
36. Mayberg HS, Liotti M, Brannan SK, et al. Reciprocal limbic-cortical function and negative mood: converging PET findings in depression and normal sadness. Am J Psychiatry 1999;156(5):675–82.
37. George MS, Ketter TA, Parekh PI, et al. Brain activity during transient sadness and happiness in healthy women. Am J Psychiatry 1995;152(3):341–51.

38. Baker SC, Frith CD, Dolan RJ. The interaction between mood and cognitive function studied with PET. Psychol Med 1997;27(3):565–78.
39. Mayberg HS, Lozano AM, Voon V, et al. Deep brain stimulation for treatment-resistant depression. Neuron 2005;45(5):651–60.
40. Kennedy SH, Giacobbe P, Rizvi SJ, et al. Deep brain stimulation for treatment-resistant depression: follow-up after 3 to 6 years. Am J Psychiatry 2011; 168(5):502–10.
41. Lozano AM, Mayberg HS, Giacobbe P, et al. Subcallosal cingulate gyrus deep brain stimulation for treatment-resistant depression. Biol Psychiatry 2008;64(6):461–7.
42. Lozano AM, Giacobbe P, Hamani C, et al. A multicenter pilot study of subcallosal cingulate area deep brain stimulation for treatment-resistant depression. J Neurosurg 2012;116(2):315–22.
43. Puigdemont D, Pérez-Egea R, Portella MJ, et al. Deep brain stimulation of the subcallosal cingulate gyrus: further evidence in treatment-resistant major depression. Int J Neuropsychopharmacol 2012; 15(1):121–33.
44. Puigdemont D, Portella MJ, Pérez-Egea R, et al. A randomized double-blind crossover trial of deep brain stimulation of the subcallosal cingulate gyrus in patients with treatment-resistant depression: a pilot study of relapse prevention. J Psychiatry Neurosci 2015;40(4):224.
45. Holtzheimer PE, Husain MM, Lisanby SH, et al. Subcallosal cingulate deep brain stimulation for treatment-resistant depression: a multisite, randomised, sham-controlled trial. Lancet Psychiatry 2017;4(11):839–49.
46. Bari AA, Mikell CB, Abosch A, et al. Charting the road forward in psychiatric neurosurgery: proceedings of the 2016 American Society for Stereotactic and Functional Neurosurgery Workshop on Neuromodulation for Psychiatric Disorders. J Neurol Neurosurg Psychiatry 2018;89(8):886–96.
47. Hamani C, Mayberg H, Snyder B, et al. Deep brain stimulation of the subcallosal cingulate gyrus for depression: anatomical location of active contacts in clinical responders and a suggested guideline for targeting. J Neurosurg 2009;111(6): 1209–15.
48. Riva-Posse P, Choi KS, Holtzheimer PE, et al. Defining critical white matter pathways mediating successful subcallosal cingulate deep brain stimulation for treatment-resistant depression. Biol Psychiatry 2014;76(12):963–9.
49. Riva-Posse P, Choi K, Holtzheimer PE, et al. A connectomic approach for subcallosal cingulate deep brain stimulation surgery: prospective targeting in treatment-resistant depression. Mol Psychiatry 2018;23(4):843.
50. Satterthwaite TD, Kable JW, Vandekar L, et al. Common and dissociable dysfunction of the reward system in bipolar and unipolar depression. Neuropsychopharmacology 2015;40(9):2258.
51. Smoski MJ, Rittenberg A, Dichter GS. Major depressive disorder is characterized by greater reward network activation to monetary than pleasant image rewards. Psychiatry Res Neuroimaging 2011;194(3): 263–70.
52. Keedwell PA, Andrew C, Williams SC, et al. A double dissociation of ventromedial prefrontal cortical responses to sad and happy stimuli in depressed and healthy individuals. Biol Psychiatry 2005;58(6): 495–503.
53. Schaefer HS, Putnam KM, Benca RM, et al. Event-related functional magnetic resonance imaging measures of neural activity to positive social stimuli in pre- and post-treatment depression. Biol Psychiatry 2006;60(9):974–86.
54. Zellner MR, Watt DF, Solms M, et al. Affective neuroscientific and neuropsychoanalytic approaches to two intractable psychiatric problems: why depression feels so bad and what addicts really want. Neurosci Biobehav Rev 2011;35(9):2000–8.
55. Sesack SR, Grace AA. Cortico-basal ganglia reward network: microcircuitry. Neuropsychopharmacology 2010;35(1):27.
56. Dichter GS, Kozink RV, McClernon FJ, et al. Remitted major depression is characterized by reward network hyperactivation during reward anticipation and hypoactivation during reward outcomes. J Affect Disord 2012;136(3):1126–34.
57. Schlaepfer TE, Bewernick BH, Kayser S, et al. Rapid effects of deep brain stimulation for treatment-resistant major depression. Biol Psychiatry 2013; 73(12):1204–12.
58. Bewernick BH, Kayser S, Gippert SM, et al. Deep brain stimulation to the medial forebrain bundle for depression-long-term outcomes and a novel data analysis strategy. Brain Stimul 2017;10(3): 664–71.
59. Fenoy AJ, Schulz P, Selvaraj S, et al. Deep brain stimulation of the medial forebrain bundle: distinctive responses in resistant depression. J Affect Disord 2016;203:143–51.
60. Fenoy AJ, Schulz PE, Selvaraj S, et al. A longitudinal study on deep brain stimulation of the medial forebrain bundle for treatment-resistant depression. Transl Psychiatry 2018;8(1):111.
61. Coenen VA, Panksepp J, Hurwitz TA, et al. Human medial forebrain bundle (MFB) and anterior thalamic radiation (ATR): imaging of two major subcortical pathways and the dynamic balance of opposite affects in understanding depression. J Neuropsychiatry Clin Neurosci 2012;24(2): 223–36.

62. Grossman F, Potter WZ. Catecholamines in depression: a cumulative study of urinary norepinephrine and its major metabolites in unipolar and bipolar depressed patients versus healthy volunteers at the NIMH. Psychiatry Res 1999;87(1):21–7.
63. Charney DS. Monoamine dysfunction and the pathophysiology and treatment of depression. J Clin Psychiatry 1998;59(Suppl 14):11–4.
64. Herkenham M, Nauta WJ. Efferent connections of the habenular nuclei in the rat. J Comp Neurol 1979;187(1):19–47.
65. Sutherland RJ. The dorsal diencephalic conduction system: a review of the anatomy and functions of the habenular complex. Neurosci Biobehav Rev 1982;6(1):1–13.
66. Celada P, Puig MV, Casanovas JM, et al. Control of dorsal raphe serotonergic neurons by the medial prefrontal cortex: involvement of serotonin-1A, GABAA, and glutamate receptors. J Neurosci 2001; 21(24):9917–29.
67. Condés-Lara M. Different direct pathways of locus coeruleus to medial prefrontal cortex and centrolateral thalamic nucleus: electrical stimulation effects on the evoked responses to nociceptive peripheral stimulation. Eur J Pain 1998;2(1):15–23.
68. Sartorius A, Henn FA. Deep brain stimulation of the lateral habenula in treatment resistant major depression. Med Hypotheses 2007;69(6):1305–8.
69. Vollmayr B, Henn FA. Stress models of depression. Clin Neurosci Res 2003;3(4–5):245–51.
70. Shumake J, Edwards E, Gonzalez-Lima F. Opposite metabolic changes in the habenula and ventral tegmental area of a genetic model of helpless behavior. Brain Res 2003;963(1–2):274–81.
71. Morris J, Smith K, Cowen P, et al. Covariation of activity in habenula and dorsal raphe nuclei following tryptophan depletion. Neuroimage 1999; 10(2):163–72.
72. Sartorius A, Kiening KL, Kirsch P, et al. Remission of major depression under deep brain stimulation of the lateral habenula in a therapy-refractory patient. Biol Psychiatry 2010;67(2):e9–11.
73. Ramasubbu R, Anderson S, Haffenden A, et al. Double-blind optimization of subcallosal cingulate deep brain stimulation for treatment-resistant depression: a pilot study. J Psychiatry Neurosci JPN 2013; 38(5):325.
74. Filkowski MM, Mayberg HS, Holtzheimer PE. Considering eligibility for studies of deep brain stimulation for treatment-resistant depression: insights from a clinical trial in unipolar and bipolar depression. J ECT 2016;32(2):122.
75. Insel T, Cuthbert B, Garvey M, et al. Research domain criteria (RDoC): toward a new classification framework for research on mental disorders. Am J Psychiatry 2010;167(7):748–51.
76. Widge AS, Malone DA Jr, Dougherty DD. Closing the loop on deep brain stimulation for treatment-resistant depression. Front Neurosci 2018;12:175.
77. Merkl A, Schneider GH, Schönecker T, et al. Antidepressant effects after short-term and chronic stimulation of the subgenual cingulate gyrus in treatment-resistant depression. Experimental neurology 2013;249:160–8.

Nerve Stimulation for Pain

Mark Corriveau, MD, Wendell Lake, MD, Amgad Hanna, MD*

KEYWORDS

• Neuromodulation • Peripheral nerve stimulation • Peripheral nerve field stimulation
• Transcutaneous electrical stimulation

KEY POINTS

- Nerve stimulation is a reversible technique that is used successfully for the treatment of traumatic neuropathic pain, complex regional pain syndrome, and craniofacial neuropathic pain.
- Nerve field stimulation targets painful regions rather than a single nerve and has expanded indications, including axial low back pain.
- Appropriate patient education and motivation are crucial prior to surgery.
- Ongoing research is necessary to provide high-level evidence for the use of nerve stimulation.
- Most electrodes are primarily designed for spinal cord stimulation, hence the need to develop nerve electrodes dedicated for nerve stimulation.

INTRODUCTION

Chronic neuropathic pain is a common pathology that offers significant management challenges. Although the pain alone may be debilitating, many patients face additional challenges, including an inability to work or high doses of narcotic pain medicine. Although physicians have long been aware of electrical stimulation's potential for pain relief, the use of neuromodulation for the treatment of neuropathic pain was not introduced to clinical practice until the 1960s. This type of pain is rarely curable but nerve stimulation has shown increasing promise as a means by which to decrease patient discomfort and minimize the need for oral pain medication. As interest in the field has grown, the applications of nerve stimulation have continued to broaden.

A critical element to the success of nerve stimulation is appropriate patient selection. Nerve stimulation requires significant patient involvement and feedback in regard to maintenance and follow-up to maximize the benefit of the procedure. Additionally, it is paramount that patients understand the benefits and the limitations of nerve stimulation so they have appropriate expectations. With appropriate patient selection and good communication between the physician and patient, nerve stimulation has proved a valuable treatment of chronic neuropathic pain.

HISTORY OF NERVE STIMULATION

Although the use of electricity to treat neuropathic pain is a relatively modern concept in clinical practice, it has roots dating back to the first century. In 15 CE, a Roman court physician Scribonius Largus noted that patients with gout experienced some relief of their pain when exposed to the electric shock experienced by placing their feet in a pool of torpedo fish.[1] Ultimately, he began recommending electric shock treatment with torpedo fish for a variety of painful ailments, including headaches.[2] Records exist indicating that such uses of electric fish persisted for decades and were used on American plantations. In the mid-nineteentth century, the German-English physician Julius Althaus was the first physician to experiment with the effects of the direct application of electricity to a peripheral nerve, noting diminished sensitivity in the associated distribution. Later, in the early twentieth century, a device that applied

Disclosure: The authors have nothing to disclose.

Department of Neurosurgery, University of Wisconsin Hospitals and Clinics, 600 Highland Avenue, Madison, WI 53792, USA
* Corresponding author.
E-mail address: ah2994@yahoo.com

Neurosurg Clin N Am 30 (2019) 257–264
https://doi.org/10.1016/j.nec.2018.12.008

transcutaneous electrical stimuli called Electreat was developed and marketed not only for the control of pain but also for a wide variety of other health issues.[1,2]

It was not until the mid-twentieth century, however, that physicians began to explore in a dedicated manner the applications that direct nerve stimulation may have to the treatment of chronic pain. The stimulus for these advances was the publication in 1965 of the landmark article by Melzack and Wall[3] proposing the gate control theory of pain. This theory proposes that the conscious perception of pain is not a simple on-and-off switch regulated by a single stimulus but that large and small fibers have variable effects on transmission cells in the substantia gelatinosa. Whereas large heavily myelinated fibers have a positive effect on substantia gelatinosa (SG) cells and thereby facilitate inhibition of transmission neurons, small nociceptive Aδ and C fibers have the opposite effect. The investigators hypothesized that it was the balance between these 2 systems that regulated the transmission of nociceptive stimuli. Therefore, if this balance were altered, painful sensation with innocuous sensory information, it may be possible to suppress the transmission of pain.[3]

This led to the development of several methods for delivering electrical stimuli to peripheral nerves later in the 1960s. Although Electreat had already been introduced decades earlier, this technology was refined to involve surface metal electrodes placed over the course of peripheral nerves just proximal to painful areas.[4] Subsequent investigation into the efficacy of this so-called transcutaneous nerve stimulation in the 1970s indicated an average decrease in pain by 40% on the visual analog scale in a wide variety of patients.[5] With further refinement over the course of the next several decades, this method ultimately became the modern transcutaneous electrical nerve stimulation (TENS) unit. Patrick Wall, who coauthored the initial article on gate control theory, partnered with William Sweet of Massachusetts General Hospital to pioneer a second method of electrical pain control, percutaneous stimulation. In 1967 they published an article in which 8 patients with chronic pain were treated with percutaneous stimulation for 2 minutes with electrodes placed near the suspected affected nerve. The etiology of pain in these patients varied widely, from trauma to malignancy-related pain, but all patients experienced a reportedly "not unpleasant" tingling sensation in the distribution of the stimulated nerve. During stimulation, previously painful stimuli were found innocuous in the region of the tingling. Prior to assessing the results clinically patients, Wall and Sweet assessed the effect of the stimulator by inserting it into their own infraorbital nerves.[6] Although this technique is no longer used to provide long-term pain relief, it was an important proof of concept in regard to the gate control theory and spurred continued research into the area.

The precursor to modern implantable peripheral nerve stimulation (PNS) was developed around this same time. Again, it was Wall and Sweet who performed the first surgery for an implantable PNS. They operated on a 26-year-old woman with symptoms consistent with what would now be called complex regional pain syndrome (CPRS). This incipient case used silastic split-ring platinum electrodes wrapped around both the ulnar and median nerves. Similarly, early case series investigating PNS primarily used bipolar cuff-type electrodes attached to a subcutaneous radiofrequency (RF) generator.[1,2,7] Although this type of electrode was ultimately abandoned given side effects of perineural fibrosis and nerve strangulation, it served as the basis from which modern paddle-type electrodes evolved.

REVIEW OF THE PUBLISHED LITERATURE

Early Literature

Once the concept electrical stimulation for pain control had been established, several physicians began investigating the efficacy of stimulators in a more controlled and systematic fashion. One of the first trials to do this was published by Campbell and Long[4] in 1976; 23 patients were selected who underwent trial stimulation with either a transcutaneous electrode or percutaneous electrode. Although all 23 had some relief of pain with a brief 30-minute to 60-minute trial, only 9 of the 23 experienced moderate or significant relief of pain at 9 months' to 17 months' follow-up. The investigators, however, made the astute observation that patients with a traumatic neuropathy constituted a majority of successes, whereas patients with low back pain/sciatica or metastasis-related pain fared poorly with implanted stimulators. This conclusion has proved consistent in several additional studies over the following decades.

Just a few years later, Law and colleagues[8] published a series of 22 patients, bearing in mind the results of Campbell in 1976. They exclusively selected patients with chronic pain secondary to posttraumatic neuropathy. Intraoperatively, a multiple button cuff electrode was wrapped around the nerve of interest proximal to the region of pain. Patients were then woken up from anesthesia and different settings were tested and optimized prior to final implantation of the receiver. Patients were followed for 9 months to 88 months, with 62% reporting "useful" pain relief, defined as use of only the stimulator for pain control.

These more promising results were soon validated by Waisbrod and colleagues[9] in 1985. Again, these investigators focused on patients with posttraumatic neuropathies of an extremity; 19 patients were recruited after undergoing percutaneous stimulation of the affected nerve proximal to the area of pain. Only patients who experienced 50% or greater pain relief from the trial underwent subsequent permanent implantation of a cuff electrode and RF generator. At 11.5 months postprocedure, 58% of patients reported complete pain relief whereas an additional 21% had "meaningful" pain relief, defined as cessation of oral pain medication. These early studies established several important concepts, including the use of temporary trial stimulation prior to placement of a subcutaneous RF stimulator as well as anatomic placement of the electrode proximal to the patient's pain. It is now well established that a proximal location is necessary to obtain the best results.

During these early trials, several investigators sought to establish a means by which to predict those patients that would most benefit from implantable nerve stimulators. In the 1970s, response to a TENS unit was used as a selection criterion for the placement of a permanent PNS. Unfortunately, several investigators found that there was no difference in the rate of long-term success with implanted stimulators between those who did and those who did not receive temporary benefit from a TENS unit.[10–12] In 1975, Kirsch and colleagues[10] published an article evaluating different electrostimulation techniques, including transcutaneous stimulation and PNS. This allowed them to evaluate for correlations between success with these 2 modalities, and again none was found.

Other investigators believed that perhaps percutaneous electrical nerve stimulation as a more targeted therapy may prove a better predictor of long-term success with a permanent device. This too failed to bear out in clinical evaluation. Because of this, most practitioners now evaluate patients with repeated selective nerve blocks prior to a trial of nerve stimulation with an external pulse generator. If the latter results in meaningful pain relief, then the final step with implantable pulse generator (IPG) placement is performed.

Recent Literature

Despite the success of these early trials, it was still several years before PNS began to grow in popularity. Several larger trials were eventually published validating the results of the studies performed in the 1980s as well as expanding the indications for nerve stimulation. In 1996 Hassenbusch and colleagues[13] published an article including 32 patients with CPRS, with symptoms exclusive to the distribution of a single peripheral nerve. Of these, 30 patients experienced greater than 50% reduction in pain with a trial stimulator and underwent permanent placement. These patients were followed for 2 years to 4 years, with 63% experiencing positive results, and an average drop of 4.8 points on the visual analog pain scale. This was followed shortly by the work of Cooney in 1997, who also reported excellent pain relief with PNS in patients with CPRS.[14]

Recently, literature has begun to focus on not only the technical results of nerve stimulation but also the socioeconomic impact as well. In 2000 Novak and McKinnon[15] reported on 17 patients with neurogenic pain who underwent PNS implantation. Consistent with earlier results, 65% had good or excellent pain relief. In addition, 12 of the initial 17 patients had stopped working due to their pain, and, of these, half were able to return to work with their PNS during the follow-up time period. Strege and colleagues[16] similarly reported 5 of 24 patients who were able to return to their baseline level of activities after implantation. One of the largest series of patient to date was published by Mobbs and colleagues[17] in 2007. Of the 45 patients initially included, 41 ultimately underwent surgery for placement of a stimulator. Again, 61% of these patients reported greater than 50% relief of their pain, with 47% reporting significant improvement in their daily activities and 63% reducing or eliminating their use of opiates.

Therefore, by the late 2000s, nerve stimulation had become a validated method for management of chronic pain in patients with traumatic neuropathies and CPRS. Studies consistently demonstrated efficacy of 60% or greater for significant pain relief. Additionally, they highlighted the effect of stimulation on not only the subjective experience of pain in these patients but also the positive impact it could have on their daily level of functioning and ability to return to work. Given such promising results, it is not surprising that practitioners have sought to expand the use of these devices to other pathologies.

Wall and Sweet inadvertently pioneered the use of PNS for craniofacial pain when they inserted electrodes into their own infraorbital nerve region. In 2006, however, Slavin and colleagues[18] were one of the first groups to formally investigate stimulation of trigeminal branches for the treatment of trigeminal pain. They implanted 3 infraorbital and 4 supraorbital nerve stimulators demonstrating long-term relief of pain in several of the cases. In 2008 Amin and colleagues[19] expanded on this work, implanting 10 permanent supraorbital nerve stimulators and achieving an average reduction of 50% in opioid use for control of frontal headaches. Pain secondary to postherpetic neuralgia has also been successfully treated with PNS.[20–24] One of the most striking successes that has been achieved by PNS is with occipital nerve stimulation for headache control, this is discussed elsewhere in this series.

New Techniques

Although nerve stimulation has largely focused on the treatment of pain through stimulation of a single large nerve trunk, a new branch of this modality has recently emerged termed peripheral nerve field stimulation (PNFS). The same basic principles apply, however, with PNFS, multiple small electrode arrays are placed subcutaneously in the region of pain, rather than a single array proximal to the area of pain on a large nerve trunk. Investigators cite several advantages to this technique including a decreased risk in the development of painful fibrosis around dissected nerves as well as the ability to treat several pathologies that have been poorly managed with PNS alone. Several studies have demonstrated success with the use of PNFS not only for limb pain, but for unilateral or bilateral axial low back pain, failed back surgery syndrome, and craniofacial pain. Results to date are comparable to those achieved by PNS, with 50% to 70% of patients achieving greater than 50% pain relief with this procedure.[25–28] There were 3 large prospective studies involving the use of PNFS for chronic back pain performed between 2011 and 2014, all of which reported lasting meaningful pain relief in excess of 69%.[29] This method, therefore, represents a promising new application of nerve stimulation.

SURGICAL TECHNIQUE(S)

As with any surgical procedure, patient selection is a crucial component when considering PNS. This article presents a thorough literature review and discussion of the history and efficacy of PNS. Several investigators have compiled these results into a list of indications when considering offering nerve stimulation to patients, including components related both to pathology and psychosocial background. Pathologic indications include

- Limb pain from
  - Nerve injury (traumatic, iatrogenic, or postsurgical)
  - CPRS
  - Phantom limb pain[31]
- Axial pain (exclusive to PNFS)
  - Unilateral or bilateral chronic low back pain
  - Failed back surgery syndrome
- Craniofacial pain
  - Migraine or cluster-type headaches
  - Trigeminal neuropathic pain
  - Postherpetic neuralgia

Patient factors are important as is the underlying pathology. Patients must be motivated to be involved in their own care. Inclusion factors for these patients involve[12,29]

- A clear area of neuropathic pain. Some investigators suggest that this should be in the presence of demonstrable pathology
- Failure to respond to more conservative measures including medications, physical therapy, TENS unit, and, potentially, failure to respond to other invasive surgical methods, such as nerve decompression or neuroma resection
- Appropriate patient expectations, namely, a clear understanding that an implantable nerve stimulator is likely to moderate pain rather than completely relieve it
- Successful trial stimulation with a trial lead and external generator or with anesthetic block of a particular peripheral nerve
- Patient motivation to be involved in the care, upkeep, and programming of the device

The surgical procedure itself is typically carried out in 2 stages, a trial phase and an implantation phase. The most common type of electrode in use is a paddle-type electrode. The first phase of surgery is performed with several basic steps:

1. Isolation and exposure of the nerve of interest using standard surgical procedure. This should be proximal to the site of injury or region of pain if no identifiable injury exists (**Fig. 1**).
2. Longitudinal exposure of a length of nerve sufficient to support the paddle electrode. There are currently paddle-type electrodes that contain 4, 8, or 16 contacts, so the surgery must be tailored accordingly.
3. The nerve is dissected and lifted up allowing placement of the electrode deep to the nerve. Here it is sutured to surrounding muscle and/or fascia to prevent migration.
4. If done with sedation and local anesthesia, trial stimulation may be performed prior to tunneling to ensure appropriate positioning of the leads.

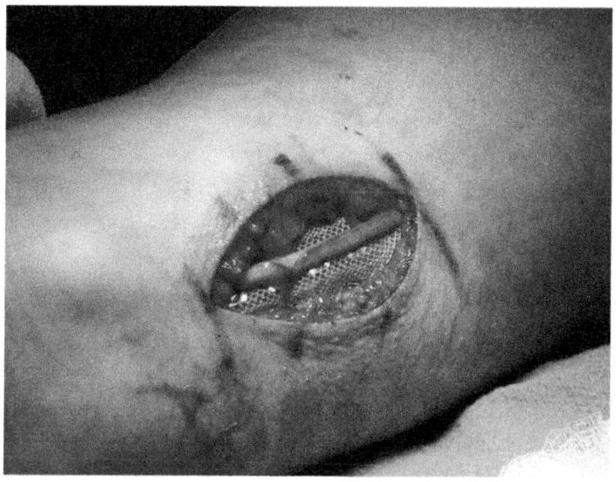

Fig. 1. A 37-year-old man with a previous crush injury to the right hand. He had residual pain in an ulnar nerve distribution in his hand refractory to conservative measures. An incision was made along the course of the ulnar nerve just proximal to the elbow to avoid placing the electrodes over a mobile segment. Here it is demonstrated that the ulnar nerve has been circumferentially dissected, and the 4-contact paddle-type lead has been secured deep to the nerve.

Otherwise, impedances should be checked if done under general anesthesia.

5. The leads are tunneled to the exterior for connection to a pulse generator for the duration of the trial period, often approximately 1 week.

Many investigators consider a successful trial a 50% reduction in patient pain symptoms. If the trial period does not yield successful results, the electrode may be removed. If, however, there is significant reduction in pain during this time period, patients are returned to the operating room for phase 2 of the operation, described in a stepwise fashion:

1. The prior incision is opened as is a second incision to allow for placement of the RF generator or the IPG. Common sites include the chest, abdominal wall, buttock, or lateral thigh depending on the involved nerve (**Fig. 2**).
2. Lead extenders may be used if necessary and are tunneled subcutaneously to the site of RF or IPG implantation. Care must be taken to position extenders with strain relief loops and to minimize strain on any wires that cross a joint.
3. Settings are usually adjusted and tailored on an outpatient basis. Initial programming begins approximately 2 weeks after placement of the device. Immediately after stimulator placement, the device is typically left in the off position to minimize changes in stimulation results due to resolving edema.
4. Some investigators recommend obtaining plain films of the lead position that may be compared with films in the future to assess for possible migration in the event that efficacy diminishes.
5. Some surgeons skip the trial period and proceed with implantation right away.

A comment should be made about RF-coupled systems versus IPGs. RF-coupled systems were the first type of implantable device, but they had the disadvantage of still requiring an external component that limited the ability to maintain stimulation in some situations, such as bathing. They were, however, eventually Food and Drug Administration (FDA) approved for use in nerve stimulation. IPGs, developed later, are almost exclusively used over RF generators, because they do not require manual input with an external component to generate pain relief. The only disadvantage in this case is that IPGs run out of battery several years after placement, requiring another surgery to replace them. Rechargeable IPGs mitigate the need for battery replacement, with some devices having lifetimes in excess of a decade. Despite that RF-coupled systems gained FDA approval decades ago, IPGs have never been FDA approved for this use, and, therefore, most modern procedures of PNS are technically performed as physician-directed indications.[2]

The description provided in this article is for open surgical placement of paddle-type electrodes, although percutaneous insertion of cylindrical and small paddle-type electrodes is growing in popularity. Given the small size and superficial nature of craniofacial nerves, percutaneously placed leads are typically chosen for these procedures. Several investigators have demonstrated successful and efficacious use of these electrodes in the extremity as well.[30] This procedure may be done exclusively with a Tuohy needle or with a minimal open approach. Petersen and Slavin[29] published an excellent overview of the surgical steps involved in percutaneous lead placement just a few years ago.

COMPLICATIONS AND CONCERNS

With few large trials involving PNS or PNFS, most of the statistics regarding complications with these procedures come from small case series. The most common complications are not surprising and include wound infection, electrode migration, and skin erosion. PNS represents a far greater body of literature than PNFS, with wound infection rates reported between 3.6% and 17.9%. Intuitively, lead migration is more common with percutaneously placed leads because there are no sutures directly anchoring the electrode array to

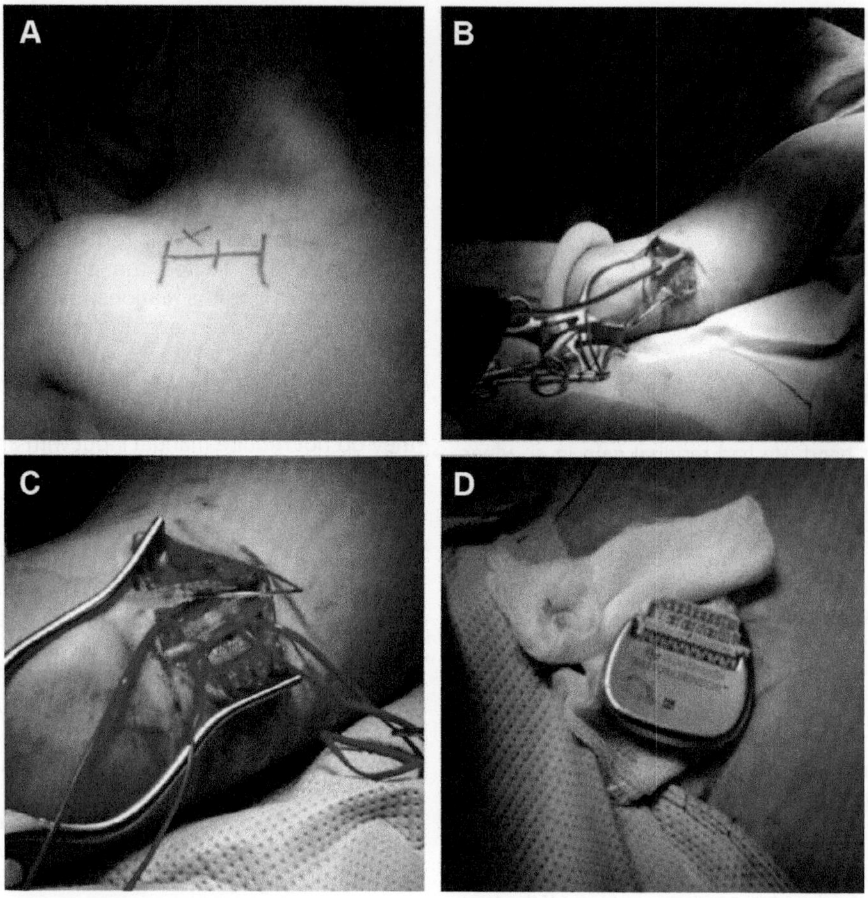

Fig. 2. (*A*) The chest incision has been marked beneath the clavicle for this ulnar nerve stimulator. (*B*) A tunneling trochar is passed in a subcutaneous fashion from the nerve to the IPG incision. (*C*) The leads are then connected to extenders and tunneled. (*D*) The leads are connected to the IPG after testing for imped. Both wounds are then irrigated and closed in a standard fashion.

muscle or fascia around the nerve, but no literature directly comparing the 2 exists. Overall, migration is reported to occur between 9% and 25%. One report even suggested a 100% rate of lead migration with percutaneously placed arrays. Although there is much more of a paucity of literature regarding complications and PNFS, a recent study of PNFS for back pain indicated an infection rate of 4.4%. Lead migration occurred in 15.6% of their patients, but erosion occurred in only 2.2%. Because percutaneous leads are placed without direct visualization of the affected nerve, it is possible to place them into the wrong tissue compartment. These electrodes, however, are characteristically placed with the assistance of fluoroscopy and more recently ultrasound, making this complication exceedingly rare.[32–38] See the article by Garrett P. Banks and Christopher J. Winfree's article, "Evolving Techniques and Indications in Peripheral Nerve Stimulation for Pain," elsewhere in this issue for further discussion of percutaneous and ultrasound-guided PNE placement.

Although not a complication in the conventional sense, failure of efficacy is perhaps the most significant outcome that can occur in this patient population, most of whom have been suffering from debilitating pain for several years and for whom nerve stimulation is their last option. Good or excellent results have been consistently achieved in 60% to 70% of patients, but the population that experiences no benefit or a worsening of symptoms constitutes only approximately 20%. As emphasized previously, the most crucial aspect of nerve stimulation is adequate counseling of the patient prior to undergoing the trial period. Establishing a confidence between practitioner and patient allows for informed decisions, open communication, and superior results.

SUMMARY

Chronic neuropathic pain is a common issue that is often refractory to medical treatment. Neuromodulation for the management of chronic pain is a technique that has its roots in the establishment of the gate control theory in 1965. Over the past 80 years it has undergone significant refinement and expansion, leading to the neuromodulation treatments available today. PNS/PNFS is now successfully used to treat traumatic nerve pain, low back pain, craniofacial pain, and a variety of other painful chronic neuropathies. Despite this success, the field is hampered by a lack of prospective randomized controlled evidence. It is crucial to pursue ongoing investigation into these techniques to provide the best evidence-based care to patients.

REFERENCES

1. Kumar K, Rizvi S. Historical and present state of neuromodulation in chronic pain. Curr Pain Headache Rep 2014;18:387.
2. Slavin KV. History of peripheral nerve stimulation. Prog Neurol Surg 2011;24:1–15.
3. Melzack R, Wall PD. Pain mechanisms: a new theory. Science 1965;150:971–9.
4. Campbell JN, Long DM. Peripheral nerve stimulation in the treatment of intractable pain. J Neurosurg 1976;45:692–9.
5. Laitinen L. Placement of electrodes in transcutaneous stimulation for chronic pain. Neurochirurgie 1976;22:517–26 [in French].
6. Wall PD, Sweet WH. Temporary abolition of pain in man. Science 1967;155:108–9.
7. Eisenberg L, Mauro A, Glenn WW, et al. Radiofrequency stimulation: a research and clinical tool. Science 1965;147:578–82.
8. Law JD, Swett J, Kirsch WM. Retrospective analysis of 22 patients with chronic pain treated by peripheral nerve stimulation. J Neurosurg 1980;52:482–5.
9. Waisbrod H, Panhans C, Hansen D, et al. Direct nerve stimulation for painful peripheral neuropathies. J Bone Joint Surg Br 1985;67:470–2.
10. Kirsch WM, Lewis JA, Simon RH. Experiences with electrical stimulation devices for the control of chronic pain. Med Instrum 1975;9:217–20.
11. Picaza JA, Hunter SE, Cannon BW. Pain suppression by peripheral nerve stimulation. Chronic effects of implanted devices. Appl Neurophysiol 1977;40:223–34.
12. Rasskazoff SY, Slavin KV. An update on peripheral nerve stimulation. J Neurosurg Sci 2012;56:279–85.
13. Hassenbusch SJ, Stanton-Hicks M, Schoppa D, et al. Long-term results of peripheral nerve stimulation for reflex sympathetic dystrophy. J Neurosurg 1996;84:415–23.
14. Cooney WP. Electrical stimulation and the treatment of complex regional pain syndromes of the upper extremity. Hand Clin 1997;13:519–26.
15. Novak CB, Mackinnon SE. Outcome following implantation of a peripheral nerve stimulator in patients with chronic nerve pain. Plast Reconstr Surg 2000;105:1967–72.
16. Strege DW, Cooney WP, Wood MB, et al. J Hand Surg Am 1994;19(6):931–9.
17. Mobbs RJ, Nair S, Blum P. Peripheral nerve stimulation for the treatment of chronic pain. J Clin Neurosci 2007;14:216–21 [discussion: 22–3].
18. Slavin KV, Colpan ME, Munawar N, et al. Trigeminal and occipital peripheral nerve stimulation for craniofacial pain: a single-institution experience and review of the literature. Neurosurg Focus 2006;21:E5.
19. Amin S, Buvanendran A, Park KS, et al. Peripheral nerve stimulator for the treatment of supraorbital neuralgia: a retrospective case series. Cephalalgia 2008;28:355–9.
20. Dunteman E. Peripheral nerve stimulation for unremitting ophthalmic postherpetic neuralgia. Neuromodulation 2002;5:32–7.
21. Johnson MD, Burchiel KJ. Peripheral stimulation for treatment of trigeminal postherpetic neuralgia and trigeminal posttraumatic neuropathic pain: a pilot study. Neurosurgery 2004;55:135–41 [discussion: 41–2].
22. Kouroukli I, Neofytos D, Panaretou V, et al. Peripheral subcutaneous stimulation for the treatment of intractable postherpetic neuralgia: two case reports and literature review. Pain Pract 2009;9:225–9.
23. Stidd DA, Wuollet AL, Bowden K, et al. Peripheral nerve stimulation for trigeminal neuropathic pain. Pain Physician 2012;15:27–33.
24. Yakovlev AE, Peterson AT. Peripheral nerve stimulation in treatment of intractable postherpetic neuralgia. Neuromodulation 2007;10:373–5.
25. Feletti A, Santi GZ, Sammartino F, et al. Peripheral trigeminal nerve field stimulation: report of 6 cases. Neurosurg Focus 2013;35:E10.
26. McRoberts WP, Wolkowitz R, Meyer DJ, et al. Peripheral nerve field stimulation for the management of localized chronic intractable back pain: results from a randomized controlled study. Neuromodulation 2013;16:565–74 [discussion: 74–5].
27. Mironer YE, Hutcheson JK, Satterthwaite JR, et al. Prospective, two-part study of the interaction between spinal cord stimulation and peripheral nerve field stimulation in patients with low back pain: development of a new spinal-peripheral neurostimulation method. Neuromodulation 2011;14:151–4 [discussion: 5].
28. Verrills P, Vivian D, Mitchell B, et al. Peripheral nerve field stimulation for chronic pain: 100 cases and review of the literature. Pain Med 2011;12:1395–405.

29. Petersen EA, Slavin KV. Peripheral nerve/field stimulation for chronic pain. Neurosurg Clin N Am 2014;25:789–97.
30. Reverberi C, Dario A, Barolat G, et al. Using peripheral nerve stimulation (PNS) to treat neuropathic pain: a clinical series. Neuromodulation 2014;17: 777–83 [discussion: 83].
31. Soin A, Fang ZP, Velasco J. Peripheral neuromodulation to treat postamputation pain. Prog Neurol Surg 2015;29:158–67.
32. Carayannopoulos A, Beasley R, Sites B. Facilitation of percutaneous trial lead placement with ultrasound guidance for peripheral nerve stimulation trial of ilioinguinal neuralgia: a technical note. Neuromodulation 2009;12:296–301.
33. Chan I, Brown AR, Park K, et al. Ultrasound-guided, percutaneous peripheral nerve stimulation: technical note. Neurosurgery 2010;67:ons136–9.
34. Gofeld M, Hanlon JG. Ultrasound-guided placement of a paddle lead onto peripheral nerves: surgical anatomy and methodology. Neuromodulation 2014; 17:48–53 [discussion].
35. Huntoon MA, Burgher AH. Ultrasound-guided permanent implantation of peripheral nerve stimulation (PNS) system for neuropathic pain of the extremities: original cases and outcomes. Pain Med 2009;10: 1369–77.
36. Skaribas I, Alo K. Ultrasound imaging and occipital nerve stimulation. Neuromodulation 2010;13:126–30.
37. Slavin KV. Technical aspects of peripheral nerve stimulation: hardware and complications. Prog Neurol Surg 2011;24:189–202.
38. Trentman TL, Zimmerman RS. Occipital nerve stimulation: technical and surgical aspects of implantation. Headache 2008;48:319–27.

Evolving Techniques and Indications in Peripheral Nerve Stimulation for Pain

Garrett P. Banks, MD*, Christopher J. Winfree, MD

KEYWORDS

- Peripheral nerve stimulation • Pain • Neurosurgery • Chronic pain

KEY POINTS

- Peripheral nerve stimulation plays an important role in treating chronic refractory pain syndromes that manifest in limited distributions and overlap with areas of neurologic innervation.
- Careful patient selection along with treatment trialing is an essential part of the workup owing to the subjective nature of symptoms.
- Recent advancements in stimulation technology allow for less invasive placement procedures, less noticeable stimulation, and the use of external pulse generators.

INTRODUCTION

Peripheral nerve stimulation (PNS) is the direct electrical stimulation of named nerves outside of the central neuraxis to alleviate pain in the distribution of the targeted peripheral nerve.[1] The technique works by directly stimulating the nerve responsible for the conduction of painful information from the area in which the patient is experiencing symptoms. Since it was first shown by Sweet and Wall that stimulation of the peripheral nervous system could ameliorate pain,[2] neural stimulation has been used by many practitioners for treating various etiologies of pain. These treatments have shown efficacy in treating a large variety of neuropathic,[3,4] musculoskeletal,[5] and visceral refractory pain[6] pathologies, and although not first line, these therapies are an important part of the treatment repertoire for chronic pain. These methods can be used either in isolation or in addition to techniques such as spinal cord stimulation or deep brain stimulation to tailor patient-specific treatments.

THE MECHANISM OF NEUROSTIMULATION

Our understanding of neurostimulation for pain has been improving since Sweet and Wall first described their success in the reduction of pain using PNS.[2,7] Although we still have much to learn regarding how the physiology works, the process is generally thought to capitalize on the inhibition and activation of pain-related neural circuitry, including ascending pathways in the dorsal horn nucleus and the modulatory pathways of the autonomic system.[8] Additionally, the treatment of pain using neurostimulation has been shown to not simply work by directly sending electrical signals to the areas of interest. Rather, the process involves modulation of several neurotransmitters, such as gamma-amino butyric acid and adenosine. Interestingly, the original mechanism, gate theory, used to explain why stimulation leads to pain relief suggested the necessity of paresthesias to induce analgesia, but new research has shown that high-frequency stimulation (~10 kHz) and burst spinal cord stimulation can provide at least similar, if not greater, pain relief even if the

Disclosure Statement: The authors have nothing to disclose.
Department of Neurosurgery, Columbia University, 710 West 168 Street, 4th Floor, New York, NY 10032, USA
* Corresponding author.
E-mail address: gpb2111@cumc.columbia.edu

Neurosurg Clin N Am 30 (2019) 265–273
https://doi.org/10.1016/j.nec.2018.12.011

stimulation is not readily perceivable. Because these high-frequency paradigms, which are now also being used in PNS, successfully produce analgesia despite patients not being consciously aware of stimulation, it suggests that we still do not fully understand the mechanistic underpinnings of electrical stimulation for pain.[9,10]

PREOPERATIVE ASSESSMENT

- Psychological screening of patients with medically refractory pain should be done as part of evaluation for PNS.
- The type of stimulation should be the least invasive, yet still efficacious, modality available.
- Diagnostic trials should be used when possible to raise the likelihood of success for those implanted.

Although neural stimulation for pain is efficacious, it is important to note that these patients must first be screened carefully. The first requirement for establishing candidacy is that the patient must have had failed first-line medical conservative therapies. To be eligible for neurostimulation, patients should have demonstrated inadequate response to medications, noninvasive treatment options, and minimally invasive pain management strategies, as appropriate to their specific pathology.[11] Once all conservative options are exhausted, patients should next undergo psychological testing.[12] Because many psychological characteristics and psychiatric pathologies can greatly exacerbate chronic pain, psychological evaluation can be useful for determining if psychological (or psychiatric) treatment is first warranted before exploring surgical options.

The most important factor in determining the type of stimulation that best addresses a patient's pain is the anatomic distribution of the patient's pain. For any given neurostimulation treatment, the chosen modality should specifically target the area where pain is experienced, and more invasive modalities should not be chosen over less invasive approaches that are just as efficacious and easier to implement. After selection of an appropriate modality, most institutions implement a trial before the permanent implant to determine if the implant is likely to achieve an adequate decrease in pain. Some practitioners perform a trial using a diagnostic nerve block, whereas others perform a trial using implanted temporary leads. The rationale for performing a nerve block is that, if the experienced pain improves after chemically blocking the nerve, then the correct anatomic target has been chosen as a stimulation candidate for relieving the patient's pain. Although this practice is helpful in some instances, the necessity of this step is debated.[9] The controversy is due to the unclear usefulness of a negative result. Although a successful nerve block supports treating the nerve in question, many patients have been found to benefit from neurostimulation, even if their initial nerve block was negative.

For those who do not screen patients using a nerve block, the patient must first undergo a short trial of stimulation.[13] The trial consists of implanting a patient with an electrode that is connected to an external pulse generator. The patient is then sent home with the electrode and receives stimulation for a week. The trial is considered a success if there is a 50% or greater decrease in the level of pain and if there is a meaningful improvement in their quality of life. The temporary device is then replaced with the permanent system. By using this paradigm, only patients who demonstrate benefit from trial stimulation undergo surgical implantation. Although there is no way to predict with 100% certainty which patients will ultimately benefit, the combination of judicious screening, careful patient selection, and trialing stimulation itself allows the practitioner to maximization of the likelihood of success for those who undergo electrical stimulation for chronic pain.

OPEN PLACEMENT OF PERIPHERAL NEUROSTIMULATION

Since Sweet and Wall described their success in 1967, surgeons began to use implantable neurostimulation devices as a means of treating refractory pain.[14] To perform an open implantation, the patient is provided monitored anesthesia and then prepped and draped in the usual fashion. The nerve in question is isolated and exposed by dissection and neurolysis from the surrounding tissue. Once properly exposed, a lead is placed along the nerve (**Fig. 1**). Although historically the lead has been wrapped around the nerve, this practice is no longer recommended owing to the resultant scarring and adhesions. At first, surgical descriptions of paddle lead placement along the nerve recommended the placement of a fascial layer between the electrode array and the nerve itself. This step was undertaken to dampen the stimulation intensity, because the early implantable pulse generators did not allow for fine adjustments and patients could experience dramatic changes in stimulation intensity with minor adjustments. Current pulse generators allow for much finer adjustments, obviating the need for a fascial barrier.

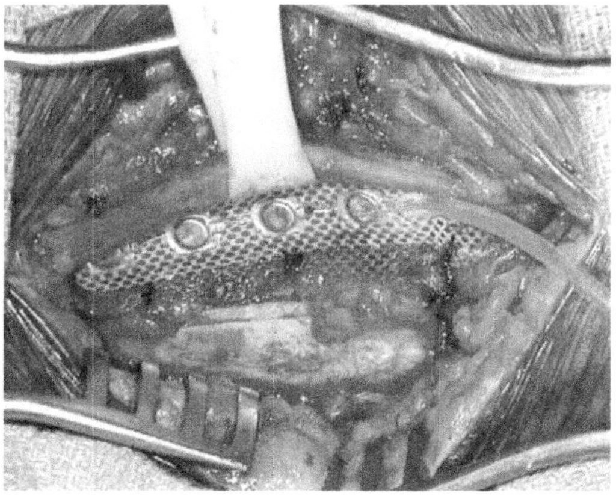

Fig. 1. Open placement of a tibial nerve stimulator. Although this intraoperative photo demonstrates a paddle lead, cylindrical electrodes may also be used. (*From* Stuart RM, Winfree CJ. Neurostimulation techniques for painful peripheral nerve disorders. Neurosurg Clin N Am 2009;20(1):115; with permission.)

The electrodes are then trialed in the operating room using an external pulse generator, and the stimulation is adjusted to ensure appropriate coverage. Once satisfactory coverage is achieved, the leads are sutured to the surrounding tissue and then attached to a disposable extension wire that is tunneled out through the skin. The extension lead is then attached to an external pulse generator and placed in a sterile sleeve. This sleeve is adhered to the outside of the body. The patient leaves the hospital that same day to trial the stimulator for approximately 1 week. If the trial is successful, the patient returns for internalization of the device. The disposable extensions are discarded and the leads are tunneled and connected to an implantable pulse generator that is placed in a subfascial pocket. The most commonly used locations to implant pulse generators are the buttocks, medial thigh, and subclavicular areas.[15]

Although the technique is efficacious and currently covered by payers such as Medicare and private insurance, open surgical exposure of the nerve for placement of the electrode is a procedure that can result in significant postoperative pain and often results in the buildup of scar tissue after multiple revisions. Also, owing to the mechanically dynamic nature of the areas where the leads are commonly placed, peripheral leads are more prone to experience mechanical failure and migration.[16]

PERCUTANEOUS PLACEMENT OF PERIPHERAL NEUROSTIMULATION

An alternative method for implanting stimulation leads is percutaneous placement. This alternative technique can be used for both trial electrode and permanent electrode placement. Similar to an open approach, the patient is provided monitored anesthesia and then prepped and draped in the usual fashion; however, instead of visualizing the nerve via surgical dissection, a needle and tunneling system is used to place a 4- or 8-contact electrode in the epifascial plane adjacent to the nerve. When placing electrodes in shallow areas with external landmarks (such as for craniofacial stimulation), fluoroscopic guidance is generally not required, but can be useful for verifying placement and for adjusting the leads. Deeper lead placement requires ultrasound guidance, as discussed elsewhere in this article.

Once again, after placement, the electrode is connected to an external pulse generator and a stimulation paradigm is chosen that results in adequate coverage. If the placement and coverage are satisfactory, then the lead or leads are anchored to the skin with a 3-0 silk to avoid strain or torque on the leads. The external pulse generator is placed in a sterile enclosed adhesive pocket, which is adhered to the patient near to where the lead exits the skin. The exit site is covered in sterile dressings and the patient is sent home for a week to trial the stimulation. Of note, the authors of this article do not regularly prescribe antibiotics for a routine stimulation trial. In contrast with the open placement method, the whole apparatus is usually removed at the end of the trial, no matter the result. If the trial was considered a success, fresh new leads are tunneled into position and connected to a pulse generator that is implanted subcutaneously.

Compared with open surgical placement of the electrode, percutaneous placement is faster, less traumatic, and usually results in markedly less postoperative pain; however, the technique historically was only well-suited for superficial targets, because the placement is performed indirectly. The main drawback of percutaneous placement in comparison with open placement is that cylindrical leads have a greater tendency to migrate.[16] There is minimal tissue friction with cylindrical leads, and only an anchor and a stitch hold the lead in place. When it occurs, lead migration tends to be along the pathway of the implantation (which is relatively easy to fix by repositioning); however, repeated revision of the lead can be burdensome for the patient.

TRIGEMINAL BRANCH STIMULATION

Craniofacial stimulation has been, and still is, one of the more successful indications for PNS owing to the inability to use spinal cord or dorsal root ganglion stimulation to treat pain in craniofacial distributions.[17] In fact, one of the original patients in the landmark series published by Wall and Sweet was able to attain chronic facial pain relief using infraorbital stimulation. Since then, PNS has been used to help many patients achieve facial pain relief. Both infraorbital and supraorbital stimulation have been found to alleviate pain in either postherpetic neuralgia or trigeminal posttraumatic neuropathic pain.[17–21]

Trigeminal branch stimulation is performed using a percutaneous lead insertion technique. The percutaneous implantation paradigm is used owing to its superficial location. Of note, although the trial implantation can be performed under conscious sedation, the permanent implant should ideally be placed under general anesthesia owing to the discomfort that results from tunneling down the neck to the area where the battery will be placed. The percutaneous entry point is marked out behind the hairline and above the zygoma for supraorbital placement or below the zygoma for infraorbital placement. The area is numbed with lidocaine and a stab incision is made. A large-gauge Tuohy needle is passed subcutaneously under fluoroscopic guidance to the supraorbital or infraorbital region, roughly 1 cm above or below the orbital rim, until the lead reaches the medial border of the orbit (**Fig. 2**). After passage of the needle, the stylet is removed and a 4- or 8-contact electrode is passed to the region of interest. For the trial, a temporary electrode is

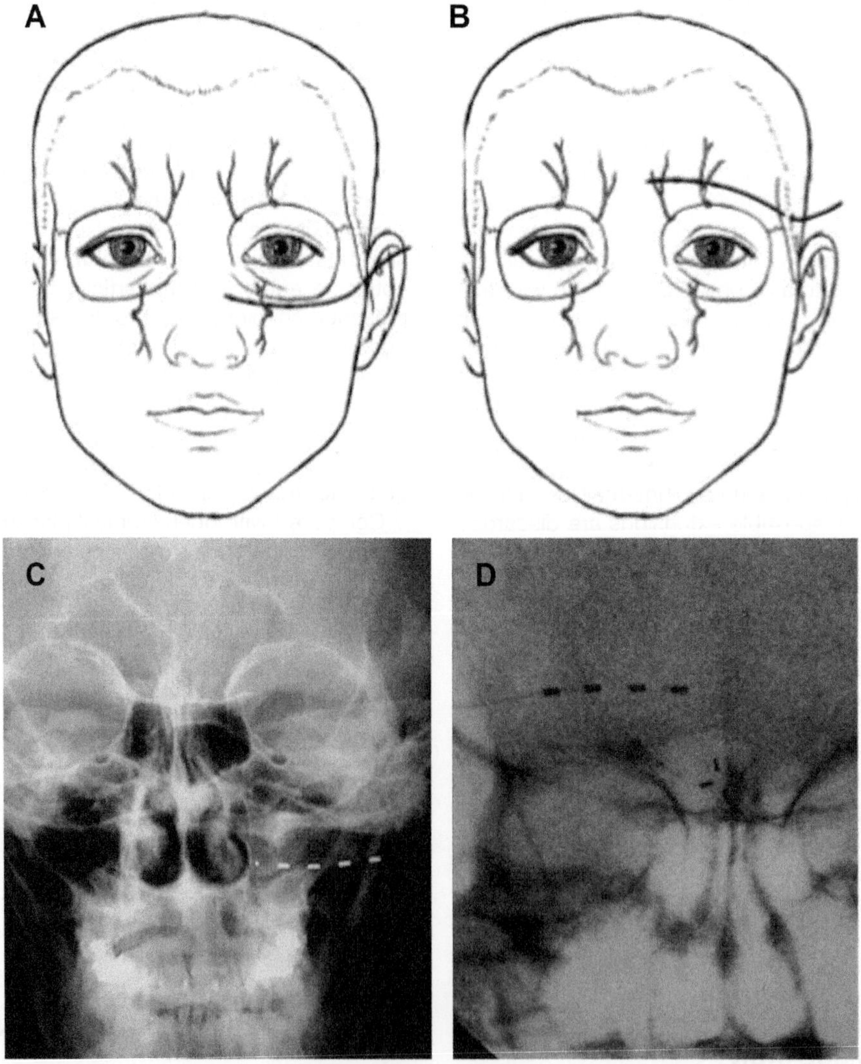

Fig. 2. (*A*, B) Where infraorbital and supraorbital electrodes are placed, respectively. (*C*, *D*) Placement of infraorbital and supraorbital electrodes on plain film radiographs. (*From* Slavin KV, Wess C. Trigeminal branch stimulation for intractable neuropathic pain: technical note. Neuromodulation 2005;8(1):8–11; with permission.)

connected to an external pulse generator to confirm coverage, and adjustments are made if necessary. The electrode is anchored in place with a silk suture, and hooked up to an external pulse generator. If the trial is successful, a permanent electrode is implanted. The permanent electrode is connected via extension wires to a pulse generator usually placed in a subcutaneous infraclavicular pocket.

Interestingly, not only does superficial pain respond well to trigeminal branch stimulation, but a variety of headache etiologies do as well. Chronic cluster headaches have been reported to respond well to supraorbital neurostimulation in patients who gained minimal benefit from nerve blocks.[22] The dual use of both supraorbital and occipital nerve stimulation has also been used to control chronic migraine headaches.[21]

STIMULATION FOR OCCIPITAL NEURALGIA

Occipital neuralgia is a condition where patients experience sharp, shooting, paroxysmal pain (although occasionally throbbing) from the occiput to the posterior scalp in the distribution of the occipital nerve.[23] The pain can be bilateral, but most patients present with unilateral pain distributions. Although the pain can occur with triggers, these episodes of pain can occur unprovoked as well. For most patients, there is a history of injury to the areas such as compression or trauma.

Like other peripheral pain pathologies, first-line therapy consists of medications such as antiepileptics or antidepressants. For refractory pain, local anesthesia, Botox, and steroid injections are able to temporarily relieve symptoms, but have limited durability. After appropriate conservative management has failed, patients may be considered for surgical therapy.

Surgical therapy for occipital neuralgia can either be ablative or stimulation based. Multiple ablative procedures have been used to treat occipital neuralgia, ranging from ganglionectomy to neurolysis and posterior partial rhizotomy.[24] These procedures vary in efficacy and carry their own specific side effects, which are usually not reversible. Alternatively, one of the main benefits of occipital nerve stimulation is that the procedure is efficacious, durable, reversible, and carries minimal side effects.

Current guidelines recommend the use of occipital nerve stimulation for medically refractory occipital neuralgia; however, this recommendation is not based on class I evidence, because there are no randomized, controlled trials of stimulation for occipital neuralgia.[25] A review of the existing literature (mostly retrospective studies) reveals that, with appropriately selected patients, occipital nerve stimulation can effectively decrease both pain (as measured on a visual analog scale) and medication use. The screening process is similar to other PNS indications, with patients requiring psychiatric evaluation and then a trial of stimulation.[26–28] Reported efficacy varies from trial to trial, but almost all patients endorsed a greater than 50% decrease in their pain at the follow-up assessment, with many experiencing little to no pain at all.[25] Of note, despite the impressive efficacy in these studies, it must be kept in mind that these are not randomized controlled trials.

The surgical technique for placing electrodes also varies from study to study, but the general principals remain the same. Patients are brought to the operating room and positioned usually in the prone position. The level of anesthesia varies from study to study, with some practitioners using general anesthesia and others using conscious sedation. The patient is then prepped and draped in the usual fashion.

The electrodes can either be passed starting at the mastoid process inferomedial across the passage of the occipital nerve or starting medially and taking the same pathway, but in reverse. The specific implanted device used varies in the literature, with some practitioners using percutaneous leads and some using paddle leads. For permanent implants, the most frequent location for the internal pulse generator is in an infraclavicular pocket. Similar to other percutaneous implantation techniques, the most common technical adverse event in the postoperative period is lead migration.[25] Evidence for and techniques for occipital nerve stimulation are covered in detail by Konstantin V. Slavin and colleagues' article, "Occipital Nerve Stimulation," in this issue.

STIMULATION FOR HEADACHE

Stimulation of the occipital nerves has also been used for the treatment of chronic headache. The technique has demonstrated efficacy in migraine, cluster headache, posttraumatic headaches, and hemicrania continua.[29] In a large trial of more than 100 patients receiving occipital nerve stimulation for chronic migraines, a 50% decrease in the number of headache days experienced by patients was seen in approximately one-half of the population treated (47.8%).[30] Approximately 70% of those treated endorsed improved quality of life at 1 year after the procedure. The implantation technique is the same as for occipital neuralgia, and the adverse event profile is also similar. Mechanical failures were the number one complication that required surgical revision, consisting of lead migration (13.9%), lead fracture (3.3%), and battery failure (3.8%).

POSTAMPUTATION LIMB PAIN

After amputation, a majority of patients (70%–80%) are left with chronic pain, which is either classified as phantom limb pain or residual limb pain. Inadequately treated pain syndromes in these patients can further impair their function, hamper their rehabilitation, and even prohibit the use of prosthetics. Unfortunately, pharmacologic treatment for postamputation pain is frequently inadequate, and carries with it both unwanted side effects and the potential for addiction. In patients with pain after amputation, PNS of the femoral or sciatic nerve has been shown to significantly reduce pain.[31] The majority of patients in a small, retrospective series who were implanted for residual limb pain experienced a significant decrease in their pain along with an improved quality of life.[32]

Recently, some groups have started placing PNS leads for postamputation limb pain percutaneously using landmarks in effort to design a less morbid methodology. The sciatic nerve can be accessed using a posterior approach, with the greater trochanter and ischial tuberosity as landmarks. The femoral nerve can be accessed using an anterior approach, with the femoral artery and femoral crease as landmarks.

Before placing the lead, a monopolar needle electrode is inserted to within 0.5 to 3.0 cm of the trunk of the femoral or sciatic nerve to deliver a test stimulation to ascertain proximity to the nerve. This testing stimulation determines if comfortable paresthesias can be produced without evoking muscle contractions or irritating sensations. If the positioning is correct, the paresthesias should manifest in the distribution of the postamputation pain. If local subcutaneous sensations are experienced, the position is likely superficial and the needle can be advanced. Alternatively, if either muscle contractions or uncomfortable sensations in the area supplied by the nerve trunk are elicited, the needle is withdrawn slightly. After a satisfactory result is achieved, the stimulation needle is removed and a fine wire needle is used to place the lead in the same trajectory under ultrasound guidance. Of note, the lead is often advanced approximately 1 centimeter less than the stimulation electrode, placing the lead slightly farther from the nerve.

Last, some groups have begun to use high-frequency stimulation for postamputation pain.[33] This technique uses alternating current at a frequency of 5 to 30 kHz to produce a reversible conduction block of the nerve implicated in the patient's postamputation pain. In a recent study, stimulation resulted in an average of a 75% decrease in pain at 3 months after implantation. Although the study only included 7 patients, it demonstrated the possibility of effectively treating postamputation pain with high-frequency stimulation.

PERIPHERAL NERVE/FIELD STIMULATION

When patients suffer from pain not clearly localized to a specific nerve's distribution, stimulation of the peripheral nerve innervating the area in question is not an option. For these patients, if their pain is relatively limited in total surface area, the location itself can be stimulated. This technique is called peripheral nerve/field stimulation (PNFS), and is performed by directly placing electrodes subcutaneously in the area of pain. For this procedure, the method is similar to placing a percutaneous peripheral nerve lead, but the leads are implanted in relationship to the area of pain rather than the nerve.[11] Cylindrical leads are classically used for this technique owing to the simplicity of implantation (although some practitioners have reported using paddle leads as well.)

When implanting electrodes for PNFS stimulation, the depth is very important, because electrodes implanted too shallow will cause a stinging or burning sensations and may result in erosion, and electrodes implanted too deep will cause unintended muscle stimulation and twitching.[16] Similar to other nerve stimulation techniques, stimulation is first trialed, and a permanent implant is placed if the trial is considered a success.

PNFS has been published on extensively in the literature, with studies demonstrating a decrease in lower back pain,[34,35] chronic abdominal pain, inguinal neuralgia, chronic pancreatitis-related pain, and pain after liver transplantation.[6,36] PNFS has even been able to improve thoracic and chest wall pain when implanted at the site of pain.[37] However, although the technique has been shown in many case series to be beneficial, the method is no longer reimbursed in the United States. Owing to difficulty in attaining reimbursement, PNFS has largely fallen out of favor as a treatment for refractory chronic pain, at least in the United States.

ULTRASOUND-GUIDED PERIPHERAL NERVE STIMULATION

Historically, one of the main drawbacks of percutaneous implantation was that the positioning of electrodes near deeper targets was technically difficult. Recently, to attain the minimal morbidity benefits of percutaneous placement, practitioners have begun to use ultrasound guidance during the placement of electrodes for deeper targets.

After the patient is administered local anesthesia and antibiotics, the patient is draped in the usual fashion. A small skin nick is made and a 14-gauge epidural needle is passed to the target using ultrasound guidance. The needle is advanced until it is a few millimeters past to the nerve. A standard 8-contact percutaneous epidural neurostimulation electrode is then passed through the needle until resistance is met. The needle is then withdrawn while keeping the electrode in place (**Fig. 3**). After stimulation demonstrates paresthesias in the correct location, the lead is anchored in the skin for trials or to the superficial fascia for permanent

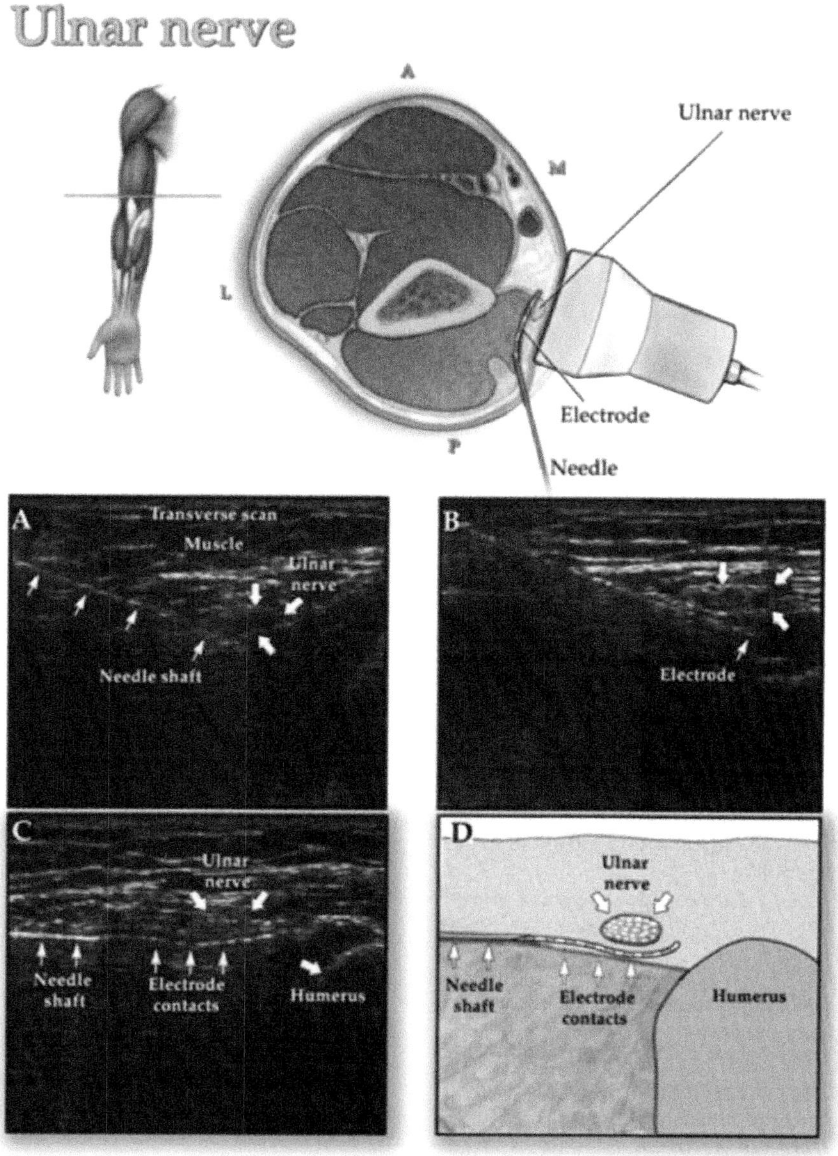

Fig. 3. Ultrasound-guided placement of a lead near the ulnar nerve. (*Top*) A slice through the arm at 12 cm proximal to the epicondyle. (*A*) The needle approaching the ulnar nerve, which is highlighted by *block arrows*. (*B*) The electrode emerging from the needle tip. (*C*) The deploying of the electrode lead with the needle being removed. (*D*) Depiction of the finished construct. (*From* Huntoon MA, Burgher AH. Ultrasound-guided permanent implantation of peripheral nerve stimulation (PNS) system for neuropathic pain of the extremities: original cases and outcomes. Pain Med 2009;10(8):1371; with permission.)

implants. A strain loop is created at the anchoring site to prevent strain-related damage or migration of the lead.[38]

Ultrasound guidance has the potential to significantly alter the field of neurostimulation for pain, and the use of ultrasound-guided implantation of percutaneous leads is growing as practitioners continue to gain expertise. As experience in the field grows, deeper and more difficult targets are becoming simpler procedures that no longer require open dissection and neurolysis. Published case series have shown that it is feasible to implant stimulation electrodes adjacent to the median, radial, ulnar, peroneal, and posterior tibial nerves.[38] The increasing experience with ultrasound guidance has even lead practitioners to perform in-office ultrasound-guided placement of trial electrodes instead of requiring placement in the operating room. The preliminary results from this change in treatment paradigm are promising and may allow for PNS for chronic pain to become more accessible.[39]

EXTERNAL PULSE GENERATORS

A recently developed device using a permanently implanted electrode that communicates with an external pulse generator showed promising results in a prospective randomized trial.[40] Whereas previous PNS devices classically use an implanted pulse generator, this new device is powered by an external rechargeable device that is worn outside of the body. This new technology has also been specifically designed to address many of the limitations of PNS and PNFS, such as having leads manufactured with tines to prevent migration. The study demonstrated significantly improved pain scores in a randomized clinical trial compared with controls, along with improvements in mood, physical activity, and quality of life.

SUMMARY

PNS is an efficacious technique for alleviating chronic refractory pain that is refractory to first-line therapy. The techniques can be used either in isolation or in combination with other stimulation strategies to tailor neuromodulation therapies to a patient's specific needs. Recent technological advancements are mitigating historical limitations, making implantation strategies less morbid and more accessible. Understanding the indications, benefits, and limitations of PNS for chronic refractory pain is crucial for any practitioner treating chronic pain.

REFERENCES

1. Diwan S, Staats P. Atlas of pain medicine procedures. New York: McGraw-Hill Companies, Inc.; 2015.
2. Wall PD, Sweet WH. Temporary abolition of pain in man. Science 1967;155(3758):108–9.
3. Al-Jehani H, Jacques L. Peripheral nerve stimulation for chronic neurogenic pain. Prog Neurol Surg 2011; 24:27–40.
4. Slavin KV. Peripheral nerve stimulation for neuropathic pain. Neurotherapeutics 2008;5(1):100–6.
5. McRoberts WP, Roche M. Novel approach for peripheral subcutaneous field stimulation for the treatment of severe, chronic knee joint pain after total knee arthroplasty. Neuromodulation 2010;13(2): 131–6.
6. Paicius RM, Bernstein CA, Lempert-Cohen C. Peripheral nerve field stimulation in chronic abdominal pain. Pain Physician 2006;9(3):261–6.
7. Melzack R, Wall PD. Pain mechanisms: a new theory. Science 1965;150(3699):971–9.
8. Lee AW, Pilitsis JG. Spinal cord stimulation: indications and outcomes. Neurosurg Focus 2006; 21(6):E3.
9. Slavin KV, Colpan ME, Munawar N, et al. Trigeminal and occipital peripheral nerve stimulation for craniofacial pain: a single-institution experience and review of the literature. Neurosurg Focus 2006;21(6): E5.
10. De Ridder D, Plazier M, Kamerling N, et al. Burst spinal cord stimulation for limb and back pain. World Neurosurg 2013;80(5):642–9.e1.
11. Deogaonkar M, Slavin KV. Peripheral nerve/field stimulation for neuropathic pain. Neurosurg Clin N Am 2014;25(1):1–10.
12. Campbell CM, Jamison RN, Edwards RR. Psychological screening/phenotyping as predictors for spinal cord stimulation. Curr Pain Headache Rep 2013; 17(1):307.
13. Mekhail NA, Mathews M, Nageeb F, et al. Retrospective review of 707 cases of spinal cord stimulation: indications and complications. Pain Pract 2011; 11(2):148–53.
14. Campbell JN, Long DM. Peripheral nerve stimulation in the treatment of intractable pain. J Neurosurg 1976;45(6):692–9.
15. Weiner RL. The future of peripheral nerve neurostimulation. Neurol Res 2000;22(3):299–304.
16. Slavin KV. Technical aspects of peripheral nerve stimulation: hardware and complications. Prog Neurol Surg 2011;24:189–202.
17. Ellis JA, Mejia Munne JC, Winfree CJ. Trigeminal branch stimulation for the treatment of intractable craniofacial pain. J Neurosurg 2015;123(1):283–8.
18. Dunteman E. Peripheral nerve stimulation for unremitting ophthalmic postherpetic neuralgia. Neuromodulation 2002;5(1):32–7.

19. Johnson MD, Burchiel KJ. Peripheral stimulation for treatment of trigeminal postherpetic neuralgia and trigeminal posttraumatic neuropathic pain: a pilot study. Neurosurgery 2004;55(1):135–41 [discussion: 141–2].
20. Slavin KV, Wess C. Trigeminal branch stimulation for intractable neuropathic pain: technical note. Neuromodulation 2005;8(1):7–13.
21. Amin S, Buvanendran A, Park KS, et al. Peripheral nerve stimulator for the treatment of supraorbital neuralgia: a retrospective case series. Cephalalgia 2008;28(4):355–9.
22. Narouze SN, Kapural L. Supraorbital nerve electric stimulation for the treatment of intractable chronic cluster headache: a case report. Headache 2007; 47(7):1100–2.
23. Slavin KV, Nersesyan H, Wess C. Peripheral neurostimulation for treatment of intractable occipital neuralgia. Neurosurgery 2006;58(1):112–9 [discussion: 112–9].
24. Acar F, Miller J, Golshani KJ, et al. Pain relief after cervical ganglionectomy (C2 and C3) for the treatment of medically intractable occipital neuralgia. Stereotact Funct Neurosurg 2008;86(2):106–12.
25. Sweet JA, Mitchell LS, Narouze S, et al. Occipital nerve stimulation for the treatment of patients with medically refractory occipital neuralgia: congress of neurological surgeons systematic review and evidence-based guideline. Neurosurgery 2015; 77(3):332–41.
26. Kapural L, Mekhail N, Hayek SM, et al. Occipital nerve electrical stimulation via the midline approach and subcutaneous surgical leads for treatment of severe occipital neuralgia: a pilot study. Anesth Analg 2005;101(1):171–4. table of contents.
27. Palmisani S, Al-Kaisy A, Arcioni R, et al. A six year retrospective review of occipital nerve stimulation practice–controversies and challenges of an emerging technique for treating refractory headache syndromes. J Headache Pain 2013;14:67.
28. Magown P, Garcia R, Beauprie I, et al. Occipital nerve stimulation for intractable occipital neuralgia: an open surgical technique. Clin Neurosurg 2009; 56:119–24.
29. Brewer AC, Trentman TL, Ivancic MG, et al. Long-term outcome in occipital nerve stimulation patients with medically intractable primary headache disorders. Neuromodulation 2013;16(6):557–62 [discussion: 563–4].
30. Dodick DW, Silberstein SD, Reed KL, et al. Safety and efficacy of peripheral nerve stimulation of the occipital nerves for the management of chronic migraine: long-term results from a randomized, multicenter, double-blinded, controlled study. Cephalalgia 2015;35(4):344–58.
31. Rauck RL, Kapural L, Cohen SP, et al. Peripheral nerve stimulation for the treatment of postamputation pain–a case report. Pain Pract 2012;12(8): 649–55.
32. Rauck RL, Cohen SP, Gilmore CA, et al. Treatment of post-amputation pain with peripheral nerve stimulation. Neuromodulation 2014;17(2):188–97.
33. Soin A, Shah NS, Fang ZP. High-frequency electrical nerve block for postamputation pain: a pilot study. Neuromodulation 2015;18(3):197–205 [discussion: 205–6].
34. Verrills P, Mitchell B, Vivian D, et al. Peripheral nerve stimulation: a treatment for chronic low back pain and failed back surgery syndrome? Neuromodulation 2009;12(1):68–75.
35. Kloimstein H, Likar R, Kern M, et al. Peripheral nerve field stimulation (PNFS) in chronic low back pain: a prospective multicenter study. Neuromodulation 2014;17(2):180–7.
36. Stinson LW Jr, Roderer GT, Cross NE, et al. Peripheral subcutaneous electrostimulation for control of intractable post-operative inguinal pain: a case report series. Neuromodulation 2001;4(3):99–104.
37. Goroszeniuk T, Kothari S, Hamann W. Subcutaneous neuromodulating implant targeted at the site of pain. Reg Anesth Pain Med 2006;31(2):168–71.
38. Huntoon MA, Burgher AH. Ultrasound-guided permanent implantation of peripheral nerve stimulation (PNS) system for neuropathic pain of the extremities: original cases and outcomes. Pain Med 2009;10(8): 1369–77.
39. Reddy CG, Flouty OE, Holland MT, et al. Novel technique for trialing peripheral nerve stimulation: ultrasonography-guided StimuCath trial. Neurosurg Focus 2017;42(3):E5.
40. Deer T, Pope J, Benyamin R, et al. Prospective, multicenter, randomized, double-blinded, partial crossover study to assess the safety and efficacy of the novel neuromodulation system in the treatment of patients with chronic pain of peripheral nerve origin. Neuromodulation 2016;19(1): 91–100.

Brain-Computer Interfaces in Quadriplegic Patients

Morgan B. Lee, BS[a,b,c,*], Daniel R. Kramer, MD[a,b,c], Terrance Peng, BS, MPH[a,b,c], Michael F. Barbaro, BA[a,b,c], Charles Y. Liu, MD, PhD[a,b,c], Spencer Kellis, PhD[a,b,c], Brian Lee, MD, PhD[a,b,c,d]

KEYWORDS

- Brain-computer interfaces (BCI) • Neuromodulation • Brain-machine interfaces (BMI)
- Functional electrical stimulation (FES)

KEY POINTS

- BCI aim to restore function to quadriplegic patients through virtual prosthetics, physical prosthetics, and FES systems.
- State-of-the-art invasive neural recording devices read from primary motor cortex or posterior parietal cortex to control a range of effectors.
- Future BCI will build on the research successes of motor BCI and incorporate sensory feedback, creating a closed-loop system.

INTRODUCTION

Spinal cord injury affects approximately 17,000 people per year in the United States, with a prevalence of 280,000 people.[1] The loss of function suffered by these patients is life altering. Quadriplegic patients require lifelong assistance to interact with their world. Brain-computer interfaces (BCI), have the potential to restore function to these patients in a meaningful way.

BCI aims to restore function to patients affected by neurologic injury by connecting the brain to an effector that can perform functions that were lost. Progress in the ability to read from the brain and decode motor intent has facilitated success in early human clinical trials.[2–4] Robust virtual and physical prosthetics aim to restore naturalistic function, with goals including speed, complexity, and somatosensory feedback.[5–7]

This review summarizes the progress that has been made in BCI. Advances in each component of the BCI system bring us closer to a solution that can move from clinical trials to widespread adoption as a standard of care technology.

MOTOR BRAIN-COMPUTER INTERFACES

The goal of a BCI is to restore motor and sensory function for persons who have lost a limb or suffered a neurologic injury, such as stroke, spinal cord injury, or amyotrophic lateral sclerosis.[8]

The fundamental components of a motor BCI include a sensor to record neural signals; a decoder to interpret movement intention; and an effector, such as a robotic limb, wheelchair, or a computer cursor, which interacts with the external environment (**Fig. 1**).[9,10] A pioneering study published in 1999 by Chapin and colleagues[2] demonstrated

Disclosure Statement: The authors have nothing to disclose.

[a] Department of Neurological Surgery, Keck School of Medicine of USC, University of Southern California, 1200 North State Street, Suite 3300, Los Angeles, CA 90033, USA; [b] USC Neurorestoration Center, Keck School of Medicine of USC, University of Southern California, 1975 Zonal Ave, Los Angeles, CA 90033, USA; [c] T&C Chen Brain Machine Interface Center, California Institute of Technology, 1200 E California Boulevard, Pasadena, CA 91125, USA; [d] Department of Biology and Biological Engineering, California Institute of Technology, 1200 E California Boulevard, Pasadena, CA 91125, USA

* Corresponding author. Department of Neurological Surgery, Keck School of Medicine of USC, University of Southern California, 1200 North State Street, Suite 3300 Los Angeles, CA 90033.
E-mail address: morganle@usc.edu

Neurosurg Clin N Am 30 (2019) 275–281
https://doi.org/10.1016/j.nec.2018.12.009

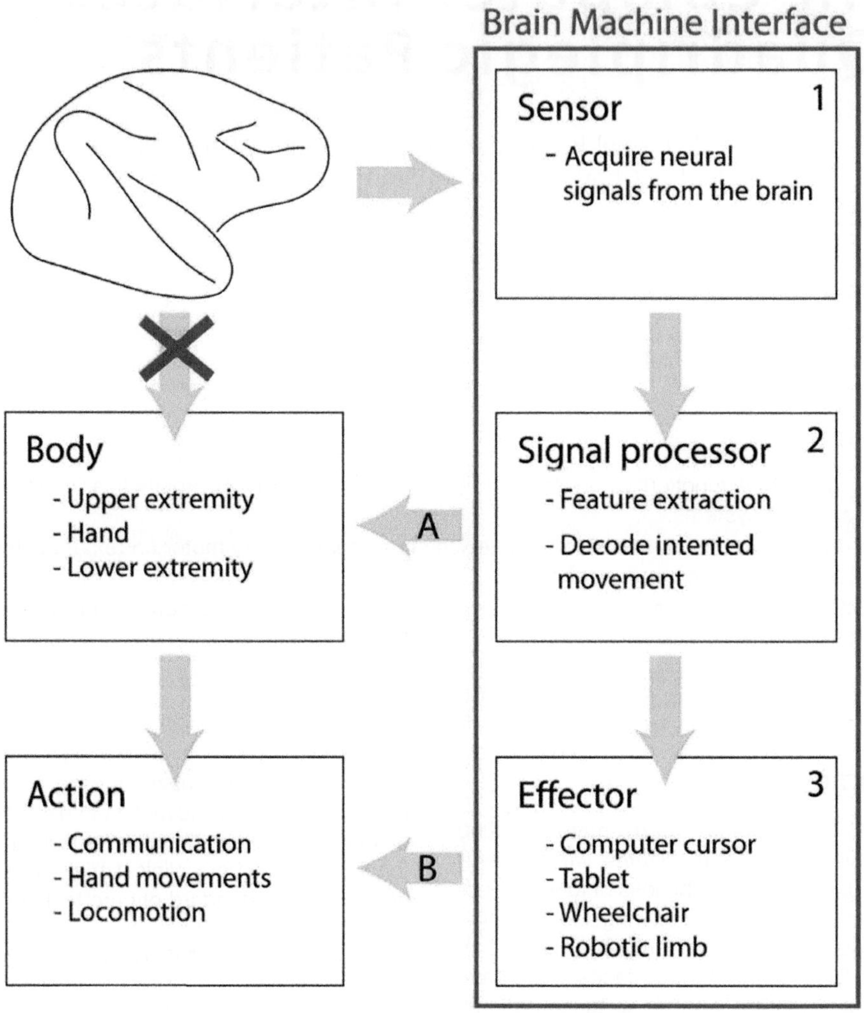

Fig. 1. Schematic representation of a brain-machine interface. The terms BCI and neuroprosthetic are also used when referring to this system. When the connection between brain and body is disrupted by neurologic injury or limb amputation, a BCI can bypass this interruption using a sensor, signal processor, and effector. The sensor (1) records neural signals from the brain. The signal processor (2), or decoder, interprets the neural signal to determine motor intention. This intention is directed to the body (A) using functional electrical stimulation or to an effector (3). The end result is an intended action restored to the patient. (*From* Lee B, Liu CY, Apuzzo MLJ. A primer on brain-machine interfaces, concepts, and technology: a key element in the future of functional neurorestoration. World Neurosurg 2013;79(3-4):460; with permission.)

that motor cortex recordings from a mouse could be decoded to control a robotic arm. Since then, significant progress has been made in all of the components of BCI: sensors, decoders, and effectors.

BCI have been created with neural signals derived from recording modalities covering a range of spatiotemporal resolutions, including electroencephalogram, electrocorticography (ECoG), and microelectrode arrays (MEAs). MEAs can record single unit activity from individual neurons. The other two modalities record field potentials, which represent the aggregate activity of thousands of neurons. These devices are less invasive than MEAs and cover a larger cortical area at the cost of lower quality neural signals. MEAs provide the highest quality neural signals in today's BCI.

One of the most commonly used MEAs in human BCI research is the 4 mm $\times$ 4 mm, 96-channel MEA from Blackrock Microsystems (Salt Lake City, UT).[8] These arrays have been implanted in primary motor cortex (M1)[3,11,12] and the posterior parietal cortex (PPC)[4] of nonhuman primates and humans to control upper extremity motor BCI.

The BrainGate group conducted the first human trial of motor BCI starting in June 2004. Hochberg and colleagues[3] recorded from a Blackrock 96-channel MEA implanted in the arm area of M1 in a patient with tetraplegia following cervical spinal cord injury. They achieved two-dimensional movement of a cursor on a screen and subsequently used this "neural cursor" to direct the movement of a robotic limb.

EXTERNAL EFFECTORS IN MOTOR BRAIN-COMPUTER INTERFACES

The effector used in a motor BCI system is virtual or physical. Quadriplegic patients in particular stand to benefit from an array of effector options, because they have lost more than the function of one limb.

Virtual effectors include keyboards that have been optimized for communication speed. Using advanced decoding techniques, Pandarinath and colleagues[7] demonstrated high-performance electronic typing. They found that the OPTI-II keyboard controlled by two MEA implants in M1 can achieve near normal type speeds. Further advances in virtual typing have created systems that are self-calibrating, which addresses the issue of MEA signal changing over time.[13]

For upper extremity restoration, the two state-of-the-art robotic limbs are the DEKA arm and the modular prosthetic limb (MPL).[8] The DEKA arm is produced by DEKA Integrated Solutions Corporation (Manchester, NH). It was created as part of the Defense Advanced Research Project Agency Revolutionizing Prosthetics project. The DEKA arm was created with upper limb amputees in mind and comes in three configurations to suit different levels of amputation: radial configuration, humeral configuration, and shoulder configuration.[14]

Although originally designed for upper extremity amputees, the advanced functionality of the DEKA arm has allowed it to be used as an effector in motor BCI systems in quadriplegic patients. The DEKA arm was used by the BrainGate team in their second clinical trial, BrainGate2, in which two tetraplegic patients completed a task requiring three-dimensional reach and grasp. Both patients were implanted with Blackrock MEAs in M1.[11]

The MPL was built by the Johns Hopkins University Applied Physics Laboratory through the Defense Advanced Research Project Agency Advanced Revolutionizing Prosthetics project. At only 9 lb, it was designed to mimic the weight of a natural arm and features 17° of freedom.[8] Along with more advanced motion, the MPL has built-in sensors that have the potential to provide somatosensory feedback. Sensors are able to detect force, vibration, temperature, and contact.[6]

Collinger and colleagues[12] demonstrated the utility of the MPL in a patient with tetraplegia from spinocerebellar degeneration. Using recordings in M1, the patient was able to achieve seven-dimensional movements, including three-dimensional translation, three-dimensional orientation, and one-dimensional grasping.

BEYOND M1 FOR MOTOR BRAIN-COMPUTER INTERFACES

Motor BCI began with recordings from M1, but further work has demonstrated the utility of recording from the PPC. Aflalo and colleagues demonstrated that recordings from the PPC can also be used to control a cursor and robotic arm in a tetraplegic subject. The patient had two MEAs implanted into a reach area and a grasp area in PPC. Building on previous nonhuman primate work,[15,16] they demonstrated that PPC represents motor intention and could be used in a BCI. The signals decoded from PPC allowed the patient to control the robotic arm with enough dexterity to drink a beverage unassisted.[17] Advantages found using the PPC recording site include fast decoding of intended movement, the ability to record and use goal and trajectory, and the representation of both limbs in one hemisphere.[4]

NATIVE EFFECTORS IN MOTOR BRAIN-COMPUTER INTERFACES

Quadriplegic patients have sustained an injury that blocks the natural connection from brain to body. BCI discussed previously read the intention of the brain to control external effectors. Functional electrical stimulation (FES) uses a native effector: the patient's own musculature.

FES has been used without neural control for applications beyond the upper extremity, requiring control signal from other functional muscles or the use of an external controller. In the lower extremities, standing[18,19] and walking[20] are of interest. Stimulators used to improve urinary continence in spinal cord injury patients are also under the domain of FES,[21] as are phrenic nerve stimulators that have the potential to help ventilator-dependent quadriplegic patients.[22]

An FES BCI system is a motor BCI that truly restores the connection between the body and the brain. Much like earlier motor BCI, signal is recorded from either M1 or PPC. Rather than controlling a prosthetic limb or virtual effector, stimulation is used to reanimate the targeted limb. Muscles are activated using either noninvasive surface electrodes or invasive intramuscular electrodes.

Pfurtscheller and colleagues[23] demonstrated that electroencephalogram could be used to control FES in the first human BCI FES system. Grasping was controlled by beta bursts that were recorded when the patient imagined moving his foot. To achieve more functional movements, higher quality

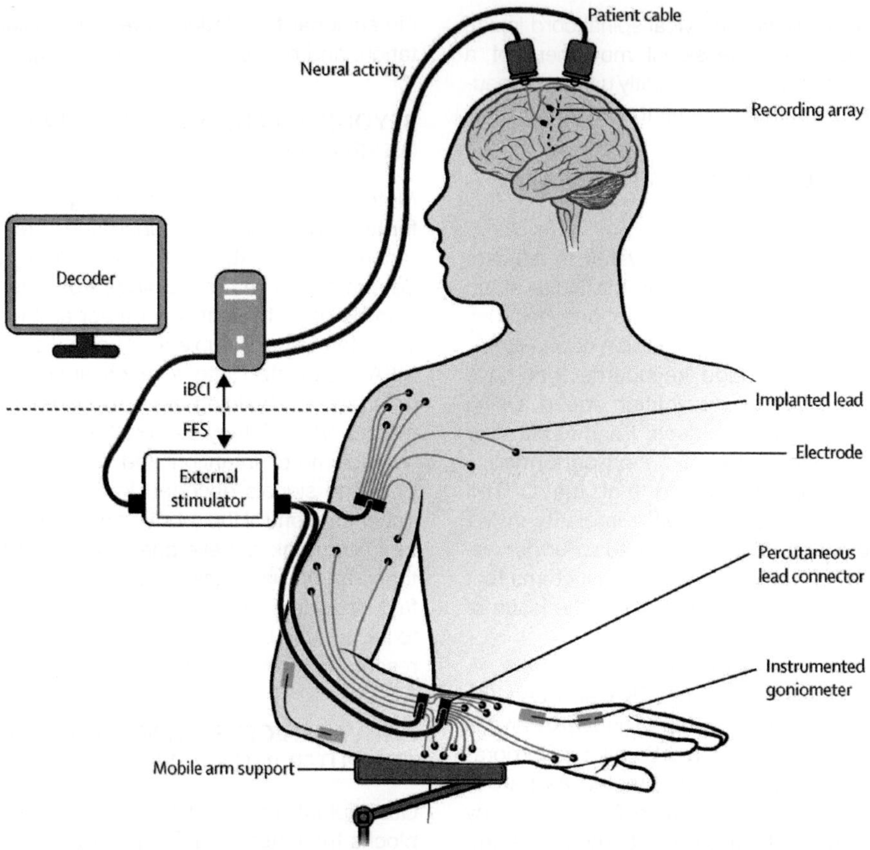

Fig. 2. Schematic of a BCI with FES. Motor intention is recorded from motor cortex using two MEAs and interpreted using an external decoder. This information is used to control an external stimulator connected to implanted electrodes in the upper extremity. (*From* Ajiboye AB, Willett FR, Young DR, et al. Restoration of reaching and grasping movements through brain-controlled muscle stimulation in a person with tetraplegia: a proof-of-concept demonstration. Lancet 2017;389(10081):1823; with permission.)

neural signal from MEA is needed. Bouton and colleagues[24] from Battelle Memorial Institute and Ohio State University was the first group to demonstrate fine cortical control of an FES in humans. Using a Blockrock MEA in M1 and a noninvasive neuromuscular electrical stimulation sleeve, a patient with quadriplegia achieved six wrist and hand movements and was able to complete functional tasks. Further work from Friedenberg and colleagues[25] achieved more fine control of the upper extremity. Graded muscle contraction was achieved using MEAs in M1 and noninvasive FES.

As part of the BrainGate2 trial, Ajiboye and colleagues[26] restored reaching and grasping to a patient who had lost voluntary control of their arm following a spinal cord injury. This BCI was controlled by two Blackrock MEAs in M1. The FES system was invasive, with 36 percutaneously implanted electrodes and a controllable mobile arm support (**Fig. 2**). BCI with FES was able to restore reaching and grasping to the patient's own arm, allowing them to drink coffee and eat with a fork.

SENSORY BRAIN-COMPUTER INTERFACES: CLOSING THE MOTOR/SENSORY FEEDBACK LOOP

Current motor BCI systems rely exclusively on visual feedback; however, it is difficult to make smooth and accurate movements without cutaneous and proprioceptive feedback.[27] The ultimate goal of BCI is to provide natural, intuitive control over the effector, and sensory information is an essential component of this experience (**Fig. 3**).

Somatosensation plays a vital role in motor function,[28–30] and work has already begun to incorporate artificial sensory feedback into BCI systems.[5,27,31–33] O'Doherty and colleagues[31] used microwire arrays in M1 of nonhuman primates to control a virtual robotic arm, and intracortical microstimulation (ICMS) of primary somatosensory cortex (S1) to provide sensory feedback. This study demonstrated that the monkeys could use the artificial sensory information

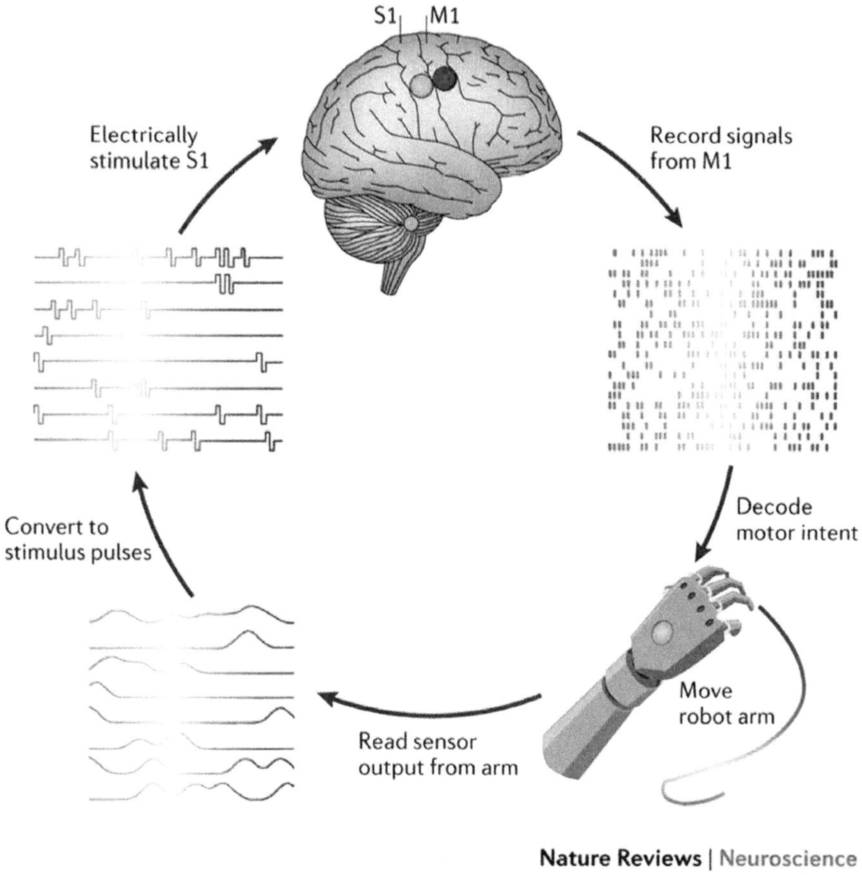

Fig. 3. Schematic of a motor sensory BCI system. Neural signals are recorded from M1. Signals are decoded to determine motor intention and used to control a robotic arm. The robotic arm includes sensors that deliver somatosensory feedback to S1. The sensor output is converted into stimulation pulses that provide the patient with information about the ongoing activity. This feedback allows the motor intention to be adjusted as needed, creating a closed-loop BCI system. (*From* Bensmaia SJ, Miller LE. Restoring sensorimotor function through intracortical interfaces: progress and looming challenges. Nat Rev Neurosci 2014;15:313; with permission.)

delivered through stimulation of S1 to discriminate information about visually identical objects. Also in nonhuman primates, Klaes and colleagues[32] used microwire arrays in PPC to control a virtual prosthetic arm and a Blackrock MEA in S1 to deliver ICMS feedback. They were able to deliver discriminable percepts and use ICMS as target feedback in a "handbag" task where no visual feedback was provided.

Human studies have provided further information about the quality and location of the sensory percepts. This work is an important step in the quest to create a closed-loop BCI, because only human subjects can describe the experience of the sensory feedback. Flesher and colleagues[33] used two 32-channel Blackrock MEAs to deliver ICMS to the hand region of S1 in a patient with tetraplegia from a spinal cord injury. They mapped the location and quality of evoked sensation and found that stimulation amplitude correlated positively with perceived intensity. Armenta Salas and colleagues[27] used ICMS in two 48-channel Blackrock MEAs implanted into S1 of a patient with spinal cord injury to evoke sensation in the hand and arm region. The location and quality of the evoked sensations were mapped, and perceived sensations were found to depend on the frequency and amplitude of stimulation. Both cutaneous and proprioceptive sensations were elicited by varying the stimulation parameters.

Although MEAs have provided the highest quality neural signal for human motor BCI, selecting the appropriate modality for sensory BCI requires careful consideration. For example, the upper extremity is represented over a large area of cortex, and MEAs cover only a small portion of this area.[27] Naturalistic sensory restoration would require access to a larger cortical area than MEA can safely cover. For this reason, ECoG arrays have been studied for sensory BCI, because they can safely cover a larger cortical surface, providing more useful percepts.[5] Lee and colleagues[5] used 64-channel mini-ECoG grids to deliver electrical stimulation to S1 in nine patients with epilepsy undergoing intracranial monitoring. They found that these mini-ECoG grids could potentially provide more complete hand coverage than was observed in prior MEA studies. The sensations evoked were mostly artificial in quality but also reliable and discriminable. Intensity of the sensations could be modulated by varying frequency, amplitude, and pulse width of the stimulation.

The future of sensory BCI requires further characterization and optimization of evoked percepts. Sensors on complex, multimodal effectors need to be mapped and paired with the corresponding cortical stimulation locations and parameters to provide meaningful feedback. Combining sensory and motor BCI in a closed-loop system has the potential to provide patients with a highly effective and intuitive BCI.

SUMMARY

BCI provide an opportunity to restore function to patients with a variety of neurologic injuries, including spinal cord injury. Substantial progress has been made in BCI hardware and software that make clinically useful devices closer than ever. Recordings from M1 and PPC in human cortex have been successfully used to control effectors.[4,10] The effectors that have been developed offer different ways a patient can interact with their world. These options include virtual devices, advanced physical prosthetics, and FES systems that restore function to the patient's own limb. Restoring naturalistic function will also incorporate somatosensation. Closing the motor/sensory feedback loop will allow for intuitive control of effectors, and prosthetics, such as the MPL, have been engineered with next step in mind. Moving forward, a range of highly optimized effectors will provide the best possible treatment options for different physical and neurologic injuries.

BCI will someday be a mainstay of treatment of quadriplegic patients. Existing clinical BCI are well established therapies for epilepsy,[34–36] movement disorders,[37,38] and chronic pain.[39–41] The success of these early clinical BCI has paved the way for BCI. The path through regulatory processes, funding, and hospital infrastructure to support complex neurologic devices has been forged. BCI are an exciting next step in the frontier of neuromodulation.

REFERENCES

1. Eckert MJ, Martin MJ. Trauma: spinal cord injury. Surg Clin North Am 2017;97(5):1031–45.
2. Chapin JK, Moxon KA, Markowitz RS, et al. Real-time control of a robot arm using simultaneously recorded neurons in the motor cortex. Nat Neurosci 1999;2:664.
3. Hochberg LR, Serruya MD, Friehs GM, et al. Neuronal ensemble control of prosthetic devices by a human with tetraplegia. Nature 2006;442:164.
4. Aflalo T, Kellis S, Klaes C, et al. Decoding motor imagery from the posterior parietal cortex of a tetraplegic human. Science 2015;348(6237):906–10.
5. Lee B, Kramer D, Salas MA, et al. Engineering artificial somatosensation through cortical stimulation in humans. Front Syst Neurosci 2018;12:1–11.
6. Armiger RS, Tenore FV, Katyal KD, et al. Enabling closed-loop control of the modular prosthetic limb through haptic feedback. Johns Hopkins APL Tech Dig 2013;31(4):345–53.
7. Pandarinath C, Nuyujukian P, Blabe CH, et al. High performance communication by people with paralysis using an intracortical brain-computer interface. Elife 2017;6. https://doi.org/10.7554/eLife.18554.
8. Lee B, Attenello FJ, Liu CY, et al. Recapitulating flesh with silicon and steel: advancements in upper extremity robotic prosthetics. World Neurosurg 2014; 81(5–6):730–41.
9. Wolpaw JR, Birbaumer N, McFarland DJ, et al. Brain–computer interfaces for communication and control. Clin Neurophysiol 2002;113(6):767–91.
10. Brandman DM, Cash SS, Hochberg LR. Review: human intracortical recording and neural decoding for brain–computer interfaces. IEEE Trans Neural Syst Rehabil Eng 2017;25(10):1687–96.
11. Hochberg LR, Bacher D, Jarosiewicz B, et al. Reach and grasp by people with tetraplegia using a neurally controlled robotic arm. Nature 2012;485:372.
12. Collinger JL, Wodlinger B, Downey JE, et al. High-performance neuroprosthetic control by an individual with tetraplegia. Lancet 2013;381(9866):557–64.
13. Jarosiewicz B, Sarma AA, Bacher D, et al. Virtual typing by people with tetraplegia using a self-calibrating intracortical brain-computer interface. Sci Transl Med 2015;7(313):313ra179.
14. Resnik L, Klinger SL, Etter K. The DEKA Arm: its features, functionality, and evolution during the Veterans Affairs Study to optimize the DEKA arm. Prosthet Orthot Int 2014;38(6):492–504.
15. Gnadt JW, Andersen RA. Memory related motor planning activity in posterior parietal cortex of macaque. Exp Brain Res 1988;70(1):216–20.
16. Mulliken GH, Musallam S, Andersen RA. Forward estimation of movement state in posterior parietal cortex. Proc Natl Acad Sci U S A 2008;105(24): 8170–7.

17. Feltman R. After years of paralysis, a man drinks a beer with the help of a mind-reading robot. The Washington Post 2015. Available at: https://www.washingtonpost.com/news/speaking-of-science/wp/2015/05/21/after-years-of-paralysis-a-mind-reading-robot-helps-a-man-drink-a-beer/?noredirect=on&utm_term=.ec2e7559cb7f.
18. Nataraj R, Audu ML, Kirsch RF, et al. Comprehensive joint feedback control for standing by functional neuromuscular stimulation: a simulation study. IEEE Trans Neural Syst Rehabil Eng 2010;18(6):646–57.
19. Fisher LE, Miller ME, Bailey SN, et al. Standing after spinal cord injury with four-contact nerve-cuff electrodes for quadriceps stimulation. IEEE Trans Neural Syst Rehabil Eng 2008;16(5):473–8.
20. Dutta A, Kobetic R, Triolo RJ. Ambulation after incomplete spinal cord injury with EMG-triggered functional electrical stimulation. IEEE Trans Biomed Eng 2008;55(2 Pt 1):791–4.
21. Radziszewski K. Outcomes of electrical stimulation of the neurogenic bladder: results of a two-year follow-up study. NeuroRehabilitation 2013;32(4):867–73.
22. DiMarco AF, Onders RP, Ignagni A, et al. Phrenic nerve pacing via intramuscular diaphragm electrodes in tetraplegic subjects. Chest 2005;127(2):671–8.
23. Pfurtscheller G, Müller GR, Pfurtscheller J, et al. Thought'–control of functional electrical stimulation to restore hand grasp in a patient with tetraplegia. Neurosci Lett 2003;351(1):33–6. Available at: http://www.ncbi.nlm.nih.gov/pubmed/14550907.
24. Bouton CE, Shaikhouni A, Annetta NV, et al. Restoring cortical control of functional movement in a human with quadriplegia. Nature 2016;533(7602):247–50.
25. Friedenberg DA, Schwemmer MA, Landgraf AJ, et al. Neuroprosthetic-enabled control of graded arm muscle contraction in a paralyzed human. Sci Rep 2017;7(1):8386.
26. Ajiboye AB, Willett FR, Young DR, et al. Restoration of reaching and grasping movements through brain-controlled muscle stimulation in a person with tetraplegia: a proof-of-concept demonstration. Lancet 2017;389(10081):1821–30.
27. Armenta Salas M, Bashford L, Kellis S, et al. Proprioceptive and cutaneous sensations in humans elicited by intracortical microstimulation. Elife 2018;7:1–11.
28. Cramer SC, Lastra L, Lacourse MG, et al. Brain motor system function after chronic, complete spinal cord injury. Brain 2005;128(12):2941–50.
29. Kikkert S, Kolasinski J, Jbabdi S, et al. Revealing the neural fingerprints of a missing hand. Elife 2016;5:1–19.
30. Sainburg RL, Poizner H, Ghez C. Loss of proprioception produces deficits in interjoint coordination. J Neurophysiol 1993;70(5):2136–47.
31. O'Doherty JE, Lebedev MA, Ifft PJ, et al. Active tactile exploration using a brain-machine-brain interface. Nature 2011;479(7372):228–31.
32. Klaes C, Ying S, Kellis S, et al. A cognitive neuroprosthetic that uses cortical stimulation for somatosensory feedback. J Neural Eng 2015;2(2):147–85.
33. Flesher SN, Collinger JL, Foldes ST, et al. Intracortical microstimulation of human somatosensory cortex intracortical microstimulation of human somatosensory cortex. Sci Transl Med 2016;1–11. https://doi.org/10.1126/scitranslmed.aaf8083.
34. Johnson RL, Wilson CG. A review of vagus nerve stimulation as a therapeutic intervention. J Inflamm Res 2018;11:203–13.
35. Sun FT, Morrell MJ. The RNS System: responsive cortical stimulation for the treatment of refractory partial epilepsy. Expert Rev Med Devices 2014;11(6):563–72.
36. Salanova V, Witt T, Worth R, et al. Long-term efficacy and safety of thalamic stimulation for drug-resistant partial epilepsy. Neurology 2015;84(10):1017–25.
37. Lyons KE, Pahwa R. Deep brain stimulation and essential tremor. J Clin Neurophysiol 2004;21(1):2–5.
38. Weaver FM, Follett K, Stern M, et al. Bilateral deep brain stimulation vs best medical therapy for patients with advanced Parkinson disease: a random ized controlled trial. JAMA 2009;301(1):63–73.
39. Kumar K, Taylor RS, Jacques L, et al. Spinal cord stimulation versus conventional medical management for neuropathic pain: a multicentre randomised controlled trial in patients with failed back surgery syndrome. Pain 2007;132(1–2):179–88.
40. Deer T, Slavin KV, Amirdelfan K, et al. Success using neuromodulation with BURST (SUNBURST) study: results from a prospective, randomized controlled trial using a novel burst waveform. Neuromodulation 2018;21(1):56–66.
41. Kumar K, Taylor RS, Jacques L, et al. The effects of spinal cord stimulation in neuropathic pain are sustained: a 24-month follow-up of the prospective randomized controlled multicenter trial of the effectiveness of spinal cord stimulation. Neurosurgery 2008;63(4):762–70.

Printed and bound by CPI Group (UK) Ltd, Croydon, CR0 4YY
08/05/2025
01864745-0018